CHILD PSYCHIATRY AND THE LAW

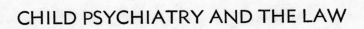

Child Psychiatry and the Law

Edited by
DIANE H. SCHETKY, M.D.
and
ELISSA P. BENEDEK, M.D.

BRUNNER/MAZEL, Publishers • New York

Library of Congress Cataloging in Publication Data

Main entry under title:
Child psychiatry and the law.

Includes bibliographies and index.
1. Juvenile courts—United States.   2. Children—Legal status, laws, etc.—United
States.   3. Forensic psychiatry—United States.   4. Child psychiatry—United
States.   I. Schetky, Diane H., 1940-   II. Benedek, Elissa P.   [DNLM: 1. Jurisprudence. 2. Forensic psychiatry—In infancy and childhood. 3. Juvenile delinquency.
4. Child advocacy.   W740 S327c]

KF9794.C52   345.73'08   80-12463
ISBN 0-87630-231-2

Publishde by
BRUNNER/MAZEL, INC.
19 Union Square
New York, New York 10003

*To our patients in appreciation for what we
have learned from them*

FOREWORD

The most significant influence on the practice of child psychiatry in the past decade has been the expanding influence of law and in particular the development of the rights of minors.

This volume provides the first comprehensive compilation of the pertinent issues by informed, experienced, psychologists, psychiatrists, social workers and lawyers. Knowledge and experience in human service law tend to be compartmentalized and uneven. It is difficult for the scientifically oriented professions because there is no presumption of a general theory or paradigm. Law is a product of the human mind accumulated slowly from multiple sources and is dependent on the momentum, rate, and channels of culture flow and the procedures inherent in the skeleton of the legal process. Reality consists of the word, the written law, the interpretations of judges, and attorneys, and the ascertained facts allowed by the rules of evidence. Each legal action is a unique event imbedded in a ritualized procedure.

For the student or newcomer to the field, Chapters 3, 4, 5, and 11 provide a bridge from the familiar and known procedures of clinical examination and diagnosis to the same but attitudinally different procedures appropriate for the written report or oral testimony of the expert witness. Chapters 3, 4, and 5 are succinct presentations of the variations appropriate for the child psychiatrist entering the foreign arena of the adversary legal process. The purpose of examination is changed. The role and status of the examiner as expert witness are different from those as decision maker, adviser, or healer. Completeness of procedural protocol, style of examination, objectivity of tests, conservative use of inference, and practical matters of fees, time, and relationships to judges and attorneys are addressed. Chapter 11 strongly advises the child psychiatrist to conduct a comprehensive and detailed diagnostic examination even though fulfilling a different role as expert witness. The reader must be sensitive to the conflict between identifying all of the clinical and developmental vulnerabilities of a potential patient and addressing the more narrow goal of relevant testimony to a legal action.

Chapters 2 and 18 are overview chapters that provide an academic introduction to the study of the child psychiatry-law interface. Chapter 18 represents a broad, clinically sympathetic, and legally accurate perspective on the continuous pervasive interaction of law and psychiatry beginning with the premise that the patient-doctor relationship is both a clinical and legal concept with diverging implications. Chapter 2 is targeted to the rights of minors as a rapidly developing special area of concern, and sketches out the ramifications beginning with a historical reference to and critique of the Juvenile Court, and then addressing the issue of children in need of supervision, known also as troubled youth, or non-criminal misbehavior, followed by attention to custody, neglect, the legal rights of families, hospitalization, and the relationship of rights and the legal process.

Chapter 12 will be comprehended easier if read after and in conjunction with Chapters 2 and 18. The complex question of juvenile court reform and the legal and clinical fate of the troubled youth who are involved in non-criminal misbehavior is being energetically addressed in torturous debate in almost every state. The hours of debate are exceeded only by the confusion of opinions. This chapter teases out the significant threads of the chaotic debate and identifies some of the sources of diversity. But a bewildering heterogeneity of adolescents, parents, juvenile court judges, correctional facilities, treatment services, schools, and community practices is involved and so far an effectively rational solution is lacking. The sections on Truancy, Disobedience of School Authorities, and Runaways are better reserved until the reader is ready to penetrate deeper into the maze of behavior covered by a legal typology based on ubiquitous superficial behaviors that may reflect much or little of clinical relevance.

The experience of each child psychiatrist and each lawyer tends to be compartmentalized to a considerable degree by the opportunities in their practices. Professionals are usually drawn into the law-psychiatry issues by individual cases or by specific jobs. Chapters 6, 7, 8, 10, and 13 provide authoritative references, reviews, guides, and bibliographies for child custody, child abuse, sexual misuse of children, adoption, and the juvenile murderer. These chapters are best appreciated and utilized when read with case in hand.

Chapter 9, although intimately involved with the question of adoption, has a broader scope in its discussion of termination of parental rights, and exemplifies the process of the evolution of new legal rights out of longstanding instances of inadequate, incompetent or insufficiently budgeted human services. In this case, foster care, once a heralded solution, has become an equally heralded type of abuse of children by the State. Some of the new solutions, e.g., adoption, subsidized adoption, or permanent foster care, are blocked by the parental rights of the natural parents. Balancing and trading off the rights of parents and the rights of children are the crux of the problem. In all of this volume there is not an operational definition of a right, but this chapter clearly equates rights and needs. "He/she [the child] also possesses the rights, that is, the overpowering need, to have parents to call his/her own on a continuing basis. . . ." For dissent one can return to the discussion in Chapter 2 where it is advocated that courts declare children have "enforceable rights" and a distinction is made between the advocacy of legal rights and the vision of "what a humane and farsighted society ought to do for its own sake and for the sake of its offspring." Rights and needs are probably different species of concepts, but in this age of the power of legal advocacy, it is the clever clinical advocate who transforms developmental needs into constitutional rights.

Chapters 14 and 17 are beautiful presentations of recent clinical experience that defines new legal issues with poignant compassionate examples. The discussions of problems in use of the preparation of the child as a witness and the related issue of psychic trauma to children are most valuable and original additions to the traditional array of legal issues, and will be secondarily rewarding to read as a spinoff of creative, sensitive clinical research.

Laws were more consistent, understandable and enforceable when the minor child was considered a non-person. The topics of Chapter 15, competency and responsibility, were confusing enough for adults, particularly as the learning, developmental, genetic, and biochemical theories of behavior identified multiple determinants of judgment that repeatedly contradicted the simplistic concept of rationality. To some extent, the entire practice of psychiatry is a determination and manipulation of the ever changing and ever relative developmental competencies and responsibilities of the individual from gestation to death. Now that the law has embarked on the delineation of the enforceable constitutional rights of minors, it must of necessity attend to the reciprocal problem of responsibilities. Inevitably, this has led to the transfer of many juveniles to the criminal court jurisdiction and has tended to contaminate the "best interest of the child" juvenile justice process with the criminal law processes of indictment, trial, conviction, and punishment. At this point, the law is only beginning to reflect the confusing problem engendered by competency of child determinations. Many years of civil and criminal litigation with accumulation of case law will be needed to define the problems. Solutions will be more difficult as the problems become clearer, and therefore more complex. Chapter 15 plunges bravely into these issues, but the reader should not expect resolution.

The most direct influence of law on child psychiatry comes through the legal paths to hospitalization. Until 1970 this was not a major consideration, but in some states it is now virtually impossible to hospitalize children. Neither situation is desirable. Despite the rhetoric of community mental health or the mixed motivated deinstitutionalization policy, there are thousands of children who desperately need residential care of a variety of types, including long-term hospitalization. It is difficult enough to meet this service need without having to surmount impossible legal obstacles. Chapter 16 presents a lucid, authoritative, reasonably well balanced discussion of commitment proceedings. Every reader will have his own disagreements and it would be a valuable discipline to put them in writing since almost everyone will have the opportunity of participating in the revision of commitment law. Presumably, most could agree that there should be a process that facilitates hospitalization when needed and presumably each child psychiatrist favors the protection and delineation of the constitutional rights of minors. From that point on, however, most every aspect of the legal process is subject to debate.

For example, there is not enough recognition given to the distinctions between the mentally ill and the mentally retarded and even less to the problem of the mentally ill retarded. Futhermore, the attorney is usually acting as if the admission process is like a space shuttle entering into the window of an earth orbit. In fact, the admission of a minor to a hospital is not a precise operation, is not intended to be, and will never be precisely defined. To talk of being error-free is to discuss another world. On the contrary, admission is always seeking for a "best path compromise," given many conflicting clinical influences. The rights of the minor are but one highly significant factor.

Then, again, the constitutional attorneys are vividly impressed with the potential for errors and abuse in the mental health service system, but appear blind to the potential for errors and abuse that will be inherent in an underfunded, understaffed, and undertrained judicial review and legal advocacy system.

FRANK T. RAFFERTY, M.D.
Medical Director,
The Brown Schools
Austin, Texas

CONTENTS

INTRODUCTION

The child psychiatrist is increasingly being called upon to give advice in legal matters involving children. This increased demand for service is related to several factors. Foremost is the increased number of children now being seen in the court system. In 1975 alone, 1,000,000 children were involved in divorce proceedings, in contrast to 431,000 children in 1960 (3). Similarly, the ranks of children involved in juvenile delinquency and status offenses are swelling. Secondly, judges, attorneys, and case workers are becoming more aware of the psychological needs of children and are turning to child psychiatrists and psychologists for guidance in making recommendations or decisions in keeping with the child's best interests.

Child psychiatry has failed to keep pace with ensuing demands for service. Most training programs have lagged in developing curricula in child forensic psychiatry despite the fact that such training is mandatory and is documented by the Council on Medical Education Guidelines. A 1975 study by McDermott (1) revealed many practicing child psychiatrists felt ill equipped to do court evaluations or testify in court. That same survey revealed that judges wished for forensically trained child psychiatrists.

Further problems in rendering consultations arise from the frequently strained relations between psychiatrists and attorneys. Philosophical differences are rooted in the physician's commitment to healing and the attorney's commitment to winning. Both, however, are committed to helping the child/client/patient. It is just that their perception of what is "help" often differs. Additionally, child psychiatrists may find the adversary system, which may pit child against family or child psychiatrist against child, is problematic in their attempts to develop a therapeutic alliance and bring families together. Polier (2), commenting on the reasons why law and psychiatry have remained so egocentric in their deal-

xiii

ings with one another, cites the fact that historically law is well established both by tradition and practice whereas psychiatry, a relative newcomer, is viewed suspiciously by the lay world as the stepchild of the medical profession. She notes that lawyers are quick to attack psychiatry for its impreciseness, yet they do not expect similar standards for their own profession where "extreme variations in justice that exist are often dependent upon which judge sits and which lawyer takes the case" (2). She further notes that psychiatry with its special ethos and process of self-exclusion has "created its own ghetto walls." The end result is that all too often transactions between lawyers and psychiatrists are "done at arm's length and with mutual suspicions" (2, p. 6).

Often overlooked are the common goals shared by law and psychiatry. To again quote Polier (2, p. x):

> Law and psychiatry are both rooted in the longings, aspirations, and fears prevalent in our world. Law is the work of many men who have sought answers to the question of how people can live together in a society and handle their fears of one another. It has been used to control and placate both those without power and those demanding more power. It has also been the instrument through which men seeking justice have sought to reshape institutions.

> Law has become one of the major instruments through which our society seeks to accomplish social change. In comparable fashion psychiatry has become not only the source of special service for the mentally ill but a resource for solving and preventing many of the personal and interpersonal problems that plague our society.

This volume is an interdisciplinary effort which reflects the fact that it is possible for attorneys and psychiatrists, in spite of traditional divisiveness, to work together toward fostering better understanding of one another's goals in the interest of better understanding the child. This book was conceived in hopes of providing a solid theoretical and practical background in child forensic psychiatry for practicing child psychiatrists, child psychologists and attorneys working with and for children to enable them to function more effectively in their roles. It is also intended to be read by other professionals, such as judges, social workers and case workers, who work at the interface of child psychiatry and the law. It is hoped that it will give them greater appreciation of some of the difficult issues at hand, as well as guidelines for dealing with these issues.

This is the first text of its kind to deal solely with the subject of child forensic psychiatry. As such, it attempts to encompass those areas most likely to be encountered in the practice of child psychiatry or psychology. Obviously, it is not all inclusive and, unfortunately, given the rate of progress in this area, it may soon be out-of-date.

The book is divided into four sections:

Part I provides the reader with general background information necessary to undertake an evaluation for the courts. A historical perspective on child forensic psychiatry is provided followed by an overview of the juvenile justice system, and discussions on the conduct of the forensic evaluation, use of psychological testing, and testifying in court. The sections which follow deal with specific issues in depth.

Part II deals with a most significant aspect of juvenile work—child custody, dependency and neglect cases, which are all too often overlooked amidst the clamor and publicity that are focused on juvenile delinquents and status offenders. These cases involve children who come to the court not because they have committed any offenses but rather through acts of commission or omission on the part of their parents, or as children caught in parental divorce. Thus, the court is acting in its role as protector of children. When parents default, the court moves in as parens patriae to provide the child with the custody and care to which he/she is entitled. The other instance in which the court is likely to become involved is as arbitrator or decision maker for divorcing parents where custody of children is at issue.

Part III of the book deals with the difficult arena of the juvenile offender. Here the psychiatrist is called upon to evaluate, treat, plan and offer prognosis for a troubled and troubling segment of the population. A core body of knowledge of general medicine, neurology, child and adult psychiatry is again put to the test by the adversary system. Additionally, the legal guidelines in this area are being closely reevaluated and, in some instances, are radically changing.

Part IV of the book deals with some very special issues which are not easily categorized—personal injury vis-à-vis psychiatric trauma qualifying the child as a witness, competency, insanity, civil commitment and confidentiality. Though the topics are divergent, it is clear that a basic knowledge of child development and of legal principles in each specialized area is essential to conduct the child forensic evaluation.

The authors recognize that in a text such as this important areas will be neglected or covered lightly. Thus, problems such as mental retardation, malpractice, the right to refuse treatment and ethics are only addressed indirectly. There is much work yet to be done.

REFERENCES

1. McDERMOTT, J. F., JR. (1975). Certification of the Child Psychiatrist. *J. Amer. Acad.,* Ch. 4, p. 196. Vol. 14, No. 2, Spring, 1975.
2. POLIER, J. W. (1968). *The Rule of Law: The Role of Psychiatry.* Baltimore: John Hopkins Press.
3. NATIONAL CENTER FOR HEALTH (1976). HEW Pub. 78-1120, Vol. 27, #5, p. 5.

CONTRIBUTORS

ELISSA P. BENEDEK, M.D.
Training Director, Center for Forensic Psychiatry, Ypsilanti, Michigan; Clinical Professor of Psychiatry, University of Michigan, Ann Arbor.

RICHARD S. BENEDEK, J.D.
Attorney, private practice, Ann Arbor, Michigan.

ANDRE P. DERDEYN, M.D.
Professor of Psychiatry and Pediatrics and Director, Division of Child and Adolescent Psychiatry, University of Virginia Medical Center, Charlottesville.

JAMES ELLIS, J.D.
Associate Professor, School of Law, University of New Mexico, Albuquerque.

ARTHUR H. GREEN, M.D.
Director, Child Abuse Crisis Nursery and Intervention Program and Faculty at Psychoanalytic Center for Training and Research, Columbia University College of Physicians and Surgeons, N.Y.

DOROTHY OTNOW LEWIS, M.D., F.A.C.P.
Research Professor of Psychiatry, Division of Child Psychiatry, New York University School of Medicine.

RUTH G. MATARAZZO, Ph.D.
Professor of Medical Psychology, Department of Medical Psychology, University of Oregon Health Sciences Center, Portland.

CAROL C. NADELSON, M.D.
Associate Professor of Psychiatry, Harvard Medical School; Psychia-

trist and Director of Medical Student Education in Psychiatry, Beth Israel Hospital, Boston.

SANDRA G. NYE, J.D., M.S.W.
Illinois Guardianship and Advocacy Commission, Chicago.

JOSEPH J. PALOMBI, M.D.
Associate Director Division of Child Psychiatry and Assistant Professor of Psychiatry, University of Connecticut Health Center, Farmington.

THEODORE A. PETTI, M.D.
Assistant Professor of Child Psychiatry and Program Director of Children's Psychiatry Intensive Care Service, Western Psychiatric Institute and Clinic, University of Pittsburgh.

ALVIN A. ROSENFELD, M.D.
Director of Training in Child Psychiatry and Assistant Professor of Psychiatry, Stanford University Medical School, Stanford.

HELEN L. SACKS, M.S.W.
Assistant Clinical Professor of Social Work, Child Study Center, Yale University School of Medicine, and Administrative Director, Psychiatric Clinic, Superior Court for Juvenile Matters, New Haven.

HERBERT S. SACKS, M.D.
Clinical Professor of Pediatrics and Psychiatry, Child Study Center, Yale University School of Medicine, New Haven, and Commissioner, Connecticut Juvenile Justice Commission.

DIANE H. SCHETKY, M.D.
Private practice, Wilton, Connecticut and Assistant Clinical Professor of Psychiatry, Child Study Center, Yale University School of Medicine, New Haven.

DAVID L. SLADER, J.D.
Attorney private practice, Portland, Oregon.

LENORE C. TERR, M.D.
Associate Clinical Professor of Psychiatry, Langley Porter Neuropsychiatric Institute, University of California at San Francisco.

PATRICIA M. WALD, LL.B.
Judge, United States Court of Appeals for the District of Columbia Circuit, Washington, D.C.

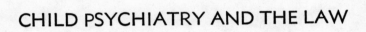

CHILD PSYCHIATRY AND THE LAW

Part I
INTRODUCTION TO FORENSIC CHILD PSYCHIATRY

1

HISTORICAL DEVELOPMENT OF FORENSIC CHILD PSYCHIATRY

DIANE H. SCHETKY, M.D. and ELISSA P. BENEDEK, M.D.

The relationship between child psychiatry and the law is as old as the child guidance movement itself, which had its origin in the public's concern over juvenile crime at the turn of the century. Under the financial support of Mrs. Drummer and others from Chicago's Hull House, the Juvenile Psychiatric Institute was organized in Chicago in 1909. Located within the newly formed Cook County Juvenile Court, it was to become the laboratory for the investigations into the study of juvenile delinquency. Its Director, William Healy, neurologist by training, stressed the need for obtaining an adequate medical history and physical exam on the child. Healy's work was notable for his application of psychoanalytic principles to the treatment of delinquency and for the emphasis he put on understanding the child's total situation. The latter provided the impetus for multidisciplinary research as well as a model for the team approach, i.e., the triad of psychiatrist, psychologist and social worker which is still used in child guidance clinics. In 1915 he published *The Individual Delinquent*, the first book of this kind, in which he stressed the need to get to know the individual, utilize knowledge from all disciplines and utilize any person or group who might be able to help the patient (11).

Prior to the creation of the juvenile court, children were considered property of their parents, could be fully exploited in the labor market and, if charged with misconduct, were subject to the same criminal proceedings as adults. The historians of social change in our country are quick to note that in the latter part of the 19th century there were laws protecting animals in the United States before there were laws protecting children. The first juvenile court was created in Chicago in 1899

3

when the Illinois legislature passed the Juvenile Court Act and by the late 1920s, all but two states, Maine and Wyoming, had enacted laws founded on the Illinois model. In 1951, Wyoming followed suit and Maine joined the nation in 1959.

The philosophy of the early juvenile court in an atmosphere of benevolence was to strive to understand the total child and respond to him "as a wise, merciful father handles his own child whose errors are not discovered by the authorities" (16). The juvenile court viewed its role as preventative, helping the child and protecting him from criminal procedures. The aura of reform and optimism is reflected in the writings of Julian Mack (16), one of the early juvenile court justices who saw the court's role as "not so much to punish as to reform, not to degrade but to uplift, not to crush but to develop, not to make him a criminal but a worthy citizen" (p. 107). He pleaded that "there be attached to the court, as there have been in a few cities, a child study department where every child, before hearing, shall be subjected to thorough psycho-physical examination. In hundreds of cases, the discovery and remedy of defective eyesight or hearing or some slight surgical operation will effectuate a complete change in the character of the lad" (16, p. 120).

In 1916, disillusioned by the lack of facilities and funds available to treat delinquents, Healy left Chicago to head the Judge Baker Center in Boston where he was joined by Augusta Bronner, a psychologist, in his research. Other psychiatric clinics soon developed, including the Boston Psychopathic Hospital (1912) and The Phipps Psychiatric Clinic (1913) directed by Adolf Meyer who endorsed Healy's multidisciplinary approach to the evaluation of patients. In 1924, the American Orthopsychiatric Association was founded and two years later it opened its doors to nonphysicians becoming an interdisciplinary forum for the understanding and treatment of delinquency. The publication of Aichhorn's *Wayward Youth* (1), with its psychoanalytic interpretation of delinquent behavior, which was to have significant impact on the treatment of delinquents, occurred in 1925.

Important contributions to the epidemiology of juvenile delinquency were made by the Gluecks (7, 8), who attempted to delineate environmental factors that might predispose children to delinquency. Robins (19) later followed this same line of investigation and provided important follow-up data on children with delinquent behavior. Merton attempted to explain social deviance on grounds of socioeconomic difference as an adaptation to a malignant environment (17, 18). Intrapsychic factors and parental attitudes as contributors to delinquency were described in the writings of A. Freud (5), Johnson (13), Friedlander (6) and Greenacre (9). While the nature versus nurture controversy continues, recent epidemiological research by Lewis et al. (14, 15) on genetic and biological factors brings us back to the wisdom of Healy who stressed the need to get a total picture of the child and maintain some perspective.

The juvenile court did not live up to its promise and disillusionment was bound to follow. Healy and Bronner became discouraged by the failure of the courts to follow out their recommendations and the Gluecks (8) in a follow-up study concluded that a loose relationship between court and clinic, which was only used as a diagnostic center, availed little for the successful treatment of delinquents. Rather, they urged that the clinics develop a treatment component if good results were to be achieved. Years later, Fortas (In re Gault) charged that "in most juvenile courts the child receives the worst of both worlds: that he gets neither the protection accorded to adults nor the solicitous care and regenerative treatment postulated for children" (12). Similarly, in 1976, Stone charged that "the court's only function in many cases is to funnel children from unsuitable homes to unsuitable placements" (21, p. 156). He comments on the failure of collaboration between the legal and mental health systems and the reluctance on the part of psychiatric facilities to accommodate delinquent youths. He concludes that "the practice and paucity and poverty of dispositional options is seen to distort, corrupt and betray the whole system" (21, p. 147).

It is beyond the scope of this chapter to critique all the shortcomings of the juvenile court, which will be done in more depth in Chapter 2. However, we do wish to discuss the past failures in the training of child psychiatrists to function in this area and explore what is being done to remedy the situation (2).

Prior to 1972 there was no formal requirement for a training experience in either child or adult forensic psychiatry (3). The 1972 Guide for Residency Programs in Psychiatry and Neurology spelled out a detailed experience in Forensic Psychiatry and Adult Psychiatry for the resident: "Inevitably, the psychiatrist must relate to the law. His education should include seminars relative to the legal aspects of psychi? as well as opportunities to testify in court under the guidance to experienced psychiatrist who can instruct him in the rules of fr and court procedures" (10). Thus, those residents interested fr rensic area learned from their own experience and mist their consultation with colleagues.

Although the Liaison Council on Medical Education, the accrediting body for child psychiatry programs, now mandates an experience in forensic child psychiatry, that mandate is generally ignored. The evolution of forensic child programs has been haphazard. There is currently no generally accepted core curriculum in forensic child psychiatry. Ordinarily, this subspecialty is taught in elective programs which are fortunate to have a staff member with special interest, expertise and training in the field. Sadoff's comprehensive survey of training programs in forensic psychiatry revealed 15 training centers with a program for psychiatric residents and medical students in the area of law and psychiatry, 13 of which have provisions for post residency training programs (20). It would seem that subspecialization in forensic child psychiatry would be available in only a few of these programs.

In our opinion, all child psychiatry training programs must comply more fully with the L.C.M.E. standards. A knowledge of forensic child psychiatry is as important to the modern, well-trained child psychiatrist as is child psychopharmacology or behavioral therapy with children. Such training should encompass both didactic and experiential components.

In addition, such training should be multidisciplinary and should involve other professionals as both teachers and students. More specifically, in addition to the usual child psychiatry team, would-be lawyers and law students would also be involved in this multidisciplinary training approach. This early familiarity would hopefully breed respect, empathy and perhaps an understanding of the philosophical bases of these two different, but complementary, professions, as well as the development of a common language.

Didactic work might cover such areas as the history and philosophy of the law in respect to children and their families. It would also cover more important and critical arenas of forensic collaboration, such as the juvenile court, divorce, child custody, child abuse and neglect. The experiential component might be a series of visits and consultations to important community agencies and services where psychiatrists and attorneys traditionally act. Those agencies might include the juvenile court, the family court, the Legal Aid Society, and the Detention Home. Visits and consultations would be designed to enable the student to see the system in action, to observe other colleagues' performance in the ʾgm and to discuss the pragmatic problems facing child psychiatrists foreʾ̣urt workers, judges, attorneys, child psychiatrists and other per-ʾʾ̣nally, in our opinion, the student ought to complete an actual ʾʾ̣ation and assume responsibility for his/her work. The evaluation might be done for the juvenile court, the child protective services, the family court or other agencies. Not all forensic evaluations lead to court appearances and testimony; however, an experience in testifying either about a case or as an exercise has a special value which serves to test the student's familiarity with the law and relative testimony in a particular area and also allows multidisciplinary students to experience a variety of roles—judge, defense attorney, prosecutor, expert witness and juror. Those few programs that do offer mock trial experiences to residents report enthusiastic responses (2, 3, 4).

A videotape of such a trial enhances its effectiveness if it is used to desensitize the resident student and as a means for evaluation and critique. In fact, residents report that the critique of the mock trial is as valuable for them as the actual experience. Our residents and fellows view the mock trial as a rite of passage.

It is important to provide remedial experiences in forensic child psychiatry to those fellows who have completed their training. A review of recent programs sponsored by the American Psychiatric Association, the American Academy of Child Psychiatry and the American Academy of Psychiatry and the Law reveals an increasing number of such programs offered to membership. Such training is often multidisciplinary in design and when adequately planned and structured affords practicing psychiatrists and attorneys opportunities to talk to each other about professional concerns and responsibilities outside the arena of the courtroom. We would hope that such collaborative experiences will increase.

REFERENCES

1. AICHHORN, A. (1925). *Wayward Youth*. New York: Viking Press.
2. BARR, N. & SUAREZ, J. (1965). The Teaching of Forensic Psychiatry in Law Schools, Medical Schools and Psychiatric Residences in the United States. *Amer. J. Psych.*, 122:612-616.
3. BENEDEK, E. (1975). Forensic Training for Child Psychiatrists. *Bull. Amer. Acad. of Child Psych.*, 12:721-737.
4. COHEN, S., FOLBERG, H., & SACK, W. (1977). Meeting a Training Need: An Interdisciplinary Seminar of Family Law and Child Psychiatry. *Amer. Acad. of Psych. and Law*, Vol. 5, 3:336-343.
5. FREUD, A. (1965). *Normality and Pathology in Childhood*. New York: International Universities Press, Inc.
6. FRIEDLANDER, K. (1949). Latent Delinquency and Ego Development. In *Searchlights on Delinquency*, K. Eissler (Ed.). New York: International Universities Press, Inc.
7. GLUECK, S. & GLUECK, E. (1930). *Five Hundred Criminal Careers*. New York: Knopf.
8. GLUECK, S. & GLUECK, E. (1943). *The Commonwealth Fund*. New York.
9. GREENACRE, P. (1950). Problems of Acting Out. *Psychoanal. Quart.*, 19:455-465.
10. Guide to Residency Programs in Psychiatry and Neurology, Residency Review Committee for Psychiatry and Neurology. Presented to the American Board of

       Psychiatry and Neurology, Council on Medical Education of the American Medical Association, 1972, p. 13.

11. HEALY, W. (1915). *The Individual Delinquent. A Textbook of Diagnosis and Prognosis.* Boston: Little, Brown.

12. In re Gault 387 U.S. 1.

13. JOHNSON, A. (1948). Sanctions for superego lacunae of adolescence. In *Searchlights on Delinquency*, K. Eissler (Ed.). New York: International Universities Press, Inc.

14. LEWIS, D. & BALLAS, D. (1976). *Delinquency and Psychopathology.* New York: Grune & Stratton.

15. LEWIS, D., SHANOK, S., PINCUS, J., & GLASER, G. (1979). Violent Juvenile Delinquents: Psychiatric, Neurological, Psychological Abuse Factors. *J. Amer. Acad. Ch. Psych.,* 18:307-319.

16. MACK, J. (1909). The Juvenile Court. *Harvard Law Review,* 23:104-122.

17. MERTON, R. (1938). Social Structure and Anomie. *Amer. Sociol. Rev.,* 3:672-682.

18. MERTON, R. (1957). *Social Theory and Social Structure.* New York: Free Press, 225-245.

19. ROBINS, L. (1966). *Deviant Children Grown Up.* Baltimore: Williams & Wilkins.

20. SADOFF, R. (1979). Survey of Forensic Training Programs. *Amer. Acad. of Psych. and the Law,* 4:1, Jan.

21. STONE, A. (1976). *Mental Health and the Law: A System in Transition.* New York: Jason Aronson.

2

INTRODUCTION TO THE JUVENILE JUSTICE PROCESS: THE RIGHTS OF CHILDREN AND THE RITES OF PASSAGE

PATRICIA M. WALD, LL.B.

At the turn of the century, the juvenile court movement came into being. Its motivations were exemplary; it aimed to provide a nonpunitive setting in which a wayward child and his parents could discuss their problem, be counseled by a wise patriarchal juvenile judge, and go away redeemed, not to sin again. When it became necessary to remove the child from the home, he/she was to be cared for by tender and trained surrogate parents who would lead him/her to law-abiding ways. It was a noble experiment, indeed, designed to protect children from the stigmatizing label of "criminal" and from the contamination of incarceration with hardened adult offenders. The child was deemed not legally capable of committing a crime; he/she was in need of counsel, education and help. It was not what he/she did that was important but why he/she did it and how he/she could be prevented from doing it again. As a result procedures were informal and discursive; counsel was either not required or in some cases not permitted; the formalities of "due process" like notice, the right to cross examine witnesses, the right not to answer questions if they would incriminate oneself—these rights were considered irrelevant to a "helping" process. The goal was "treatment" of the child and his/her family.

Sixty-five years later in 1967 a Presidential Crime Commission reported:

At the time this chapter was written, Patricia Wald was Assistant Attorney General for Legislative Affairs, Department of Justice. The views expressed here are entirely her own.

9

the great hopes originally held for the juvenile court have not been fulfilled. It has not succeeded significantly in rehabilitating delinquent youth, in reducing or even stemming the tide of juvenile criminality, or in bringing justice and compassion to the child offender (19).

Half of the juvenile court judges surveyed in 1966 had not graduated from college; 75 percent handled juvenile cases only on a part-time basis. Juvenile court resources were sparse; probation officers typically earned $4,000-5,000 a year and supervised 70-80 cases simultaneously. Juvenile court hearings usually lasted 15-20 minutes. Psychologists and psychiatrists were infrequent participants in the juvenile court process. Treatment resources—family counseling, foster and group homes, residential facilities or even outpatient clinics for emotionally disturbed youngsters—were nearly nonexistent.. Particularly disillusioning was the state of the training schools to which juveniles were sent to be rehabilitated:

> Institutionalization too often means storage—isolation from the outside world—in an overcrowded, understaffed, high-security institution with little education, little vocational training, little counseling or job placement or other guidance upon release. Programs are subordinated to everyday control and maintenance... 'There are things going on, methods of discipline being used in the state training schools of this country that would cause a warden of Alcatraz to lose his job if they used them on his prisoners' (19).

The President's Crime Commission went on to indict the juvenile courts for being overambitious in their outreach to take charge of truants, runaways, and those beyond control of their parents when they did not have the knowledge or the resources to help such children. It also endorsed far stricter due process controls for juveniles accused of law offenses, including notice of the specific offense, the right to counsel —irrespective of parents' means—and rights against self-incrimination. At the same time, it voted to place increased discretion on court intake workers and on police to dismiss nonserious cases against juveniles, and in the court itself to make an individualized determination of what sanctions should be applied to a juvenile divisions in police departments, more resources for juvenile courts, youth service bureaus to coordinate community services for children and families, and more humane and enriching institutional experiences (19).

At just about the time the Crime Commission published its findings a series of legal decisions were beginning to come from the courts. Often these decisions cited the findings of the Crime Commission for the proposition that the consequences of being found guilty in a juvenile court were in fact just as onerous as in an adult criminal court and hence the same legal rights were due a child as an adult. But the decisions can be traced even more directly to the advent of a new breed of aggressive legal services lawyer available for the first time in meaningful numbers to parents and juveniles involved with the law. These lawyers did not hesitate to challenge existing notions and precedents about the benevolence of the juvenile court. They signalled the start of the juvenile rights movement.

We are now almost a decade and a half into that movement. During that time, there has been a steady and concerted attempt by legal advocates to make courts declare that children in certain circumstances have enforceable rights against their parents, their schools, their physicians, and agencies of the state. There is an important difference between this latter day juvenile rights movement and predecessor reform movements that concentrated on making children's situations better through compulsory education, child labor laws, and welfare benefits. The former were motivated and controlled by adults with a particular vision of what a humane and farsighted society ought to do for its own sake and for the sake of its offspring. There was no hint of sharing power with the next generation. The legal rights movement, on the other hand, has had as one of its overriding themes insistence on an increasing share of power for young persons in vital decisions affecting their lives. Additionally, it has reflected a profound cynicism with respect to what state authorities and juvenile "experts" could and would do when a juvenile was placed in their custody. The difference is a critical one, perhaps even a revolutionary one.

RIGHTS OF DELINQUENTS AND WAYWARD CHILDREN

The first cases in the juvenile legal rights movement attacked the failure of the juvenile court to afford due process to children accused of wrongdoing who were threatened with removal from home and placement in state institutions. A series of Supreme Court cases in the mid-sixties and early seventies declared that children in delinquency proceedings needed their own counsel notice of the charges, a right to confront their accusers and to be warned that they might incriminate themselves (7), a right to be adjudicated guilty only on the same "beyond a reasonable doubt" basis as an adult offender (22), and the right not to be put in double jeopardy by being tried in both a juvenile court and an adult court (2). One court has recently extended that parallel to the right of a juvenile to raise the insanity defense and to be declared incompetent to stand trial (3). The Supreme Court refused, however, to rule that juveniles have a constitutional right to a jury trial in delinquency proceedings (14). The Supreme Court agonized about these rulings, recognizing that the actual workings of state juvenile court systems revealed inadequacies in funding, skilled personnel and rehabilitative potential. Yet the Court exhibited understandable reluctance to admit the entire juvenile court experiment was ultimately a failure. The Justices wanted to encourage the states to keep trying to make the separate juvenile court system work because their instinct was that children ought to be treated differently from adults. Their bottom line was that juveniles must be given almost the same procedural due process as adults before their lives could be seriously interfered with by the state on the grounds that they had violated the law.

One critical point should be noted about these early decisions in contrast to later ones; all of them dealt with the conflict between the state and the child; the parent was not a formal party to the dispute. Indeed the so-called status offender jurisdiction of the juvenile court, i.e., truancy, ungovernability, runaways, has been affected in only a limited way by these decisions. The Supreme Court has several times refused the invitation to rule on children's rights in such proceedings (6). There is a strong movement afoot to abolish, or at least curb, juvenile court jurisdiction over status offenders, but the fight has been waged primarily in the state legislatures and in Congress. Many recent state codes have restricted the power of juvenile courts to send such children to state institutions or even to keep them temporarily in secure detention where they would be mixed with delinquents. The Juvenile Justice Delinquency and Prevention Act of 1974 (11a) expressly made Federal subsidies conditional on states not mixing youthful offenders with adult criminals and on a plan to remove status offenders from secure institutions within a certain number of years. A quite passionate debate is still being waged on whether we are doing troubled youngsters who truant, runaway, or habitually disobey their parents a favor or merely perpetrating another rejection of them by leaving them alone. Should the state back up parents by using coercion and threats of compulsory treatment or removal from home in order to keep adolescents under control? Should the state monitor children until they reach the age society thinks is proper for them to make their own mistakes or possibly ruin their lives? Advocates of abolition of all juvenile court jurisdiction state these Persons in Need of Supervision (PINS) offenders invariably wind up being treated badly and corrupted insidiously by court processing. They add that involuntary services just don't work and they suggest better voluntary services are the only answer. The skeptics of abolition—including a large number of juvenile court judges—say that refusing help even when it is less than totally adequate consigns troubled children to the fate of the streets, prostitution, petty crime and drug addiction.

The PINS dilemma involves a conflict between parents' rights and children's rights of the most troublesome kind. It has so far not been amenable to final resolution by the courts. The 1974 Juvenile Justice Delinquency and Prevention Act and the Runaway Youth Act have spurred the establishment of new alternatives to institutionalization for such offenders. State codes are increasingly limiting the nature of the available dispositions. But we are probably unlikely to get a more definitive legal solution for a while.

Beginning in the early seventies, a new kind of juvenile rights case emerged: class action suits brought to correct inhumane conditions in children's training schools or detention centers. These cases argued constitutional and statutory rights of incarcerated children to minimum restrictions on mail and visiting privileges, humane living conditions, decent educational and vocational opportunities, and freedom from physical and sexual abuse while in confinement (15, 16). Limited budgets, low political priority, rural locations, and difficulties in recruiting personnel were the usual defenses raised in such suits to explain admittedly inferior conditions of confinement. Although many state and Federal courts have recognized confined children's rights to have a decent environment, endless arguments continue about what constitutes minimal standards and how fast and how soon the state should have to meet them.

Activist judges who wrote such decisions have been widely criticized —as well as defended—for getting the courts into matters better left to the legislatures and for ending up as social service administrators themselves. Thus, although the legal rights of juveniles to decent residential care have been established in the lawbooks, there is wide disagreement about how far the courts can mandate the details of such care or whether they can insist state legislators pay for this care. One may safely predict there will be a cautious attitude in the future about these lawsuits—now that the judiciary has seen how long and hard it is to get results after their decisions have been handed down. Many of these lawsuits begun almost a decade ago are still in the courts.

Lately, there has been a decided trend to tougher attitudes toward violent or habitual serious juvenile offenders. Some states have altered their juvenile law to permit waivers to adult courts of children from age 13 on. Other states are moving toward a system of fixed penalties for specific crimes committed by juveniles. In this kind of system, juveniles' claims on due process rights will be even stronger but their claims for special treatment after conviction will be diminished. They could end up with little more than the rockbottom standard of the 8th amendment that forbids confinement of juveniles and adults alike in conditions that amount to "cruel and unusual punishment." There may, however, always be a powerful argument that the state owes a greater duty to an undeveloped mind and body over whom it exerts total control than to a mature adult. Just what the contours of such a duty are is, at this moment in the history of the juvenile justice process, unclear.

RIGHTS OF CHILDREN IN NEGLECT AND CUSTODY DISPUTES

The campaign to define rights for juveniles in neglect and custody proceedings has proven even more difficult than defining rights for delinquents. Changes in disputed child custody, abuse and neglect cases —the traditional fare of domestic relations and family courts— have been far less dramatic. In this type of case, the state is customarily proceeding against the parent rather than the child or, in disputed custody cases, one parent is proceeding against the other. Until recently, the child's interests were presumed to be in accord with the state's interests in abuse and neglect cases and to be adequately protected by the neutral judge in custody disputes. The most significant development in these cases in the past decade has been a requirement, in many jurisdictions, for separate counsel to represent the child's interests in abuse and neglect cases. Rarely is this requirement for counsel called for in custody cases (13). Some lower courts have said that the state must sustain a high burden of persuasion before it can remove children from their homes without first offering the families assistance in solving their economic or psychological problems. The landmark work of Goldstein, Solnit and Freud, *Beyond the Best Interests of the Child* (10) has escalated the awareness that children should not be left in foster care indefinitely (20) and that a court should make the least drastic intervention possible in the child's life when deciding what to do in such cases. In child custody disputes, judges now tend to pay greater attention to the articulated choices of the child from an early age.

The push toward more deliberate and measured state interference in the family under the abuse and neglect rubric was mounted in large part by poverty and civil rights lawyers who saw the impact of these laws fall unfairly on poor and minority families whose mores did not always fit the tastes of state social workers or court personnel. Juvenile rights as such, except for the right to be represented by independent counsel, were not, however, the primary focus in the changing direction of abuse and neglect law. It was rather the right of the parent, climaxed by the Supreme Court's declaration in *Stanley* v. *Illinois* (21), that a natural father had such a right with regard to his illegitimate child, that was being vindicated. This right of family integrity, so strongly supported by coalitions of minority and poverty advocates, on some occasions seems to conflict with the juvenile's rights. This conflict, in turn, may result in inner tensions and priority fights in local and national child advocacy organizations.

In sum, the kind of knotty, multiple problem situations presented by child custody fights and—more intractably—by neglecting and abusive parents do not lend themselves to easy legal solutions. Each such tragedy is unique and solutions—if they exist at all—lie more often in resources for the beleaguered family, education on how to parent, or fostering of changes in the attitude of the parents toward each other and toward the child. More recently, it appears that, certainly in urban centers, the threat of premature or unthinking intervention in salvageable family structures is relatively infrequent. The danger of returning a neglected or abused child to be reexploited is greater. The services provided such parents are too sparse, episodic and fragmented. They are often irrelevant. The state's ultimate solution—removal from the home—generally spells a dubious future for the child.

Conscientious juvenile and family judges are chronically frustrated by their inability to mandate the right services for the family or the right placement for the neglected or abused child. They blame inadequate budgets and unresponsive bureaucrats. They also frequently vocalize irritation with the war of child mental health "experts" in such cases. Right now, these expert witnesses seem to be lined up on both sides of virtually any issue involving proper treatment or disposition of children. They may casually contradict one another first to the amazement then to the gradual cynicism of the courts. How much do court hearings in which parents testify negatively about their children traumatize these children? Do parents resent and reject children when their efforts to institutionalize them fail? Are children actually asking to be dealt with authoritatively when they object and rebel? When can children make informed and responsible decisions about their own lives? Up to what point is arguably abusive treatment by one's own kith and kin preferable to sanitized—but nonabuse—treatment at the hands of strangers? Perhaps there are no hard and fast answers or even consensus about questions such as these. Minimally, however, it does seem there might be more exchange and possibly even some joint principles worked out between child-oriented professions and lawyers. Thus, a judge—untutored in this area—cannot now recognize whether an expert witness is giving a truly objective summary of the state of the art or merely an offbeat opinion one of the parties found on the nineteenth try. All "experts" have equal access to the judge and those who have the best "courtroom manners" may prevail. There ought to be exploration of ways a conscientious judge could obtain a neutral summary of the thinking in the field and a map of where the experts fit on the terrain. The adversary process now is costly and confusing and too often totally misleading. More cooperative work needs to be done on assuring that the social sciences contribute the best and most complete thinking they are capable of to these critical child-related decisions.

LEGAL RIGHTS IN THE FAMILY

By far the thorniest area in juvenile law concerns the child's rights inside his/her own family, and the degree to which courts will interfere with family autonomy in decision-making. It is also the area about which traditional poverty and civil rights juvenile advocates feel most uncomfortable. Indeed, one sometimes sees them on opposite sides of the same juvenile rights case. Many of these intrafamily cases involve decisions about medical and psychiatric care for the child. Their precursors may be found in the Jehovah's Witness blood transfusion cases where courts were called upon to decide under a neglect and abuse rubric whether the child's life should be saved at the expense of the parent's religious beliefs. The child's interests in survival—represented by state or hospital authorities—have usually won out in these cases.

The newer cases are more complex. They may pose the parents' rights to opt for the natural death of a child instead of life in a severely handicapped state and conversely the right of adolescents themselves to make such a choice. They also challenge the right of parents to make critical medical decisions that affect the lives of their children, such as kidney transplants from one child to another, where the parents' interests may be in conflict with the interests of the individual child. *The New*

York Times (Nov. 26, 1978) recently carried two illustrative examples. In the first case, parents of a Down's syndrome child refused to consent to a heart operation which could help, but might also weaken, their child. Without the operation, the doctors said the child would die by the age of 30. The parents said he would never be able to live independently and once they were gone, he would be abandoned and warehoused. The state—on behalf of this child—is appealing the court's refusal to consent to the operation. The second item told of the death of a 13-year-old girl who refused a marrow transplant from her sister because of her own and her parents' religious beliefs; she was upheld by the court in that refusal. We can expect more of these cases as parents and even adolescents become aware of their rights to die and to allow their children to die in certain circumstances. Medical authorities themselves are generally the instigators of these suits, probably from a natural desire to protect themselves from malpractice as well as from a genuine desire to see the child given the best chance to survive. The principles on which such cases must be decided are not yet agreed upon. One lawyer, also an expert in child psychology, suggests that the choice should definitely be with the parents or the mature adolescent—even where the choice means death—unless the result of the operation or procedure will be a *substantial* chance at a reasonably normal life (8).

Parental decisions to subject children to medical experimentation and to undertake high risk procedures such as psychosurgery or electroshock have also been held subject to judicial oversight. Some child advocates would extend the range of challengeable treatment decisions to prolonged drug therapy or aversive regimes for behavioral modification. The unsettled issue is which among critical decisions affecting a child's life demand some oversight by a court (or possibly by some other objective third party such as a peer review or human rights review committee attached to a hospital or institution) either because the parent isn't informed enough or because the parent is too close to an inherently conflicting situation to make a decision "in the best interests of the child."

For the second term in a row, the Supreme Court in 1979 considered the dilemma of whether parents on the advice of doctors may "voluntarily" institutionalize children in mental facilities without a prior judicial or administrative hearing (11). The court was obviously troubled; the Justices are parents themselves. The integrity of the family decision-making process was pitted against the terrible harms that unhappy families can intentionally or unwittingly do to their children. What bothered most lay people—and the Justices—was the notion that the child's protector in such a situation would be a stranger/lawyer and those the child was being protected against were his blood relatives. Even if a lawyer convinced a court that the child did not need institutionalization, where would the child go?

A divided Court decided to uphold the family decision in such cases, provided that the decision to institutionalize was supported by that of an independent admitting physician. It furthermore allowed the same result where the initiative to institutionalize was made by a social worker for a child already in state custody. It said that children did indeed have a "liberty interest" in staying free of confinement but that such an interest was adequately protected by the combination of family or social worker decision-making vindicated by a medical concurrence that institutionalization was necessary. It was enough for due process that the doctor made a medical rather than a legal-type inquiry, just as they had previously ruled that a child could be expelled or suspended from school only after the school principal made some kind of appropriate inquiry—but not necessarily a full-fledged trial—into the child's alleged misconduct (9).

The *Parham* decision represented a resounding victory for parental authority. It is difficult to envision very many—if any—situations short of abuse or neglect, where courts will now intervene to monitor family decisions about the medical or psychiatric treatment of children if professional support is present. Legislative changes are still possible but, in light of the political strength of family-rightists, not likely.

A still different kind of juvenile legal issue is presented by the abortion-contraceptive-VD-drug-treatment cases involving adolescents. Here the juveniles are typically asking for the right to make their own decisions about their own bodies without parental veto. The Supreme Court has now said that parents cannot be given by law the right to say a definitive "No" to abortions their daughters want (18). They have also said that states cannot make it a criminal offense to sell contraceptives to adolescents (14). More recently, however, the court has decided that a state law can provide for a requirement that a minor seek court approval for an abortion when parental consent is not forthcoming (1).

These decisions pose new legal problems for doctors and health providers dealing with adolescents. Also complicating matters for these child-care workers are the many state laws allowing juveniles to seek VD, drug treatment, or contraceptive information and help on their own. No longer is the informed consent, or lack thereof, of the parents necessarily enough. If the child is old enough to have an opinion, he/she may have to be consulted. If the parent and the child disagree, where does the doctor go—to court? In cases where the child's consent is enough by statute, the criteria for insuring that consent is informed may be more stringent in a juvenile's case than in an adult's. Adults have successfully sued institutional doctors and superintendents for unnecessarily prolonging hospitalizations—children may be able to do the same. And many state laws put the doctor in the position of broker between child and parent—he/she must decide when it is in the child's best interests or will jeopardize his/her health and safety to notify a parent about ongoing treatment. If he/she makes a bad call, either parent or child may cry foul and sue for malpractice. Finally, children have privacy rights and inappropriate disclosure of their medical records can invite lawsuits. There is little question that the advent of juvenile legal rights in the area of medical care has complicated the caregiver's profession.

JUVENILE RIGHTS AND JUVENILE PROCESSES

The juvenile legal rights movement has, of course, had significant implications for the juvenile court and juvenile justice system. Yet, many of the landmark juvenile cases have actually arisen in nonjuvenile courts. Thus, concern with fundamental issues affecting juveniles has permeated the entire American judicial system, and juvenile experts may be called upon to enter any of several state or federal judicial forums.

The juvenile justice system itself has in recent years been subjected to intensive study. The most ambitious project sponsored by the American Bar Association and the Institute of Judicial Administration spent six years, culminating in over 20 volumes on every facet of the process. Its recommendations are legion but their philosophical thrust is directed toward more procedural rights, more regularized procedures, less sentencing discretion for judges and more restrictions on juvenile correctional administrators, less emphasis on treatment and rehabilitation and more controls on state intervention with neglected children and status offenders. Many now question whether a separate juvenile justice system has any continuing justification, especially when adequate resources continue to be denied to implement individualized treatment for young clients.

In short, for almost two decades now there has been a tug-of-war between the opponents and proponents of the juvenile justice process. On the one hand, opponents claim it has little to offer troubled children or their parents. On the other hand, proponents still dream of a specialized forum for juveniles which can provide help and guidance instead of punishment. They continue to fight for more resources and the power to intervene where needed to help children and families.

The reason is that neither the juvenile court nor the juvenile justice system has yet been allowed to show whether it can deliver high grade services that are of significant help to juveniles or their families. The juvenile justice system is truly in midpassage.

REFERENCES

1. *Bellotti* v. *Baird*, 99 S.Ct. 3035 (1979).
2. *Breed* v. *Jones*, 421 U.S. 519 (1975).
3. *Causey, In re*, 47 U.S. Law Week 2304 (1978).
4. *Carey* v. *Pop. Ser. Int'l.*, 431 U.S. 678 (1977).
5. *Dumpson* v. *Daniel M.*, N.Y. L.J. (October 16, 1974).
6. *E.S.G.* v. *State*, 447 S.W. 2d 225 (Ct Civ App Tex) (1969) cert. den. 398 U.S. 956 (1970).
7. *Gault, In re*, 387 U.S. 1 (1967).
8. GOLDSTEIN, J. (1977). Medical Care for the Child at Risk, 86 Yale L.J. 645.
9. *Goss* v. *Lopez*, 419 U.S. 565 (1975).
10. GOLDSTEIN, J., FREUD, A., & SOLNIT, A. (1973). *Beyond the Best Interests of the Child*. New York: Free Press.
11. *J.L.* v. *Parham*, 99 S.Ct. 2493 (1979).
11a. JUVENILE JUSTICE AND DELINQUENCY PREVENTION ACT OF 1974: 88 Stat. 1109 as amended 91 Stat 1048 (1977).
12. JUVENILE JUSTICE STANDARDS PROJECT (1977). Tentative Draft, Standards relating to Abuse and Neglect.
13. JUVENILE JUSTICE STANDARDS PROJECT (1978). Lawyering for Children. 87 Yale L.J. 1126.
14. *McKeiver* v. *Penn.*, 403 U.S. 528 (1971).
15. *Morales* v. *Turman*, 383 F. Supp. 53 (E.D. Tex, 1971).
16. *Martarella* v. *Kelley*, 349 F. Supp. 1130 (S.D. Miss., 1977).
18. *Planned Parenthood* v. *Danforth*, 428 U.S. 52 (1976).
19. President's Commission on Law Enforcement and the Administration of Justice, Task Force Report on Juvenile Delinquency and Youth Crime (1967) Chapter 1.
19a. Runaway Youth Act, Pub. L. 93-415, Title III, 88 Stat. 1129 (1974); 42 U.S.C. § 5701 *et seq.* (1976).
20. *Smith* v. *Org. Foster Families*, 431 U.S. 816 (1977).
21. *Stanley* v. *Illinois*, 405 U.S. 645 (1972).
22. *Winship, In re*, 397 U.S. 358 (1970).

3
INTRODUCTION TO
COURT EVALUATIONS

DIANE H. SCHETKY, M.D.

This chapter will describe the author's approach to the psychiatric evaluation of parents and children done expressly for the court and will offer practical advice on facilitating the process. The professional who chooses to do this type of evaluation should be prepared to make an investment of time and emotional commitment since one is frequently asked to participate in decisions which have lifelong implications for both child and parent. To be an effective expert witness, one must accumulate and process a vast amount of information and translate it into terms which are intelligible and useful to the court. This chapter breaks the psychiatric evaluation down into component parts: 1) communicating with the attorney; 2) the clinical evaluation; 3) the written report.

COMMUNICATING WITH ATTORNEYS

Choosing a Psychiatrist

In contrast to the usual psychiatric evaluation, the parent or child seen for a court evaluation is rarely self-referred. Most likely sources for such referrals are attorneys, child care agencies, the court, and other physicians. The attorney who refers a client to a psychiatrist is likely to be doing so to help his case rather than his client per se (3, 4). He or she seeks the best available talent but may find the ideal forensic child psychiatrist to be as elusive as the mythical perfect parent. Good child psychiatrists are likely to be busy psychiatrists and may not have schedules which lend themselves to court work. Some are quite willing to prepare a report on a child but shrink from testifying in court, reacting as if they themselves are on trial. For some, this attitude may stem from ignorance as to what

21

is expected of them when testifying. For many, however, the realities are that their schedules lack the flexibility to accommodate court hearings. A common resistance is that too much time is wasted in warming benches in court corridors. Although waits are inevitable, if given sufficient notice, the child psychiatrist can block out time, bill for it, and put waiting time to good use catching up on reading and writing or becoming more familiar with court processes and personnel. The courteous attorney will try to give the witness a close estimate of how much time will be involved (even offering a choice of times when feasible) and get the witness in and out of court as quickly as possible.

Since the attorney will have to establish the witness' expertise, credentials such as training, licensure, board certification, and clinical experience are important. Equally important, however, is the question of how the psychiatrist relates to patients, writes a report, and performs in court. A full professor may undermine a case by equivocating or hesitating to call a patient psychotic to her face, whereas a trainee with less impressive credentials but more presence may come across as a more decisive and credible witness. The attorney should not preclude using the inexperienced witness, but should plan on spending more time with him or her in pretrial preparation and going over anticipated lines of questioning. Other desirable attributes in an expert witness include a good command of written and spoken English, the ability to take a firm stand and not be intimidated by cross-examination. Finally, the child psychiatrist who ventures into court work must possess inordinate patience and the ability to live with irresolution and postponement of hearings on short notice, and with not always having his/her opinions followed. Considering the investment the expert witness puts into a case, follow-up by the attorney regarding disposition of the case, as well as feedback on testimony, is usually appreciated, although it is rarely volunteered.

Working with the Attorney

The child psychiatrist can work most effectively with the attorney if he/she has some appreciation of the framework within which the attorney operates, namely, the adversary system. In this way, potential conflicts between the two fields may be kept in historical perspective rather than being perceived in terms of interpersonal conflict. It is important to be mindful of the boundaries of one's respective roles lest the psychiatrist be tempted to play attorney or vice versa. The expert witness is only being asked for his or her opinion and relevant facts and will do well to maintain some humility with respect to the limits of his or her knowledge and ability to predict the future. Restraint with respect to not exceeding available data also serves to enhance credibility.

Adequate communication between psychiatrist and attorney is essential but often difficult to establish owing to their respectively demanding schedules. Some basic questions to be covered with the referring attorney are: 1) Who does the attorney represent? 2) What is it he or she wants to know? 3) How will the report be used and how extensive should it be? 4) Does he or she anticipate that you will be needed to testify in court? 5) To whom should the report be sent and when? 6) Who will be paying for the evaluation and how much? In some districts the juvenile court is obligated to pay for an evaluation it has ordered but there is most likely a limit on how much it will pay per evaluation. If the client is paying for the evaluation, it is prudent to either have fees paid in advance or held in trust by the attorney. A client is not going to be inclined to pay for an evaluation which he or she deems unfavorable and in custody evaluations one side is likely to emerge as the loser. One issue to be prepared for with prepayment of fees is that at the cross-examining the other attorney may infer that the expert witness' opinion has been bought. A statement to the effect that one's time rather than opinion is being paid for usually disposes of this argument.

The psychiatrist should discuss with the attorney how he or she intends to prepare the client for the evaluation and offer the attorney advice if indicated. The attorney should refrain from coaching his or her client as this only clouds the issues at hand. For example, a 15-year-old girl accused of being an accomplice to a murder had been told by her attorney to "act contrite," which only complicated the psychiatrist's task of deciding how much guilt she was experiencing over the act.

If there is any question of a client's being psychotic or incompetent, permission should be obtained from the client's guardian to proceed with the evaluation. In a recent Oregon case, a chronic schizophrenic woman was evaluated at the request of the court with respect to her ability to care for her two-year-old son who had never lived with her (7). In the course of the evaluation she claimed the child was not hers because she could not remember giving birth to him. In spite of her abdication of motherhood, her attorney appealed the termination of her parental rights on grounds that the evaluating psychiatrist had failed to get the permission of the woman's guardian to see her. Further, the court did not have the authority to order her to submit to a psychiatric evaluation. The Court of Appeals held that, in determining what is best for the child, the juvenile court has the authority to order a psychiatric or medical evaluation of the parent where results of the evaluation will be an aid to making that evaluation.

To expedite the evaluation process, the psychiatrist should request the attorney to have the client sign necessary release forms for all relevant reports and enlist the attorney's help in assembling background information prior to the evaluation. Results of previous psychiatric evaluations are extremely important, as are recommendations and whether or not they were followed. Information regarding past psychiatric treatment is considered privileged and need not be released unless the client wishes it to be. Results of psychological evaluations are also important and may spare costly duplication of efforts. When an arrest is involved, police reports may also be an important source of information. If the examiner has not had access to important pieces of information, the report should state this fact.

Some attorneys fear that sharing previous evaluations with the psychiatrist may create a bias, but a competent psychiatrist should be able to arrive at an independent opinion and feel free to differ with those offered by colleagues. Further, he or she is in a much better position if he or she has had time to process the information rather than being confronted with it for the first time in court. Generally, the more information the psychiatrist has the better able he or she is to render an opinion. Unfortunately, the law in some states and as interpreted by some courts does not see eye to eye with this position and the attorney may insist that the expert base his or her opinion solely on firsthand information. The strictest hearsay rule requires that "opinion of a medical expert as to physical or mental condition of some person involved in the proceeding, or as to the cause or effect of some disease or injury with which such person is afflicted, based upon information from third persons out of court, is inadmissible" (1). The rationale for this rule is that hearsay testimony does not provide the cross-examining attorney with the opportunity to test the reliability of that evidence. Many juvenile courts today ignore the rule or permit exceptions to it and in the author's experience secondary history has usually been admissible where it is used as corroborative information but not as the sole source of history.

THE CLINICAL EVALUATION

It is highly desirable that the psychiatric evaluation of both parents and children be carried out by someone who is not in an ongoing treatment relationship with them. This helps to overcome the problems of confidentiality, bias, and professional narcissism with respect to prognosis. It further avoids the dilemma of testimony which could be detrimental to the doctor-patient relationship.

The Parents

Exploring the parents' understanding of the psychiatric evaluation provides the basis for informed consent and also reveals a great deal about their judgment and reality testing. When asked why they think they are being seen, many parents will respond concretely "because we were told to come here," whereas for others the question may open up a Pandora's box. Parents who are veterans of the system may view the psychiatrist suspiciously as yet another arm of the court or child protective agency which is out to get them. Others, sometimes justifiably, may pour forth tales of mistreatment at the hands of agencies. A psychotic mother being seen for possible termination of her parental rights thought that she was going to be terminated. When asked what she meant by this, she replied blandly, "Why you know, terminate—exterminate—me, just the way they do on TV." The psychiatrist should, in all cases, go over the reality based reasons for the evaluation as well as the fact that it is not confidential, and obtain written permission for release of subsequent reports. Some parents, aware of this, will put their best foot forward. Many parents, however, will surprisingly proceed to reveal extremely self-damaging material which should raise questions about their judgment and motivation.

The history as obtained from the parent is extremely important as it constitutes the primary source of background information and may also point to areas of contradiction with other sources which need to be clarified. Frequently, history will be colored by parents' defensiveness. Hence, there is a need for corroboration, especially where factual data are available. Parents' biases need not necessarily be conscious or deceitful but rather may represent their perception of events in light of their life experiences. The parents' backgrounds are explored in detail with particular emphasis on how they were parented and where they are in their emotional development. The parent-child relationship is examined simultaneously with the gathering of developmental histories on the children in question.

The parents' current and past functioning and capacity for interpersonal relationships are key areas in assessing their capacity to parent. One should also include a mental status exam and develop a diagnostic formulation since one is likely to be asked about these areas in court.

Assessment of the parent-child relationship takes into consideration history, observation of the parents' feelings and sensitivity towards the child, capacity to meet the child's needs, and inquiry into what the child means to the parent. Parenting should also be evaluated through direct observation, which will be discussed in more detail in Chapter 9. Surprisingly, little has been written about how one evaluates parenting and the spectacle of the adult psychiatrist defending his or her patient's right to her child on the grounds that she loves him or that the child will provide an incentive to rehabilitation is an all too common occurrence in the court room. More specific criteria are needed to assess what constitutes, in Winnicott's terms, a "good enough parent." The following attributes are desirable if a parent is to enhance the child's normal psychological development:

1) Capacity for empathy. Adequate experiences in infancy with an empathetic mother lay the foundation for becoming an empathetic adult, whereas deficiencies in empathetic mothering lead to lack of confidence and basic trust in adults. Parents who are out of touch with their own feelings or extremely defensive about them may be ill equipped to understand the child's feelings or provide a role model to the child as to how one handles feelings.

2) The parents must regard the child as a separate being with his or her own needs and not merely as an extension of themselves or as existing to meet their needs. The parent who is unable to make this distinction often ends up projecting his or her own feelings onto the child and abusing the child because he fails to meet these unrealistic expectations. In contrast, the parent who is able to attend to the child's needs promotes self-esteem and feelings of being loved and valued.

3) Optimal psychological development requires continuity and reasonable consistency in parenting.

4) The parent needs to act as a buffer between the child and his or her environment, shielding the child from over-stimulation or excessive frustration.

5) On the other hand, the parent should be able to help the child master aggressive instincts and learn to cope with frustrations. To do so, the parent must first provide limits which the child will gradually internalize. The child who experiences no such limits may feel unloved and is likely to be frightened by the intensity of his or her unleashed aggression.

6) Parents should be flexible and able to recognize and adapt to the

child's changing needs. For example, some mothers do well with the totally dependent infant but have difficulty tolerating the toddler's burgeoning independence.

7) Finally, the parent provides a model through his or her own behavior. The parent who is physically abusive teaches the child that anger implies a right to hit and that conflicts are resolved through physical force. In contrast, the parent who is able to discipline and resolve disputes with words imparts a far more civilized model for the child to emulate.

The Child

As with adults, children who are intellectually and emotionally (age four and up) able to understand must be carefully informed of the purpose of the evaluation and the fact that it is not confidential. Even though their consent is not legally necessary to release the report, it is tactful to ask their permission to share results of the evaluation with the judge, attorney or case worker. Doing so tends to make them feel that what they have to say is important, allows them to feel they have some role in determining their fate, and helps to insure their trust in adults.

In custody evaluations, the focus shifts from traditional emphasis on diagnostic formulation to additional assessment of the child's psychological ties. These may be determined through history, direct observation, direct questioning and indirect techniques. Direct questioning requires extreme sensitivity and tact and the examiner must avoid asking leading questions. Information about the child's relationship to various family members will often emerge through puppet play, the doll house, and drawings of the family. For instance, a neglected five-year-old boy, when asked to draw a picture of his family, depicted his obese mother as a beached whale about to die and commented that the doctor would have to find her two babies a new home. Some children who have experienced parental neglect may fail to include any adults in their play and drawings, and often depict the children as having to fend for themselves or else portray them as administering to the needs of adults.

Particular attention should be paid to the child's level of development since children who have been neglected or abused, and moved around a lot, often show lags in various aspects of their development. The Denver Development Screening Test and the Goodenough Draw a Person are useful screening devices; for some children, additional psychological testing will be indicated. Ego deficits are common in this population and, though they may readily be accounted for by environmental factors, one must not overlook the possibility of central nervous system dysfunction related to earlier abuse or neglect.

Obviously, it is dangerous to generalize about the effects of abuse and neglect as there will always be the exceptional child who emerges from a deprived childhood relatively intact. Some children are constitutionally stronger and more resilient than others and manage to find means of coping with stress that might overwhelm a more vulnerable child. Other children may be adept at seeking out parental surrogates to take over where their own parents have failed.

Caution is also indicated when it comes to predicting how a child's personality will evolve over the long run. Anna Freud (6) details factors which make such clinical prediction both difficult and hazardous, stating. "There is no guarantee that the rate of maturational progress will progress on the side of ego development, that drive development will be even and whenever one side of the structure outdistances the other in growth, a variety of unexpected and unpredictable deviations from normal will follow." Further, she notes, "there is no way to approach quantitative factors in drive development, nor do we necessarily have any control over the happenings in the child's environment since they are not governed by any laws" (6, p. 92).

THE WRITTEN REPORT

The content of the psychiatric report basically conforms to the standard psychiatric evaluation with an introductory segment followed by history, observations, impressions, diagnosis, recommendations and prognosis. Length will vary according to the questions asked and the individual's style. Particular attention should be paid to recording the exact amount of time spent with the patient, the place and dates of the evaluation, and referral source, with knowledge that one will be questioned about these matters in court. It is also important to record missed or canceled appointments as these may reflect the patient's attitude towards the evaluation and therapeutic intervention in general. All sources of information should be listed, as well as mention of when they were received with respect to the evaluation in case that purported bias becomes an issue. The patient's understanding of the purpose of the evaluation should be stated along with documentation of discussions regarding lack of confidentiality, lest the patient or his or her attorney try to invoke privilege as a means of suppressing testimony.

History should be condensed into salient features but may have to be recorded from the vantage points of the child, parents, foster parents, child care agency and the court, with contradictions not uncommon. The history which is obtained from secondary sources should be presented in a separate body of information in the event that it is deemed to be inadmissible hearsay.

The material one chooses to include in the report should be viewed as building blocks upon which one formulates an opinion. Thus, one must include sufficient information to provide the premises for one's conclusions while at the same time avoiding the perils of verbosity. It is helpful in the process of writing to ask oneself how various statements will hold up under cross-examination. Vague, ambiguous terminology should be avoided, and where possible, specific examples should be offered to back up one's impressions. For instance, to merely state that a mother was poorly groomed may not suffice and her attorney could argue that her appearance reflected her welfare status rather than her inability to care for herself. A more precise description in an actual case stated, "Although only 35, she could easily have passed for 50; her hair was dirty and disheveled, her body malodorous and her extremities covered with cat scratches. She wore rhinestone glasses, dirty white sneakers, and a low-cut, floor-length, gingham gown into the cleavage of which she had stuffed her house key suspended from a long string of diaper pins." In this particular instance the woman's appearance was so bizarre that it alerted the psychiatrist to the presence of a previously undetected organic brain syndrome.

A psychiatric report will also have more credibility if fortified with direct quotations from the patient, which stand up better under cross-examination than do subjective judgments. Thus a father's statement "I want my daughter (age four) back so I can get all that love and good stuff I never had as a kid" will have far more impact that any statement the psychiatrist might make regarding his motivation for requesting custody of his daughter. Secondly, the use of direct quotations helps refresh one's memory when months to years may have elapsed between evaluation and testimony.

The psychiatric report should strive to be relevant to the legal issues at hand. To do this, the child psychiatrist must have some familiarity with the relevant legal statutes in his or her state. Further, the psychiatrist should bear in mind that the court may be much more interested in practical matters, such as recommendations and prognosis, than in theoretical formulations. One must use discretion in deciding what material to include, weighing its significance and relevance against possible harm to the parents and child. For instance, an adolescent's sexual fantasies may be of interest to the psychiatrist but have little bearing on the behavior that brought her to court. To include this material in the report is to invite questioning at the risk of considerable embarrassment to the patient. In contrast, an eight-year-old boy living with his grandmother was referred for evaluation because he repeatedly ran away during visits to his mother. Apropos his mother's wishes to regain custody of him, the boy proposed that he should run away and whoever found him should be allowed to keep him. When asked who he thought this might be, he replied poignantly that his grandmother was old and slow and that it might take her a long time but that she would ultimately claim him because he didn't think his mother would even bother to look for him. Further exploration of his feelings revealed that he harbored murderous thoughts towards his mother who had abused him as a younger child, and that he was running away in part to protect himself from acting on these impulses. Obviously, this material was relevant and needed to be shared with the court. With his permission, it was included in the report that recommended he remain with his grandmother. Unforeseen by the child psychiatrist, the report was later shared with the boy's mother by her attorney who had it copied from the court record. She was understandably upset by it, and her relationship with her son was probably further jeopardized. In retrospect, the child psychiatrist might have been better off had she insisted upon seeing the boy's mother and discussing her recommendations with her prior to the court hearing. This case serves as a reminder that all reports become public documents once acquired by the courts since the psychiatrist loses control of their distribution.

The psychiatric report should be written in language that is intelligible to the layman. Psychiatric jargon rarely impresses and, more often than not, serves to alienate and confuse the reader. Clear thinking should be reflected in lucid writing. With practice one learns to transform phrases such as "psychosexual developmental arrest at an oedipal level" to a more acceptable and meaningful "the child is still functioning emotionally at the level of a five-year-old."

In order to convey objectivity, the psychiatrist should avoid interjecting himself or herself through use of the first person into the report. A more neutral stance is also achieved through use of terms such as "the patient states" in place of the more pejorative "the patient alleges" or "claims," which infers that the patient's credibility is in doubt. Tentative words such as "suspect" or "possibly" should be avoided as they contribute little and do not hold up under cross-examination. Conversely, one does well to avoid statements such as "obviously" or "it is clear" unless the situation is truly apparent to all concerned.

Ideally, the forensic report should be uninvolved, objective, and impartial but in reality this goal is difficult to attain. Diamond (5) recommends that the psychiatrist be requested to furnish a professional viewpoint rather than neutral expertise. Numerous factors operate to create conscious or unconscious bias in the examiner, including the relationship that develops with the patient during a prolonged evaluation. Similarly, the psychiatrist may be influenced by his or her relationship with the referring attorney and the court. Additional sources of bias are the psychiatrist's personality, theoretical framework, possible need to protect the patient, and identification with authority figures or the underdog. Finally, Bazelon cautions that "Like any other man, a physician acquires an emotional identification with an opinion that comes down on one side of a conflict; he has an inescapable, prideful conviction in the accuracy of his own findings" (2, p. 21).

Perhaps the most difficult part of the evaluation is the formulation and recommendations. It is also the most important part as it is the culmination of a lengthy process of evaluation and is the part of the report which is most likely to be read. The beginner may be tempted to avoid taking a stand on issues and write tepid, nebulous reports which may spare the feelings of the involved parties, but in the process of doing so fail to render useful information to the court which may even result in the patient's being subjected to yet another evaluation. When one is truly undecided, he or she should present the pros and cons of various custody arrangements to the court. Often, however, indecisiveness reflects inadequate information and one should either request further evaluation time or state the limiting conditions which prevented a more thorough assessment.

When the results of an evaluation are unfavorable to the patient, one should phrase findings in a humane way instead of watering down testimony. Thus rather than call a mother unfit one might say, "Unfortunately, she herself was the victim of poor parenting and is, consequently, extremely limited in her ability to meet the needs of this very difficult child. She has not been able to profit from intensive efforts aimed at intervention." Recommendations should be realistic with respect to availability of services and the court's ability to expedite treatment plans. Regarding prognosis, one is generally safest adhering to the maxim that the past is the best predictor of the future, especially where nothing has occurred to suggest any evidence of change in the patient's conduct or condition.

It may be tempting to try to fortify one's final stance with quotations of research findings from the literature. However, to do so is to invite the cross-examining attorney to come forth with references countering one's sources. While the witness cannot be questioned about something he or she has not read, exposure of one's unfamiliarity with certain authors may damage the psychiatrist's stature in the eyes of the court. The best ammunition for withstanding vigorous cross-examination remains a thorough evaluation and mastery of the facts of the case.

After completing the written report, it is a good idea to make an extra copy, since the report may be requested as evidence and this way one is not left empty handed. At the conclusion of the evaluation, working notes should either be destroyed or put in good order as they may also be called into evidence.

Billing is best handled on an hourly basis since one cannot predict how long an evaluation will take. Compensation should include time spent in preparation, consultation with attorneys, travel time, and time spent in waiting and testifying in court. Fees will vary by locale and, as with attorneys, by status. One eminent forensic psychiatrist raised his fees drastically in hopes of fending off referrals whereupon he found he was more in demand than ever before. Private evaluations are inevitably costly, but fortunately forensic evaluations are becoming more readily available through clinics so that income need not be a factor in obtaining a good evaluation.

Finally, as the experienced child forensic psychiatrist can attest, the rewards of this type of work are often not financial but rather lay in the learning process that is involved and the satisfaction that comes from helping to resolve conflicts.

REFERENCES

1. 20 Am. Jur. Evidence 866.5 (Cum. Supp. 1964).
2. BAZELON, D. (1974). Psychiatrists and the Adversary Process. *Scientific American*, 230, No. 6, 18-22.
3. BENEDEK, C. & SELZER, M. (1965). Lawyer's Use of Psychiatry. *Amer. J. Psych.*, 122: 212-213.
4. BENEDEK, E. & SELZER, M. (1977). Lawyer's Use of Psychiatry. *Amer. J. Psych.*, 134 (4):435-436.
5. DIAMOND, B. (1959). The Fallacy of the Impartial Expert. *Arch. Crim. Psychodynamics*, 3:221.
6. FREUD, A. (1958). Child Observation and Prediction of Development. *Psychoanal. Study of the Child*, Vol. 13:92-124.
7. *State of Oregon* v. *McGinnis*, 1977.

4
THE CLINICAL PSYCHOLOGIST
AND THE EVALUATION OF
PARENTS AND CHILDREN

RUTH G. MATARAZZO, Ph.D.

This chapter will be devoted to an aspect of the clinical psychologist's function which is relatively unique to the profession: the use of psychological assessment techniques. No reference will be made to the clinical interview which, although ordinarily of equal importance in the psychologist's contribution to court evaluations, is well described in other chapters.

Often much interview and case history data have been obtained by a psychiatrist and/or case worker before the psychologist is contacted. It is very important that information known to the referring source—whether psychiatrist, attorney or social worker—be forwarded to the examining psychologist before the client is seen. Otherwise the psychologist must try his/her best to obtain orienting and historical information from the parent, requiring duplication of effort and unnecessary expense. Needless to say, the background information obtained from the patient is likely to be slanted or incomplete, further emphasizing the need for relatively objective historical data from the referring source. If a psychiatrist is making the referral, a copy of his/her report is helpful.

In making the referral, it is most helpful to indicate the questions to which the psychologist should address him/herself. For example, "Is it possible for this individual to become an adequate parent and, if so, what kind of treatment would be necessary?" Such questions will orient the psychologist to seek the necessary data and to answer, explicitly, what the referring source needs to know. The inexperienced person may ask for "a Rorschach" or some other specific test, giving the psychologist no clue as to what he/she should be looking for. (One referral source

33

of the author consistently asked for "a Belvedere Wechsel," meaning a Wechsler-Bellevue. It would obviously have been more appropriate to indicate what circumstances led the person to believe that an intellectual evaluation was needed—e.g., academic failure. In many situations, some additional tests might be required in order to fully answer the questions in the mind of the referring agent.)

The following discussion of psychological testing is categorized according to whether the client is a parent or child, and by intellectual and personality measures.

EVALUATION OF THE PARENT

Intellectual Functioning

This aspect of psychological assessment is not infrequently slighted because sometimes it is possible for an experienced clinician to estimate intelligence fairly accurately from an interview and because personality and/or social dynamics may be thought to be more important or interesting. Some psychologists avoid intellectual evaluations because they can be tedious and time-consuming, and he/she may prefer to spend the available professional time with the client evaluating less prosaic matters.

However, the psychologist eliminates intelligence testing at his/her peril. One cannot always accurately estimate IQ on the basis of interview. Clients with good vocabularies, good social skills or middle-class attributes, and clients who are good-looking, are more likely to be judged intelligent than those with the opposite characteristics. Patients with a serious thought disorder or of poor socioeconomic background often appear less bright than, in fact, they are. In almost every case of child abuse or neglect, the parent's level of intelligence is of potential significance, and should be carefully measured.

In potential termination of rights cases, low intelligence is one of the parental "conditions" which may render him/her unable to care adequately for a child. This is certainly true of the individual who falls within the range of mental deficiency (IQ 69 or below on the Wechsler Adult Intelligence Scale). A not atypical mentally defective mother with IQ of 66, who was examined by the author, maintained a filthy home; failed to change the children's diapers so that they were soiled, dried and resoiled; gave her infant a mixture of coffee and milk in its bottle; put fresh milk in used bottles with curdled, dried milk; and insisted that her children remain either in bed or in the playpen for most of the day.

Intervention in the form of homemaker and parent-training were to no avail. Her infant died and one of her two remaining children was placed in foster care. The father in this situation, although relatively ineffectual and seemingly complacent in the face of an intolerable situation, was found to have an IQ of 118 and some potential for treatment. A last attempt to avoid termination of rights was then recommended by training the father to be certain that the children received adequate care evenings and weekends, while they were placed in day care during his workings hours. (This recommendation was made, despite the above, deplorable conditions, because it is presumed best to make every effort to keep children with their natural parents if at all feasible.)

The above case clearly points out the importance of knowing the intelligence of *both* parents. If the father had been of less than average ability, it is unlikely that he could have assumed the extensive leadership role of both supporting the family and supervising the maintenance of adequate home conditions. Knowing the mother's IQ, it was apparent that she could not be expected to benefit from professional assistance.

In the author's experience, parents in the "borderline" range (IQ 70-79) of intelligence are also unlikely to provide adequate parenting (this group consists of those falling between approximately the 2nd and 9th percentiles of the population). Unfortunately, there are no published studies, which the author has been able to find, presenting statistical confirmation of this statement. Nonetheless, numerous case histories bear witness to the poor judgment, inconsistency, and inadequacy of parenting at this level of intelligence. Most of these individuals are barely able to maintain a semi-independent life-style, and depend upon relatives or agencies to help them through frequent, recurrent episodes of stress. An example is that of an 18-year-old, single girl who is the mother of a 1½-year-old infant. This mother has never, independently, taken care of her baby. She has either left him with her parents or stayed in the parental home while they took major responsibility for child care. The Children's Services Division later discovered that conditions in the grandparental home were, likewise, disadvantageous to the baby (they appeared to be of subnormal intelligence although somewhat more capable than their daughter). The child was eventually placed in an unrelated foster home. The mother visited him there on an erratic schedule, partly because she was confused about the bus system. She said that her new baby, one month old, was being fed a diet of Pablum, mixed in his bottle, baby food and scrambled eggs. The mother was dependent upon the baby's grandmother to take her shopping, to the doctor, or wherever she needed to go. The baby's mother tested at a Full Scale IQ of 74, placing her within the "borderline retarded" level, with reading and writing skills at the second to third grade level, accounting for her difficulty in being independent. She could not manage her welfare money effectively and was frequently taken advantage of, financially, by acquaintances. She has had only brief relationships, characterized by passive dependency on her part. In observing the mother and infant together, it was apparent that she did not know how to interact with him, and the baby responded more positively to the welfare worker whom he had seldom seen.

At the upper end of the borderline range, specific personality characteristics may ameliorate the individual's intellectual inadequacies. Good emotional balance, good home background and modeling by their own parents, good social skills, and the presence of other responsible adults are all factors which may enable them to parent with at least minimal adequacy.

Sometimes intelligence tests reveal the presence of intellectual deficits which may or may not be associated with medically verified brain damage. Whether or not the underlying cause can be traced to brain damage, the presence of functional deficits, as measured by an instrument such as the WAIS, can alert the psychologist to the likelihood that this parent suffers from significant areas of impairment. Thus, he/she may be found to have impaired judgment, organizational ability, or decision-making despite an average overall IQ score.

The Wechsler Adult Intelligence Scale (WAIS), the instrument of choice for measuring adult intelligence, is composed of six verbal subtests and five nonverbal or "performance" subtests, and yields a separate Verbal IQ and Performance IQ as well as a composite, Full Scale IQ (18). The verbal subtests consist of general information (presumably measuring the breadth of awareness of both common knowledge and more esoteric facts); comprehension (practical judgment regarding the rationale for accepted customs of society, the reason for certain laws, interpretation of proverbs, etc.); similarities (verbal abstractions); digit span (immediate memory); arithmetic (numerical reasoning ability, requiring only basic mathematical procedures); and vocabulary. The performance tests include block designs; puzzles; arrangement of comic strip-like pictures in the appropriate sequence; and picture completions (finding the essential missing detail in a picture).

The WAIS IQ is based upon statistical concepts related to the age-appropriate population mean for the individual tested, and measures related to how far the individual deviates from the mean. For example, an IQ of 100 is at the 50th percentile; an IQ of 110 is at the 75th percentile; an IQ of 120 is at approximately the 90th percentile; and an IQ of 130 is at approximately the 98th percentile. Similarly, an IQ of 90 is at the 25th percentile, an IQ of 80 at the 10th percentile, and an IQ of 70 at about the 2nd percentile. Most "normal" individuals score at approximately the same percentile on each of the subtests, although there is, of course, always some variability which is related to individual talents and background. However, when an individual obtains subtest scores which vary widely, for example ranging from the 25th to the 75th percentiles, the psychologist is alerted to the fact that the individual's functioning is disturbed. This may be on either an organic or functional basis, but it can be assumed that such an individual will be found to be grossly ineffective in some aspects of behavior or judgment, despite an overall "average" IQ. For example, wide subtest variability was noted in the case of a mother of twins who, overall, had an IQ of 109, with Verbal IQ 118 and Performance IQ 95. This wide spread of scores alerted the psychologist to a possible borderline thought disorder or mild brain damage—in any case, to grossly inefficient functioning. She was noted, during the examination, to be indecisive and immobilized in the face of stress. This was also true of her parenting pattern. She had two-year-old twins who, when with her, were markedly hyperactive, throwing toys about, climbing over furniture, purposely breaking things, and running down the hall. Although given 15 sessions of intensive, supervised training in managing them over a three-month period, she was unable to generalize from the clinic playroom situation to the waiting room or home. (In this case, there was a question of mild brain damage and/or a borderline thought disorder, suggested by the personality testing.)

A major asset of intelligence tests is that we know they are much more valid and reliable than are clinical estimates of intelligence. In this instance, reliability refers to the extent to which two individuals, using the same instrument, arrive at very nearly identical conclusions, and the extent to which, on reexamination at another time, an individual achieves a highly similar score. By validity is meant the extent to which the technique measures what we think it is measuring, and thus whether we can accurately predict, from the test scores, other indicators of the individual's behavioral capabilities.

R. G. Matarazzo et al. (11) found a reliability coefficient for the Full Scale WAIS of .91 (after a 20-week interval) with somewhat lower reliability coefficients for the individual subtests. Where a correlation of 1.0 would indicate "perfect" reliability, this coefficient is extremely high and indicates that an individual's score is highly stable. Thus we can be quite certain, under all but the most unusual circumstances, that a score obtained today will be within a few points of a retest score given a month or a year later.

It is not as easy to make statements about the *validity* of the IQ or to state exactly what predictions we can make from it. This is because many factors in addition to IQ are responsible for human achievement and/or behavior. For example, Verbal IQ has been found to correlate about .50 with school performance, and about .70 with educational attainment. Overall intelligence scores are found to correlate most highly with academic success and occupational status (10). A large study found that men whose occupations were in the professions earned median IQs of 124 to 128 (7). Those who came from the skilled trades had median IQs of approximately 100, and those with semi-skilled occupations, a median IQ of 89. Individuals with an IQ of 70 typically attain academic skill at approximately the 3rd grade level; those with IQs of 85 at about the 6th grade level; and those with IQs of 100 at about the 9th grade level (9). Of all the WAIS subtests, vocabulary is the most highly correlated with grades in school, and the performance subtests are less highly correlated with grades than are the verbal subtests. The correlations are impressive, and indicate that IQ is a significant factor in determining important aspects of one's life. They also indicate that additional factors must be operating. Thus, personality, motivation, and other variables are of extreme importance.

As mentioned above, aspects of intellectual functioning are differentially affected by both organic and functional disorders, and subtest variability on the WAIS is usually associated with significant pathology of some kind (10). For example, Reitan (12) has suggested that the Digit Symbol subtest is the one most susceptible to organic disease or insult, regardless of its type or location; that left hemisphere damage is likely to result in relatively low arithmetic, similarities and digit span performance; and that right hemisphere damage is likely to be associated with lowered digit symbol, block design and picture arrangement subtests. Researchers have attempted to differentiate psychiatric diagnostic categories on the basis of a WAIS subtest profile, but this has not been consistently successful (17). In any case, a highly variable subtest profile does alert the clinician to disturbed intellectual and personality functioning. Along with other tests of organicity and/or personality, the WAIS can give valuable clues to the kind of adjustment deficits experienced by the client. An example of this is the frequently found tendency for white sociopaths to score higher on the performance than the verbal subtests, and for many sociopaths to perform particularly well on the picture arrangement subtest. (In part, the higher performance IQ score seems to reflect the not-uncommon finding of poor reading achievement in acting-out individuals (8). Picture arrangement appears to measure social awareness or sensitivity to social cues, as shown by its inverse relationship to introversion (14) and positive relationship to extracurricular activity among college students (15). Needless to say, sociopaths, the brain damaged, or psychotics cannot be identified *solely* on the basis of WAIS performance.

Personality Functioning

Assuming that the parents are found to have intellectual ability which is adequate to learn appropriate parenting behavior, the psychologist would wish to know about their motivation, stability, and major personality dynamics. In addition to interviews of the parents and others who know them, this is probably best measured by relatively objective personality tests such as the Minnesota Multiphasic Personality Inventory (MMPI) and California Personality Inventory. The MMPI is probably the most widely used personality test, and also is the one on which the most research has been published (3). It consists of 550 true-false items, which can be answered by the patient, independently, if he/she has at least 5th grade reading ability, and is not confused due to psychosis or organic deficit. There is a recorded version available for use with nonreaders.

On the basis of empirical research, three validity scales, nine clinical scales and a measure of introversion-extroversion have been developed on these 550 items. The three validity scales measure test-taking attitude, and extreme scores on them may indicate the tendency of the patient to present him/herself in either a defensive, overly positive, "healthy" manner (e.g., "I do not always tell the truth"—False and "I gossip a little at times"—False) or to attempt to look mentally ill, seek sympathy, etc. (e.g., "I have had strange and peculiar experiences"—True, and "I am afraid of losing my mind"—True). The relationship of these validity scales to each other will influence the clinician's interpretation of the clinical scales.

The clinical scales are not simply interpreted individually, but are meaningful in their interrelationship. A common profile among character disorders is for Scales 4 and 9 to be the most elevated. Scale 4 (labeled psychopathic deviate) measures the character elements of hostility, egocentricity, poor judgment, inability to endure short-term frustration of desires in favor of long-term achievements, etc. This character picture is then energized by the high 9 (manic) score, resulting in restlessness, impulsivity, and a tendency to get into scrapes. A thinking disorder may be reflected, for example, in elevated scores on Scale 2 (depression, hopelessness, worthlessness) and Scale 8 (schizophrenia-withdrawal, strange experiences).

A not unusual profile for a neglectful mother was that obtained from a 23-year-old, unmarried woman who had always felt socially inadequate and had abused drugs since high school. She had been successively dependent on her mother and on a number of men who had befriended her for varying periods of time. As each relationship broke up, she decompensated and several times has had to undergo psychiatric hospitalization and treatment. In each relationship, or when living with friends, she left the major responsibility for her baby to others. Her validity profile suggested that she felt inadequate and unhappy, and she presented a picture of being "sick." The MMPI clinical profile suggested both a borderline thought disorder (high 8); impulsive, hypomanic behavior (high 9); and elements of a character disorder (high 4) with nonconformity, explosive anger, and little conscience or sense of responsibility. In addition, her unusually "feminine" responses on the masculinity-femininity scale suggested passivity and dependency and the use of seductive behavior to obtain attention and nurturance from men.

Often, in abusing or neglecting parents, the MMPI profile is a "defensive" or evasive one in which no clinical scales are above the normal range. However, the validity scales and the relative heights of the clinical scales usually make interpretation possible. Such "normal-appearing" profiles are most likely to be found among relatively intelligent individuals with character disorders, who are trying to cover up their deviancy.

It is not uncommon for a referring source to ask specifically for "projective" tests (e.g., Rorschach, Thematic Apperception Test, Draw-A-Person, Bender-Gestalt) in the belief that these may prove to be more revealing than any other method of personality assessment. This is an expectation which dates back to the 1950s when personality testing was in its infancy and new "projective" devices were being spawned each year. Unfortunately, research on the validity of these devices did not treat them kindly and they continue to be used primarily because some clinicians "feel" that they obtain valuable information from them (2). In an occasional individual case, this may be true. However, inasmuch as there are few data to support such assumptions, a psychologist witness would have a difficult time convincing the judge, e.g., that a child is negativistic because he gives many white space responses on the Rorschach. In contrast, much research has been done on objective personality tests, especially on MMPI code interpretations, and the clinican can refer to numerous books and studies to substantiate his/her opinions.

EVALUATION OF THE CHILD

Intellectual Functioning or Developmental Level

Not infrequently, the intelligence of the child may be an important factor in deciding whether he/she should be placed outside the family home. During infancy, developmental rate is best determined by simple instruments such as the Denver Developmental Screening Test (5), or the Boyd Developmental Progress Scale (1). These scales measure the infant's progress in motor coordination, speech, social awareness and self-help. They give a good picture of the current level of development as well as the consistency of functioning. Unfortunately, they cannot differentiate between environmental and constitutional factors contributing to the current developmental picture.

The earlier developmental tests have little relationship to later measures of IQ, although particularly low scores do not bode well for later development unless effective remedial action can be taken. For example, poor nutrition, lack of environmental stimulation, parental overprotectiveness or overcontrol, all may be contributing factors which can be counteracted by environmental or therapeutic intervention. We have noted that, on occasion, a child who is removed from a neglectful or damaging environment and placed in a good foster home may show an IQ gain of 20 or more points within a year.

Beginning at about age three, the Stanford-Binet (16) is a useful instrument which has good predictive validity in regard to later IQ. It measures primarily verbal ability, immediate memory, judgment and motor dexterity, and has items which ordinarily arouse the interest of the young child. It does not have the advantage of the Wechsler's separate subtests measuring several verbal and nonverbal abilities. With the Stanford-Binet, the examiner must start at the age level where the child passes all items, continue to the age level at which he fails all items, and compute a composite score yielding a mental age which is then converted to an IQ.

The Wechsler Intelligence Scale for Children-Revised (19) is suitable for use with the child of approximately age eight through age 15. Although there are norms beginning at age five, there are insufficient items at the lower levels to obtain a satisfactory measure. The WISC-R is the instrument of choice, however, after approximately age eight, and is essentially a downward extension of the WAIS. As such, it has many of the same diagnostic capabilities.

The child who is acting out at school and/or at home may well be a child who is not experiencing academic success. Academic achievement in "the three R's" can be quickly assessed through such instruments as the Wide Range Achievement Test (9) or the Peabody Individual Achievement Test (4). If one discovers that school achievement is indeed a problem, it is important to know intellectual capability and whether the child would be able to profit from special tutoring or whether academic demands should be lessened and other areas of achievement stressed.

Personality Functioning

It is the author's belief that the best measure of a very young child's personality and social behavior is achieved through interview, play, and observation. Additional measures which can be used with the school age child are the Rogers Personality Test (13), drawings; several Children's Sentence Completion Tests; and, with the teenager, the California Personality Inventory (6) and Minnesota Multiphasic Personality Inventory. The latter has norms for adolescents. The Rogers Personality Test, recommended for ages about seven to 14, attempts to measure the child's adjustment to peers and his family, his feelings about himself, and his typical adjustment mechanisms. It is a questionnaire which the child can take by him/herself with possibly some help from the examiner in reading an occasional word or understanding instructions. It gives some clue as to the child's view of him/herself, social adequacy with peers, and relationship to parents. Its strength is that it gets fairly directly to these significant areas. Its weakness is that it is fairly easy for sophisticated youngsters to understand the purpose of the test and to cover up feelings and behaviors if they wish to do so.

The California Personality Inventory is much like the MMPI in form, but is clinically more appropriate to the early adolescent in that the clinical scales are not standardized on an adult, psychiatrically ill population. The scales, rather than having psychiatric labels, fall under several areas of adjustment: poise, self-assurance and interpersonal adequacy;

socialization, maturity, responsibility; achievement potential and intellectual efficiency. It includes measures of intellectual and interest modes. The MMPI is described under the section covering evaluation of parents. It should be noted that there are separate norms for adolescents (3) and that personality interpretation may vary somewhat from that for adults. The sentence completions allow the child to directly express feelings, in some important areas, by writing them. This is often easier for the child than telling them directly to an adult.

The above personality tests are useful in helping to determine whether the child may be particularly rebellious, acting out and difficult to manage, thus possibly inciting the parent to abusive behavior in an attempt to exert control or jeopardizing placement in an adoptive home. Conversely, the tests may indicate that the child is depressed and withdrawn as a result of parental neglect or abuse. In our experience, however, most of the children who come to the attention of the court for neglect or abuse are infants or toddlers rather than older children. Consequently, extensive psychological testing is frequently not appropriate. One example of an early school age referral is that of a seven-year-old girl whose mother rejected her, having placed her in foster homes for extended periods on more than five occasions and taking her back apparently only to qualify for aid to dependent children. On occasion, the mother also was violent with (i.e., beat) the child, on one occasion throwing her against the refrigerator because the latter goaded her by "purposefully" disobeying, calling her bad names, and fighting with her sister. The child was reported to have difficulty at school with teachers and peers, and to give borderline academic performance. Intellectual and achievement testing indicated that the child, like her mother, was of low normal ability and achievement. Her behavior during the examination was minimally cooperative, passive-aggressive, and "trying." She told self-aggrandizing tales, and would not give serious answers to questions on the Rogers Personality Inventory. These passive-aggressive behaviors appeared to be counterparts of her mother's behavior and one could see that her mother would have particular difficulty in tolerating them.

SUMMARY

Psychological assessment is often an important adjunct to the interview in evaluation of parental adequacy. It is important in the verification of suspected intellectual deficits and emotional or mental illness. It is not infrequently helpful in verifying a character disorder because the individual's test performance is independent of his/her charm or persuasiveness. It may uncover some strengths which raise hope that parenting ability may be increased through a therapeutic program. It is often useful to examine the developmental level of the child and to reexamine after a remedial program has been completed. Special child behavior tendencies may become evident through psychological assessment—tendencies which, themselves, need remediation if the parent is to become able to alter his/her behavior in relation to the child.

If the psychologist is to be optimally effective in helping to achieve the best outcome for the child, it is important that subsequent to the examination he/she confer carefully and thoroughly with the referring source. This enables the experts to develop carefully thought out opinions which can be presented in a mutually reinforcing and consistent manner to the court. Minor differences of opinion among expert witnesses sometimes result from their not having had access to all of the same data. Usually, after discussion, the witnesses are of much the same opinion in regard to where lies the best interest of the child. However, if they do not present this in a manner which sounds consistent to the court, their effort and expertise may be less than optimally effective.

Presentation in court is done best if the expert witness can relax, be him/herself, give straightforward, direct and sincere opinions, and not allow self-confidence to be diminished by the manipulations of a cross-examining lawyer. The expert witness is on firm ground if he/she has done a thorough examination and has a solid background in his/her specialty. There is, indeed, nothing to fear but fear itself.

REFERENCES

1. BOYD, R. (1974). *The Boyd Developmental Progress Scale.* San Bernardino: Inland Counties Regional Center, Indiana.
2. BUROS, O. K. (Ed.), (1965). *The Sixth Mental Measurements Yearbook.* Highland Park, N.J.: Gryphon Press, Chapter by A. R. Jensen.
3. DAHLSTROM, W. G., WELSH, G. S., & DAHLSTROM, L. E. (1972). *An MMPI Handbook,* (rev. ed.). Minneapolis: University of Minnesota Press.
4. DUNN, L. M. & MARKWARDT, F. C., JR. (1970). *Peabody Individual Achievement Test.* Circle Pines, Minnesota: American Guidance Service, Inc.
5. FRANKENBURG, W. K. & DODDS, J. B. (1969). Denver Developmental Screening Test. Mead Johnson Laboratories, Distributor.
6. GOUGH, H. H. (1969). *California Psychological Inventory Manual,* Rev. Palo Alto: Consulting Psychologists Press, Inc.
7. HARRELL, T. W. & HARRELL, M. S. (1945). Army General Classification Test Scores for Civilian Occupations. Educational and Psychological Measurement, pp. 229-239.

8. HENNING, J. J. & LEVY, R. H. (1967). Verbal-Performance IQ Differences of White and Negro Delinquents on the WISC and WAIS. *J. Clin. Psychol.*, 23:164-168.

9. JASTAK, J. F. & JASTAK, S. R. (1965). *The Wide Range Achievement Test Manual.* Wilmington, Delaware: Guidance Associates of Delaware, Inc.

10. MATARAZZO, J. D. (1972). *Wechsler's Measurement and Appraisal of Adult Intelligence,* 5th Ed. Baltimore: Williams & Wilkins.

11. MATARAZZO, R. G., WIENS, A. N., MATARAZZO, J. D., & MANAUGH, T. S. (1973). Test-Retest Reliability of the WAIS in a Normal Population. *J. Clin. Psychol.*, 29:194-197.

12. REITAN, R. M. (1955). Certain Differential Effects of Left and Right Cerebral Lesions in Human Adults. *J. Comp and Physiol. Psychol.*, 48:474-477.

13. ROGERS, C. R. (1961). *Personal Adjustment Inventory, Manual of Directions.* New York: Association Press.

14. SCHILL, T. (1966). The Effects of Social Introversion on WAIS P. A. Performance. *J. Clin. Psychol.*, 22:72-74.

15. SCHILL, T., KAHN, M., MUEHLEMAN, T. (1968). WAIS P. A. Performance and Participation in Extracurricular Activities. *J. Clin. Psychol.*, 24:95-96.

16. TERMAN, L. M. & MERRILL, M. A. (1960). *Stanford-Binet Intelligence Scale: Manual for the Third Revision, Form L-M.* Cambridge: Massachusetts: Houghton Mifflin.

17. WECHSLER, D. (1939). *The Measurement of Adult Intelligence.* Baltimore: Williams & Wilkins.

18. WECHSLER, D. (1955). *Manual for the Wechsler Adult Intelligence Scale.* New York: Psychological Corporation.

19. WECHSLER, D. (1974). *Manual for the Wechsler Intelligence Scale for Children.* Revised. New York: Psychological Corporation.

5

THE EXPERT WITNESS

ELISSA P. BENEDEK, M.D.

Psychiatry, I suppose, is the ultimate wizardry. My experience has shown that in no case is it more difficult to elicit productive and reliable expert testimony than in cases that call upon the knowledge and practice of psychiatry.

One might hope that psychiatrists would open up their reservoirs of knowledge in the courtroom. Unfortunately, in my experience, they try to limit their testimony to conclusory statements couched in psychiatric terminology. Thereafter, they take shelter in a defensive resistance to questions about the facts that are and ought to be in their possession. They thus refuse to submit their opinions to the scrutiny that the adversary process demands (1).

In this chapter, it is our intention to help the beginning psychiatrist/ mental health professional participate in the adversary process in an informed and knowledgeable manner as an expert witness. Though many psychiatrists and mental health professionals feel that behavioral scientists should not become involved in the adversary process as expert witnesses (8), it is our opinion that society benefits when the knowledge and insights of social scientists are utilized in the courtroom. We recognize that the courtroom is not the arena in which the social scientist ordinarily practices his/her profession and that the rules governing practice there are different from those with which he/she is likely to be most familiar. However, it is our belief that one duty of the mental health professional is to act as consultant and expert witness and to formulate and present the most accurate and informative opinion that can be reached in regard to the legal question at hand. In this capacity, the expert witness recognizes that the needs of the legal system are paramount (7) vis-à-vis the therapeutic needs of a particular patient.

In previous chapters, material about the conduct of a clinical examination which may ultimately serve as the basis for expert testimony has been set forth. As noted, it is critical that the behavioral scientist discuss legal issues in question with an attorney before agreeing to conduct any forensic examination. Thus, the expert must know the legal standards, embodied by statute or case law, in his/her particular jurisdiction relative to making a recommendation as to child custody, insanity, termination of parental rights, and so forth. The questions asked in the clinical examination are designed to seek meaningful psychological insights which bear upon the legal issues. In addition to the standard diagnostic psychiatric examination, these issues must be explored during the interview.

Previous chapters have also discussed the significance of preparing a report. The expert must strive to present his/her observations in clear and understandable writing. Behavioral observations leading to the ultimate opinion of the professional are of critical importance. In the report, if at all possible, the mental health professional must also answer the specific legal question at issue. A mental status evaluation and a diagnostic formulation are ordinarily insufficient. A well written, cogent report often eliminates the need for expert testimony in the courtroom.

There are, of course, many instances where expert testimony is required despite the submission of a quality report. Thus, the clinician who works in the interface between law and psychiatry may expect to be asked to testify as an expert witness with some degree of frequency. For the novice, any discussion of the expert witness' role in the courtroom must begin with some explanation of the adversary process, particularly with respect to the trial and the function of witnesses and evidence within it. According to Slovenko (10), "In the view of many, a trial is expected to establish the truth and to explain an event. A common assumption is that a trial, if fairly conducted, will provide complete information to the public about an event of concern to it." It is Slovenko's opinion that "A trial, however, is not an investigative but essentially a demonstrative proceeding, which, according to predetermined norms and a particular mode of proof, evaluates only the evidence brought forth by the parties. It is not expected that a trial, however fair, will produce all the evidence that exists. The trial procedure is governed by certain rules which have been modified through experience" (10, p. 7). "Under the adversary system, the judge acts as arbiter to assure conformity to those rules of fair play that have evolved over the centuries. The jury then decides the issues on the basis of those facts which the judge permits them to hear" (10, p. 19).

The law permits participation of two distinct kinds of witnesses: the ordinary witness, called by various names—including lay witness or res gestae witness—and the expert witness. In general, a lay witness can testify to facts—that which he or she has directly observed. The judge or jury hears the facts presented by this type of witness, assesses them and formulates necessary conclusions. Federal Rules of Evidence, particularly Article 7 (2) of the Federal Rules of Evidence, have somewhat relaxed the role of the lay witness by allowing some natural expression in terms of opinion or inference in describing what one has seen or heard (2). However, opinion testimony of a lay witness under Rule 701 must meet two requirements: 1) The opinion must be rationally based on the witness' own perception, that is, firsthand knowledge, and 2) the opinion must be helpful either in understanding the witness' testimony or in determining a fact in issue (2).

Considerations pertaining to expert witnesses and expert opinion are, of course, entirely different. Two conditions must be satisfied before one can qualify as an expert witness: 1) The subject matter of inference must be distinctly related to a profession beyond the ordinary knowledge of the average layman, and 2) the witness must be shown to be qualified in that profession. Testimony of the expert is governed by different rules than those which apply to the ordinary fact witness. These differences are essential to performance of the expert's role. Thus, the expert may present an opinion or conclusion to the court. Furthermore, he/she may utilize facts gathered by others in forming his/her opinion (2). For example, he/she may review past medical records, speak with family members about the behavior of a patient and request that psychological testing be performed. Information actually garnered by others and communicated to the expert via medical records, family members, psychological test results, etc. may be used in forming an opinion. This latitude is not ordinarily allowed other witnesses since testimony based upon what one has learned from others is usually inadmissible because of the "hearsay" rule. After reviewing and analyzing findings of others, the expert, however, is allowed to formulate an opinion which he/she can present to the court.

An expert, by definition, is an individual who possesses information not ordinarily possessed by the lay person. This information may be obtained through specialized training, extensive experience, or professional education. Although experts typically possess formal professional degrees, some, such as mechanics or gardeners, may be qualified as experts by reason of their on-the-job experience. In all cases, however, when an individual is presented as an expert, he/she must be "qualified" and the trial judge determines whether the witness is, in fact, an expert and, therefore, entitled to provide expert testimony. Each time a professional testifies, he/she must be duly qualified as an expert, although attorneys will often stipulate to this qualification when such a ruling by the court is a forgone conclusion.

In the field of mental health, the medically trained psychiatrist has been traditionally viewed by the court as an expert able to present opinion and testimony in regard to a variety of issues. However, during the past 30 years, federal and state courts have begun to recognize that other mental health professionals possess necessary training, education and expertise to qualify as experts in the courtroom (4). The landmark federal case regarding the role of the psychologist as an expert is *Jenkins* v. *U.S.* (1962) (3). Currently, approximately 20 states have statutes which enable psychologists to testify. Other states allow psychologists to testify without specific statutory permission. The situation with respect to social workers as expert witnesses is not entirely clear. For instance, in Michigan the *Parney* case has limited the use of social workers as expert witnesses in criminal proceedings (5).

Once the mental health professional recognizes that he or she will be asked to participate in a trial as an expert witness, it is the duty of this professional to prepare adequately. This is a professional responsibility to the patient, attorney, court and oneself. Although an expert does not function as an advocate for a client, an expert does, in a sense, function as an advocate of an opinion. Thus, it is important to be able to adequately present and defend a professional opinion once it has been carefully reached.

To this end, the first step in preparation for testifying is a conference with the attorney who will be "calling" the expert. The conference is sufficiently important to be conducted in the office of either the professional or the attorney. The witness' written report should be thoroughly reviewed during the conference. This review should focus on those portions of the report which will be helpful to the attorney as he/she advocates the client's position. It should also address portions of the written report which are unclear or may present problems in the conduct of the case. Any technical language which is difficult for the attorney to understand is also bound to be difficult for the judge and jury. Thus, the expert must translate scientific terminology into lay terms. Many attorneys draw up a list of questions that they intend to ask the expert during the conduct of the trial and review these questions with the expert. This rehearsal serves two purposes. It assures the attorney that his/her questions on direct examination can be answered and that they are relevant to the specific case. It also assists the expert in conveying his/her information in a relevant, meaningful, and understandable manner. Although the attorney cannot tell the expert what to say, he/she may certainly assist in modifying language so that opinions are more skillfully presented.

During or after the conference, the expert should review all pertinent records and materials. If the expert will be expected to know specific legal standards such as those pertaining to insanity, competency to stand trial, or the child custody law in his/her particular state, the relevant statutes ought to be reviewed. In addition, if the expert has published on the subject, and especially if his/her opinion is supported by guidelines contained in such publications or the publications of others, those publications ought to be reviewed.

The date or time for testifying—giving oral testimony at the trial—may lead to some inconvenience because of one's personal schedule. Although it is possible to ask the court to change the date of the subpoena, the expert should bear in mind that many other witnesses have also been subpoenaed and the importance of one's own personal schedule may not be the paramount consideration. For this reason, it is a good idea to establish, as soon as possible, when testimony is likely to be needed and then to attempt to keep that time free. If it is at all possible to testify on the subpoenaed date, one should. In some instances, depositions, which can have the same effect as testimony, can be taken prior to trial and introduced at the trial on videotape. However, the parties must consent to this procedure. In any event, valuable time may be conserved if the expert works closely with the counsel and court regarding specific times for the actual court appearance. Although a subpoena may be issued stating a specific time to appear, one should always check with counsel to ascertain the time that testimony will actually be taken. Such planning may avoid unnecessarily wasting valuable professional time in the courtroom.

On the day of a court appearance it is sensible to dress neatly and conservatively. Although courtroom attire has been modified through the years, and even the Supreme Court allows women attorneys to wear pantsuits, the expert is judged not only by his/her presentation but by his/her appearance. The formal atmosphere of the courtroom is no place for casual sportswear or untidy dress. The witness should appear in court promptly at the time that has been agreed upon. When the expert is called as witness, he/she should take the necessary records and walk confidently to a position in front of the court clerk. The issue of necessary records is a complicated one. Many experts prefer to take minimal notes to the witness stand out of concern that any records they do bring may be used in cross-examination. Others, while recognizing this risk, nonetheless find themselves more comfortable if they bring the entire record to the stand. Still others bring no records at all, but prepare an outline of important dates and facts. In any event, a witness who ruffles through sheaves of paper looking for a specific date is likely to appear unprepared and unknowledgeable to the judge or jury.

After the witness is sworn, the process of qualification as an expert begins. For this purpose, many experienced witnesses supply counsel with a copy of their curriculum vitae. Thus, the attorney can be assured of asking questions which focus on significant aspects of education and training as well as upon special qualifications, such as forensic expertise, publications, memberships and offices in local and national organizations. Novices often express concern that they will be asked how often they have testified in court and then fail to qualify as experts because of their limited courtroom experience. Although this rarely happens to a physician or resident, it is a potential hazard to a social worker or psychologist. However, if one lays a proper foundation of expertise, it is unlikely that a lack of actual court experience will be the factor that prevents qualification as an expert.

Once in the witness chair, it is helpful to sit comfortably. Some experts suggest that it is advisable to draw upon one's experience in the doctor/patient relationship and to envision everyone in the courtroom as patients who are asking a physician to explain relevant diagnostic treatment information to them. That is to say, all testimony must be presented in nontechnical language, and explanations to the judge and jury must be made with the assumption that their prior knowledge or understanding of psychiatric theory is limited to that of lay persons. Most experts agree that anxiety is natural in this situation, but advise the novice to attempt not to exhibit anxiety too openly by his/her gestures, facial expressions or body language. Throughout the courtroom drama, the expert, while presenting and defending an opinion in a professional manner, should bear in mind that neither he/she, nor his/her opinion are on trial, although the tactics employed by counsel may suggest otherwise.

Ordinarily, the step following qualification is direct examination. During this portion of the testimony the witness will be asked to identify the patient/defendant and to explain the clinical examination on which his/her opinion is based. It is important that the expert present all relevant data in a clear, logical and coherent fashion. It is helpful to make eye contact with the judge and jury when testifying. Afterward, feedback from the judge and jurors may enable the expert to evaluate the extent to which he/she was able to provide meaningful and understandable testimony. During the course of direct examination, opposing counsel may raise a variety of objections. These are legal objections based upon technical rules of evidence. The expert should stop testifying once an objection is made and allow counsel to argue the merits of the objection and the court to rule upon it. Testimony is resumed when the judge rules on the objection. Although the expert may know some rules of evidence, his/her function in the courtroom, quite obviously, is not to inform judge or jury about relevant law, but to allow counsel to handle these matters. Even if it seems to the witness, perhaps justifiably, that he or she knows more relevant law than court or counsel, volunteering such information is ordinarily inappropriate. Judges frequently feel threatened and, accordingly, react with anger when the mental health witness behaves as if he/she were an attorney. Moreover, such behavior may, understandably, offend any judge's sense of decorum and propriety.

The attorney's strategy may be to ask the expert to present not only that material which is consistent with his/her ultimate conclusion or opinion but also to present other information which may be brought out on cross-examination. Counsel must be relied upon with respect to trial strategy and tactics. Although the expert may feel that counsel's decisions will lead to disaster, he or she must bear in mind that the conduct of the case is the attorney's responsibility. While the expert may be correct in concluding that counsel has erred, it should be remembered that attorneys must deal with a variety of considerations with which the witness is totally unfamiliar and second guessing counsel's judgment may reflect this unfamiliarity.

Following direct examination, customary procedure calls for cross-examination. This is typically the most stressful aspect of the trial for novice and experienced witness alike. The function of cross-examination is largely to discredit the witness' testimony. This may be achieved by such means as discrediting the witness him/herself, or his/her examination, ultimate opinion, or even his/her discipline. The lawyer is trained in a variety of discrediting techniques and these are part of his/her professional armamentarium.

The witness' credentials may be questioned on the basis of his/her race, sex, age, training, theoretical orientation or experience. The length and circumstances of the examination may be scrutinized as well as the witness' attitude toward the person he/she examined. The source of remuneration commonly becomes a focal point in the attempt to discredit.

It is also permissible for an attorney to pose a "hypothetical" question during cross-examination. The question ordinarily purports to summarize the clinical data. However, psychiatric facts contained in the hypothetical question may be different from those the expert has developed during his/her clinical examination. It is important to answer the hypothetical question and then to point out how the hypothetical case differs from the case that is actually being considered in court. Needless to say, these differences may be of great importance in reaching either one conclusion or another.

One specialized line of attack that mental health professionals find particularly difficult to deal with concerns the "learned treatise" (6, 9). In this form of cross-examination, the expert is asked first to authenticate a treatise as a recognized and standard authority on a subject. Then the contents of the treatise, paper, or book are read for the purpose of discrediting and contradicting the witness. The mental health professional, however, has a variety of techniques available to him/her for handling cross-examination on such a publication. These include denying authoritativeness of the publication, pointing out that it is no longer relevant and that the rate of development of scientific literature has made that particular publication anachronistic, or citing other publications which dispute a particular author's viewpoint. This technique has been amply discussed in the psychiatric literature (6, 9).

During the cross-examination material may be taken out of context. For example, only those portions of the mental status exam reflecting psychopathology may be quoted in an attempt to discredit the expert's opinion that a defendant was legally sane. The witness can remind the court of the entire statement being quoted. One question the expert is often asked is whether other data unknown at the time of the examination might cause him/her to change his/her opinion. If, in fact, that is the case, the expert should say so.

Examining counsel may demand that a question be answered by nothing more than "yes" or "no," although it is not possible for an expert to answer very many questions in that fashion. The witness may turn to the judge and say: "Your Honor, I cannot give a 'yes' or 'no' answer to that question. May I be allowed to explain?" Such requests will ordinarily be granted by the judge or the examining counsel will at least be asked to rephrase the question.

It is important for the witness to think clearly before answering any questions, particularly those posed during cross-examination. Although time spent in thought may seem interminable, good witnesses do not allow attorneys to set the pace of their answers. Here, as elsewhere, people seldom get into trouble by thinking!

Attorneys and mental health professionals agree that the expert should answer only those questions posed and that it is not his/her role to provide a mini-course in psychiatry on issues such as custody, for example, to the court or to the jury. Such expositions serve only to satisfy narcissistic needs of the witness and actually confuse judges and jurors. Thus, it is important not to talk too much. On the other hand, the real expert is always prepared to admit weaknesses. Should cross-examination reveal an area of personal or professional ignorance, it is quite appropriate to say, "I don't know." This does not discredit the bulk of one's testimony. On the contrary, it makes the expert appear much more human and knowledgeable about his/her strengths and weaknesses.

Following direct and cross-examination, procedure allows for redirect and recross-examination. These procedures generally allow counsel to clarify material previously introduced. On redirect, the attorney who called the expert can allow the witness to expand upon previous testimony and to explain it more amply. Recross allows opposing counsel essentially the same opportunity.

Throughout all of these examinations, it is imperative that the mental health professional remain cool, calm and collected. One of the best ways of discrediting testimony is to discredit the expert—to make him/her appear foolish, lose his/her temper and become angry and belligerent and, thereby, seem unprofessional. Thus, many questions posed by some cross-examiners have no real relevance to the case, but are designed solely to intimidate the expert and increase his/her anxiety.

After testimony has been completed, the expert is excused by the judge and may leave the witness stand. Of course, the expert may choose to remain in the courtroom and listen to the other testimony. However, many professionals feel that this makes the expert appear too interested in the outcome of the case and not impartial. On some occasions, an attorney may request that the expert remain in court, sit at his/her table to advise, typically with respect to cross-examination of another witness. As a general rule, it would appear advisable for the expert, after the completion of his/her testimony, to leave the courtroom.

In this brief chapter we have attempted to prepare the novice for a "different" role, that of an expert witness. We have touched upon the function of the trial and reviewed the expert's role as participant therein. We have offered some pragmatic and down-to-earth suggestions for the expert witness. Some of these are augmented with reference to the literature. Of course, there is no substitute for observation and, better still, experience. Indeed, this chapter is not intended to be such a substitute. However, we hope that the material it contains encourages mental health professionals to participate in the legal process and facilitates their doing so. Such participation can be intellectually stimulating and emotionally fulfilling. More importantly, it can be helpful to patients, courts and society.

REFERENCES

1. BAZELON, D. (1974). Psychiatrists and the Adversary Process. *Scientific Amer.*, 230: 18-25.
2. GRAY, R., & HAMMOND, S. (1978). Opinion and Expert Testimony. *Mississippi Law Journal*, 49:1-30.
3. *Jenkins* v. *United States*, 307 F2d. 637.
4. PACH, A., KUGHN, J., BASSETT, H., & NASH, M. (1973). The Current Status of the Psychologist as an Expert Witness. *Professional Psychol.*, 4:409-413.
5. *People* v. *Parney*, 74 Mich. App. 173.
6. PERR, I. (1977). Cross Examination of the Psychiatrist, Using Publications. *Bull. Amer. Acad. Psych. and Law*, 5:327-331.
7. POLLACK, S. (1974). The Role of Psychiatry in the Rule of Law. *Psychiatric Annals*, 4:8-15.
8. POYTHRESS, N. (1977). Mental Health Expert Testimony: Current Problems. *J. Psych. and Law*, 5:201-227.
9. POYTHRESS, N. Coping on the Witness Stand: "Learned Treatises." *Professional Psychology* (in press).
10. SLOVENKO, R. (1974). *Law and Psychiatry*. Boston: Little, Brown, pp. 7, 19.

Part II

CHILD CUSTODY, DEPENDENCY AND NEGLECT

6

PARTICIPATING IN CHILD
CUSTODY CASES

RICHARD S. BENEDEK, J.D. and ELISSA P. BENEDEK, M.D.

In bygone days, when custody was more or less automatically awarded to the mother upon dissolution of a marriage, the significance of expert opinion was less apparent and presumably less important than it is today. As the basis for determining custody, current psychiatric literature suggests seeking the "psychological parent," clearly a more elusive person than a mother (2). Updated laws are doing essentially the same thing, i.e., repealing age-old presumptions favoring an award of custody to the mother. While the potential for deciding custody cases properly has been increased, the judge's task has become more complex. Each custody case should be decided on its individual merits by evaluating historical and current information about a child and his or her family in the light of sound psychiatric principles and applicable law (7). The current interest in alternative custodial dispositions, such as the various forms of joint custody, is an additional complicating factor.

It seems apparent that courts are most likely to decide the custody issue correctly if relevant insights from experts are meaningfully communicated to them. Indeed, better laws are even advising the courts to make use of behavioral scientists in the resolution of custody disputes. The high rate of divorce and the number of children involved underscore the importance of obtaining an expert's opinion. Based upon current trends, it is estimated that before the turn of the century more than half of all Americans will have been directly touched by divorce (3). Under these circumstances, it is no more than reasonable to expect mental health professionals to be well equipped to provide necessary input.

ROLE OF THE EXPERT

The expert's task is to provide the judge with that knowledge that will enable him or her to reach the right result in a custody case. The mental health professional must avoid becoming so overwhelmed by the magnitude of this undertaking that he or she leaves its performance to others who are less qualified. Conversely, qualifying as an "expert," and thus being legally competent to provide so-called expert testimony, should by no means be considered conclusive proof of one's infallibility. Qualifying as an expert is frequently easily achieved, although a competent mental health professional is not ipso facto an expert in this specialized form of forensic practice. The professional who intends to make a meaningful contribution must set his or her sights higher than merely qualifying as an expert in the technical sense, yet keep in perspective the fact that predicting the future with absolute certainty can never be achieved.

Acquiring expertise is not easy. Experience, of course, is an excellent teacher. This presents something of a Catch-22 situation since it is very difficult to embark, with experience, upon anything that is entirely new. However, experience treating families and children involved in domestic controversy and thereby discovering the complexities of the problems and the elusiveness of solutions should provide valuable insight for later application in forensic work. Current psychiatric literature dealing with child custody and children of divorce must be studied. Colleagues who possess forensic expertise should be consulted both to glean theoretical knowledge and to gain actual assistance or even supervision with respect to a particular case.

The mental health professional should also possess reasonable familiarity with the laws applicable to custody cases in the particular jurisdiction involved. It must be remembered that the judge is bound by the law and that information given to him or her that cannot be applied to the law is bound to have minimum impact upon the court's decision. For example, custody disputes in Michigan are decided pursuant to the Child Custody Act of 1970 which spells out ten designated factors such as "(a) The love, affection and other emotional ties existing between the competing parties and the child" to be "considered, evaluated and determined by the court" (6). While these factors do not have to be weighed equally, each must be addressed by the court, and their sum total is deemed to constitute "the best interests of the child" which, in turn, must "control" the decision. Therefore, the testimony of a psychiatrist that his choice of custodian was based upon the premise that custody should be awarded to the mother unless she is proved to be unfit was of little value to the court.

The format of Michigan's child custody act and other similarly enlightened laws invites examination of parental strengths with respect to parenting and focus on psychological health rather than psychopathology. Stated simply, these provide the vehicle for a positive approach to determining custody. "While the criteria to be considered, expressed in terms of 10 designated factors, are sufficiently meaningful, unless the court is able to recognize the relevance of a given piece or pattern of behavior to a particular factor and then determine whether it is a strength or weakness in respect to the party's relationship with his [or her] child, the objectives of the act will quite easily be frustrated" (1, p. 831). It is in the performance of tasks such as these that mental health professionals should be able to provide invaluable assistance to the courts.

In essence, any custody determination calls for an intelligent comparison of alternatives in order to determine which is commensurate with the child's best interests. With respect to meaningful comparison, mental health professionals should possess the expertise to provide insight that would otherwise be unobtainable. Their training and skills should enable them to assess and compare the ego strengths of the parents and to balance such elements as their weaknesses with the intensity of their emotional ties with the child. Likewise, the preference of the child, a consideration that is frequently important although, ironically, often overlooked, can most satisfactorily be ascertained by a mental health professional.

BASIS OF INVOLVEMENT

While the end result of the mental health professional's participation will be information conveyed to the court, the manner in which he or she becomes involved, coupled with the extent of this involvement, will have a profound effect upon the information that can ultimately be provided. The least conflicted means of entry is at the request of the court for the express purpose of custody evaluation. In such case, the expert should insist upon interviewing both parties, the children and extended families; that is, the significant others who are likely to materially impact the raising of the child. There will be occasions when some of the relatives or friends are recalcitrant or unavailable, but the professional should make every effort to enlist their cooperation. Recently, a psychiatrist refused to see the children in connection with a custody evaluation, despite the logic of doing so. Such self-imposed limitation on collection of available data was bound to have no effect other than to diminish the value and even the credibility of the information that was ultimately provided to the court. In this case, that is precisely what occurred.

The mental health professional who becomes involved at the request of either the court or the attorneys for both parties generally receives maximum cooperation. He or she is also least likely to become suspect of being an advocate for one of the parents or to be put in a position of potential or apparent conflict. However, neither logic nor ethics require imposition of such a limitation upon one's forensic practice.

Mental health professionals frequently enter a case at the request of the attorney for one of the parties. As long as he or she is able to interview everyone involved, the professional should be able to provide exactly the same type of information as if entry had been at the invitation of the court. Under these circumstances, it is critical for the professional to make it clear to both attorney and client at the outset that his or her opinion will be based primarily upon the diagnostic interviews. This must include the admonition that it is, therefore, entirely possible that this opinion may damage the cause of the very client that secured his or her intervention. In every respect, the mental health professional must avoid even the appearance of being overtly or covertly susceptible to seduction into an intellectually compromising position.

There are occasions when a mental health professional is asked, or is able, to see only one of the parents. Sometimes this is for the purpose of supporting or refuting a specific allegation, typically one bearing upon that party's mental health. Interviewing only one parent is not necessarily undesirable, but it is imperative that the professional appreciate the limitations doing so will impose upon the opinion he or she will ultimately be able to provide. Following such an interview, the professional should be able to testify as to that party's mental health and even as to his or her parenting ability. However, without interviewing both parties, it is impossible to compare their relative strengths. Therefore, the professional must resist any pressure or temptation to offer an opinion as to which parent should be awarded custody.

Probably the most difficult basis for entry into a custody dispute is that which results from a prior relationship with a patient whom one is treating or has treated in the past. For example, a psychiatrist who has been treating a patient for a year is asked by her attorney to testify in a custody dispute. Certainly, the prior therapeutic alliance did not contemplate the possibility that the therapist might divulge information reflecting adversely on the patient. The alliance could easily be jeopardized or destroyed by this testimony or, conceivably, even by favorable testimony. Such a therapeutic relationship also makes it extremely difficult, if not impossible, for the mental health professional to be entirely objective. Even if objectivity were possible, the professional would not ordinarily be in any position to compare the parties or to give an opinion as to which should be awarded custody. During the course of a year's treatment, he or she has presumably heard a great deal about the patient's spouse, but this has been colored by the patient's perspective and cannot be relied upon as an objective basis for a custody recommendation.

Preserving a therapeutic alliance, as well as considerations of confidentiality and objectivity, dictate the exercise of extreme caution and discretion with respect to participating in a case as the result of a prior relationship with a patient who has been seen in treatment. One psychiatrist who intervened on behalf of a patient was extremely upset with the court's decision (although that decision was consistent with the opinion of several colleagues) and complained bitterly. The problem is illustrated by the conclusion of the letter that was sent in response to this criticism

> I can easily understand your desire to be supportive of your patient, but in custody cases you might consider the possibility that in the long run you would be better serving their interests by cautioning them that the court may see things differently from the way they do. I fully appreciate the fact that expert judgments may differ. However, from what you tell me, in this particular case you apparently made a judgment with respect to custody based upon the comments of a patient you have been treating for more than a year and those of her attorney and one casual observation of her husband. To the extent that you may, consciously or unconsciously, have conveyed to her the probability that others viewing the case from a more objective perspective would necessarily reach the same conclusion, this is something that you may wish to avoid doing in the future.

POINT OF INVOLVEMENT

Customarily overlooked is the fact that child custody disputes frequently arise (and often for the first time) after the divorce has been granted. It is certainly common, and not entirely without justification, to consider all custody disputes, irrespective of their point of origin, under the same umbrella. Without question, much may be said that is relevant to all such controversy. However, there are important consequences, both social and legal, unique to disputes that arise after custody has been established. While mental health professionals are often called upon to make custody recommendations in connection with pending divorces, they frequently become involved only after the noncustodial parent has filed a petition requesting the court to change the "permanent" custody that was awarded at the time the divorce was granted. In order to provide meaningful input, it is essential that one understand the implications of this particular form of custody dispute.

The general rule must certainly be that custody, once established, should be changed only under the most compelling circumstances (2). Even a neophyte should readily perceive how such a change might easily result in sudden, and virtually total, upheaval of a child's life. Furthermore, it is from the intense relationship that exists between a very young child and his or her primary love object, ordinarily the custodial parent, that he or she learns to love and trust others. Once this relationship has been disturbed, it may be extremely difficult for the child to invest in another person psychic energy comparable to that which had been cathected to the custodial parent. Thus, the possibility of being able to form normal relationships with others later in life may be significantly diminished. This danger to the child is obviously increased by repeated changes in custody. Even disturbing this parental relationship with an older child is likely to produce similar results. Therefore, mental health professionals and well informed judges have recognized for years that great restraint should be exercised when it comes to changing custody. This concept is now being incorporated into better custody laws.

It is, however, important that one not become so complacent with respect to application of the general rule of maintaining the custodial status quo that he or she loses sight of the fact that there indeed are exceptions to it. Granted, the majority of petitions to change custody are ill conceived and granting these could do considerable damage to the child. It is equally true that comparable harm may be done by failing to recognize the case in which change is appropriate. Thus, it is impossible to qualify any request for change without first carefully evaluating all of the data, and the mental health professional should certainly resist the temptation to prejudge.

It is naive to assume that in those cases where the need for change exists that this change is necessarily readily apparent. For example, one such case involved an essentially stable, custodial father. With considerable difficulty it was learned that his new spouse was physically abusing the child. Conversely, there are situations which suggest the need for change but, when thoroughly analyzed, dictate the advisability of preserving the existing arrangements. For example, a father with little schooling, a marginal employment record, and who was an atrocious housekeeper, but who, it developed, had an impressive relationship with his child, was considered preferable to the well educated and industrious mother who sought a change of custody. For years she had been displaying virtually no interest in the child and had recently married a former mental patient with a poor prognosis for adequately raising a child.

The shortcomings of the proposed placement seldom occur to the parent seeking custodial change. It is imperative that those involved in evaluating and determining the case do not fall into the identical trap of becoming so distressed by existing conditions that they fail to realistically evaluate the alternative. While considerations pertaining to custody disputes that arise once custody has been established differ somewhat from those applicable to initial custody determination, both require the same thorough analysis and intelligent comparison of alternatives.

COMPILING DATA

As previously suggested, the mental health professional who intends to participate in custody cases, including initial determination of custody and postdivorce petitions to change custody, should first become knowledgeable in the subject and, when the time comes to act, make every effort to see all of the people likely to significantly impact the raising of the child, as well as the child. Some professionals contend that experts should be able to make recommendations based solely upon review of records compiled by others, but we believe that any attempt to make a recommendation in this manner is not sound practice. Conducting a number of detailed evaluations is time consuming and expensive, yet this is equally true of good surgery. The expert who is unwilling or unable to devote the time, thought, and energy necessary for adequate preparation of a custody case is being unfair to everyone involved.

At the outset of the interview, the parent should be advised of its purpose and his or her consent to the mental health professional's sharing information with the court and attorneys should be obtained so that subsequent disclosure is neither a breach of confidentiality nor perceived as such. A "waiver" on a form drafted by an attorney should be signed. If consultations, such as those with schools, social agencies, or friends are contemplated, waivers pertaining to them should also be obtained.

It is important that the diagnostic evaluation which follows, besides containing the elements of a typical psychiatric evaluation, be specifically directed toward collecting information relevant to that issue which the expert has been asked to consider, i.e., the custody question. This means acquiring data that pertains to the relative parenting skills and attitudes of both parents and to their emotional ties to the children. While some pertinent information can undoubtedly be garnered from a typical psychiatric examination, including current and past history and mental status, the mental health professional must pose questions to each parent such as why he or she feels that an award of custody to him or her would be in the child's best interest. Routine psychological examinations give insight into parenting ability, but answers to specific questions dealing with attitudes relating to child care will provide the professional with empirical data necessary to arrive at and support a recommendation to the court.

If the parent is receptive, the mental health professional may also use this opportunity for instruction pertaining to preparing the child for his or her interview. The child will be more comfortable and the interview will be more open as well if a parent helps him or her cope with the normal anxiety induced by the prospect of such a visit. Preparation entails candid disclosure as to the purpose of the interview and requires impressing upon the child freedom to share with the interviewer special thoughts, feelings, and ideas which are traditionally considered completely personal (5).

The mental health professional cannot rely entirely upon such advance preparation by the parent. After eliciting from the child the fantasized reasons for the visit (resulting from internal conflicts, parental misinformation, or denial) the true purpose must be explained—that is, the fact that the judge will make the decision as to the parent with whom the child is going to live and that the professional is talking to him or her in order to help the judge do this. The child may be confused as to the very nature of the legal proceedings that are taking place. The interviewer should be able to set things straight as to this, although a mental health professional should remember that legal procedure is not his or her area of expertise and refrain from imparting misinformation in regard to particulars of the case. The child should be allowed to ventilate such feelings as guilt, anger, shame, and confusion which he/she may well be experiencing. The professional can explain that other children, under similar circumstances, feel pretty much the same way.

Most of the usual rules and techniques pertaining to interviewing children are applicable to these cases (8). The interview should be conducted in a relaxed and easy manner, the interviewer avoiding the posture of an inquisitor. However, it is very important that he or she be forthright and direct. Accordingly, the mental health professional must ask the child his or her preference and elicit the reasons for it, but at the same time make it clear that this choice, if the child chooses to express it, will be only one of the elements considered by the judge in reaching a decision.

It can be very difficult for a child to verbalize the desire to live with one parent as opposed to the other or the inclination to resist a parent who is vigorously pursuing custody. Some children fear the loss of the "rejected" parent's love and others worry about hurting a parent who loves them. While children should never be coerced into stating their choice of custodian, it is important to facilitate their doing so. They frequently have a definite preference as well as good reasons for it.

The matter of confidentiality should be discussed. The mental health professional must refrain from promising the child that the preference will remain confidential because, in fact, this must ordinarily be disclosed at least to the court and generally to the attorneys. Moreover, stressing the "secrecy" of the preference is likely to be interpreted by the child as meaning that he or she did something wrong by disclosing, or even having, one. Even young children can often understand that in order to impact the decision their preference must be disclosed, and that preferring to live with one parent does not mean that the other is not loved.

The discussion should be channeled in such a direction as to enable the child to reveal feelings about both parents. When a child grapples, on a conscious level, with such issues as parental preference, matters that surface are not always easily closed off. A close relationship with the mental health professional may also develop. Therefore, termination is likely to be somewhat tacky. At the outset, the interview should be structured so that the child will know how much time will be shared with the interviewer. As the interview approaches its conclusion, the child should be made aware of this fact and appropriately assisted to terminate the relationship.

Proper handling of the interviews with parents and children is not easy and the novice examiner is well advised to seek the assistance and consultation of colleagues who are experienced in making custody evaluations, reporting to courts, and acting in the capacity of expert witness. After completing all of the interviews, the mental health professional is in a position to evaluate his or her data in order to formulate a reasoned opinion and to write a report. After proceeding in this manner, the professional is also well prepared to consult with the attorneys and testify, although not infrequently the expert's participation in a case is concluded by the submission of a quality report.

THE PSYCHIATRIC REPORT

The significance of a psychiatric report should not be underestimated. In some instances, a report may be accepted in lieu of testimony (4). In these cases, this will be the only opportunity to provide information that is likely to impact the result. An impressive report sometimes makes the outcome of a trial such a foregone conclusion that the participants are persuaded to accept the recommendation without further litigation. At the very least, the act of drafting the report should stimulate a thorough, precise, and orderly analysis of the data—a worthwhile exercise prior to testifying or even before discussing the case with counsel.

The primary object of the report is to maximize the chances of the custody issue being decided correctly. This is true whether the report is examined by the court or used exclusively by the attorneys. Therefore, the main ingredient of a sound report is an organized and astute analysis of the facts leading to a consistent, if not inevitable, conclusion. The recommendation will be justifiably suspect if it is not supported by clinical information or appears inconsistent with the expert's interpretation of his or her own data. For example, in a case in which the noncustodial parent had petitioned for a change of custody, primarily at the request of the children who wanted to live with him, the psychiatrist noted "one of the things I am struck with is the considerable feeling of power these children have over where they should live. This has gotten out of control and the resultant pressure on the children is hazardous to their development." The apparently inconsistent recommendation was that custody be changed.

Discrete reference to sound psychiatric principles enunciated in books and journals is not necessarily undesirable. However, reports are frequently weakened by excessive reliance upon general rules, guidelines, or simplistic formulas appearing in the literature, to the exclusion of meaningful analysis of the facts and dynamics of the particular case.

While the temptation to overly hedge the report may be great, the mental health professional should avoid the common error of failing to take a definite position. Although high risk of error inheres in forecasting, if the professional is to make a meaningful contribution he or she must be willing to select the parent to whom he or she feels custody should be awarded and to spell out in understandable language the elements of the particular case that have led to this conclusion. Without this, the most eloquent psychiatric jargon or detailed account of mental status will ordinarily be of little or no value to the court. At the same time, however, one must avoid the temptation to be persuasive by overstating a position. Doing so impairs credibility and, more importantly, is neither fair nor professional.

FINAL PREPARATION FOR THE CUSTODY HEARING

The mental health professional who agrees to participate in a custody contest must recognize the possibility of being called upon to testify. Testifying need not, or should not, be an unpleasant experience. For the expert witness, as well as for the attorney, anxiety in the courtroom is generally justified only in the case of inadequate preparation. The professional who is knowledgeable with respect to child custody and who has completed the appropriate interviews, carefully evaluated the data, and dictated a thorough report, requires precious little additional preparation.

Prior to the hearing, just as before any court appearance, the mental health professional and the attorney seeking his or her testimony should confer. Doing so is in no way suggestive of a willingness on the part of the professional to compromise his or her position. The professional should be willing to take the initiative and arrange for this consultation. It must be borne in mind that attorneys are often naive with respect to the most fundamental psychiatric principles and cannot be expected to recognize the importance of pieces or patterns of behavior that may asume particular significance to the trained professional. Therefore, although attorneys frequently talk about "preparing the witness," maximizing the expert's effectiveness is a two-way street whereby attorney and expert prepare one another. Not only is doing this proper, it is eminently sensible and should result in an orderly and meaningful presentation of the case.

While one's comfort in court is primarily a derivative of adequate preparation, experience is also a factor. The mental health professional is well advised to observe a few custody hearings prior to testifying for the first time in this type of case. In the final analysis, the professional who has done his or her homework should realize that he or she will probably know more about the subject matter of the testimony, if not about the entire case, than anyone else in the courtroom and, accordingly, has very little to fear.

REFERENCES

1. BENEDEK, E. P. & BENEDEK, R. S. (1972). New Child Custody Laws. *Amer. J. Orthopsychiat.*, 42:825-834.
2. GOLDSTEIN, J., FREUD, A., & SOLNIT, A. J. (1973). *Beyond the Best Interests of the Child.* New York: Free Press.
3. JOHNSON, W. D. (1977). Establishing a National Center for the Study of Divorce. *Fam. Coord.*, 26 (3):263-268.
4. LICHTNER, J. (1976). An Attorney's Approach to Psychiatrists in Custody Cases. *Bull. Amer. Acad. Psych. and Law*, IV:105-113.
5. McDONALD, M. (1965). The Psychiatric Evaluation of Children. *J. Amer. Acad. Child Psych.*, 4 (4):570-612.
6. M.C.L.A. 722.21, *et seq.* (P.A. 1970, No. 91, Eff. April 1, 1971).
7. ROTH, A. (1976-77). The Tender Years Presumption in Child Custody Disputes. *J. Fam. Law*, 15:423-462.
8. WERKMAN, S. (1965). The Psychiatric Diagnostic Interview with Children. *Amer. J. Orthopsychiat.*, 35:764-771.

7

CHILD ABUSE

ARTHUR H. GREEN, M.D.

PREVALENCE

Although the maltreatment and exploitation of children have been recorded throughout history, the phenomenon of child abuse has only recently attracted the attention of child care professionals. It was not until Kempe's classic description of "The Battered Child Syndrome" in 1962 (23), that child abuse received widespread interest from physicians, social scientists, and the law. Between 1963 and 1965, the passage of laws by all 50 states requiring medical reporting of child abuse ultimately subjected the abusing parents to legal process and catalyzed the formation of child protective services throughout the nation. Psychiatric exploration of child battering and the first psychological studies of abusing parents were carried out during this period.

Because of improved reporting procedures, the striking prevalence of child maltreatment in the United States has become apparent. For example, the child abuse law in New York State became effective on July 1, 1964. During the first 12-month period, 313 cases of child abuse were reported in New York City with 16 deaths (34). In 1977, New York City statistics (35) included 5930 reported cases with 77 deaths. An additional 18,309 children were reported to be neglected. The twenty-fold increase in reported abuse over a 13-year period obviously reflects an improvement in reporting procedures as well as a real increase in the incidence of child abuse. This impression is supported by similar increases in reported child abuse throughout the country.

Light (27) has utilized Gil's 1965 survey (14) and 1970 U.S. Census statistics to project an estimated 200,000 to 500,000 cases of physical child abuse annually. A New York State Department of Social Services estimate of the percentage of severe neglect or sexual abuse cases enables Light (27) to project 465,000 to 1,175,000 such incidents across the

71

nation annually. Combining all types of maltreatment leads to an upper projection of over 1,500,000 cases per year. This figure approximates an estimate by Douglas Besharov, Director of the National Center on Child Abuse and Neglect, who calculated 1.6 million annual cases of abuse and neglect with 2,000 to 4,000 deaths (3) based upon a statistical survey carried out by the Center.

Child maltreatment is currently regarded as a major public health problem and a leading cause of injury and death in children. The proliferation of child abuse and neglect might be related to the general increase of violence in our society demonstrated by the rising incidence of violent crimes, delinquency, suicide and lethal accidents.

DEFINITION OF CHILD ABUSE

The concept and definition of child abuse have been broadened in recent years. In Kempe's pioneering paper, he and his colleagues (23) described child abuse as the infliction of serious injury upon young children by parents and caretakers. The injuries, which included fractures, subdural hematoma, and multiple soft tissue injuries, often resulted in permanent disability and death. Fontana (11) viewed child abuse as one end of a spectrum of maltreatment which also included emotional deprivation, neglect, and malnutrition. These were all designated as components of the "Maltreatment Syndrome." Helfer (20) stressed the prevalence of minor injuries resulting from abuse and estimated that 10 percent of all childhood accidents treated in emergency rooms were consequences of physical abuse. Gil (14) further extended the concept of child abuse to include any action which interferes with a child's achievement of his physical and psychological potential.

In this chapter, child abuse will refer to the nonaccidental physical injury inflicted on a child by a parent or guardian, and will encompass the total range of physical injuries. Child abuse will be differentiated from child neglect, and the term "maltreatment" will be used as a general reference to both abuse and neglect. The terms "child abuse" and "neglect" will be based on the following legal definitions stated in the New York State Child Protective Services Act of 1973.

> Definition of Child Abuse: An "abused child" is a child less than 16 years of age whose parent or other person legally responsible for his care:
> 1) inflicts or allows to be inflicted upon the child serious physical injury, or

2) creates or allows to be created a substantial risk of serious injury, or

3) commits or allows to be committed against the child an act of sexual abuse as defined in the penal law.

Definition of Child Maltreatment:* A "maltreated child" is a child under 18 years of age who has had serious physical injury inflicted upon him by other than accidental means.

A "maltreated child" is a child under 18 years of age impaired as a result of the failure of his parent or other person legally responsible for his care to exercise a minimum degree of care:

1) in supplying the child with adequate food, clothing, shelter education, medical or surgical care, though financially able to do so; or

2) in providing the child with proper supervision or guardianship; or

3) by unreasonably inflicting or allowing to be inflicted harm or a substantial risk thereof, including the infliction of excessive corporal punishment; or

4) by using a drug or drugs; or

5) by using alcoholic beverages to the extent that he loses self-control of his actions; or

6) by any other acts of a similarly serious nature requiring the aid of the family court.

A "maltreated child" is also a child under 18 years of age who has been abandoned by his parents or other person legally responsible for his care.

DETECTION

The possibility of child abuse must be considered in every child who presents with an injury. A careful history and physical evaluation of the child are warranted when one suspects physical abuse. The physical examination should include a routine X-ray survey of all children under five and laboratory tests to rule out the possibility of an abnormal bleeding tendency. The child, of course, should be hospitalized during this diagnostic evaluation.

While there is no single physical finding or diagnostic procedure which can confirm the diagnosis of child abuse with absolute certainty, the presence of some of the following signs and symptoms drived from the history taking and physical examination is suggestive of an inflicted injury:

---

* In this legal definition, "maltreatment" refers to neglect.

History

1) Unexplained delay in bringing the child for treatment following the injury.
2) History is implausible or contradictory.
3) History incompatible with the physical findings.
4) There is a history of repeated suspicious injuries.
5) The parent blames the injury on a sibling or a third party.
6) The parent maintains that the injury was self-inflicted.
7) The child had been taken to numerous hospitals for the treatment of injuries—hospital "shopping."
8) The child accuses the parent or caretaker of injuring him.
9) The parent has a previous history of abuse as a child.
10) The parent has unrealistic and premature expectations of the child.

Physical Findings

1) Pathognomonic "typical" injuries commonly associated with physical punishment, such as bruises on the buttocks and lower back; bruises in the genital area or inner thigh may be inflicted after a child wets or soils, or is resistant to toilet training. Bruises and soft tissue injuries at different stages of healing are signs of repeated physical abuse. Bruises of a special configuration such as hand marks, grab marks, pinch marks, and strap marks usually indicate abuse.
2) Certain types of burns are typically inflicted, i.e., multiple cigarette burns, scalding of hands or feet, burns of perineum and buttocks.
3) Abdominal trauma leading to a ruptured liver or spleen.
4) Subdural hematoma with or without skull fracture.
5) Radiologic signs, such as subperiosteal hemorrhages, epiphyseal separations, metaphyseal fragmentation, periosteal shearing, and periosteal calcifications.

ETIOLOGICAL FACTORS

Parental Characteristics

Numerous theories have been advanced to explain the physical abuse of children by their parents. Early investigations of the "battered child syndrome" (6, 30, 40) attempted to identify "typical" behavioral characteristics and personality traits in abusing parents which could account for their child battering. Such parents have been described as impulsive (7), immature (6) rigid, domineering, and chronically aggressive (30), dependent and narcissistic (36), isolated from family and friends (40) and experiencing marital difficulties (23). The diversity and lack of specificity of these observations failed to support the notion of a typical child abusing personality. The fact that these observations were not controlled, and were often derived from clinical interviews divorced from the parent-child interaction raised further questions about their reliability and specificity.

More penetrating impressions of the personality defects and underlying psychopathology of abusing parents have been gathered from observations during their psychiatric treatment and while interacting with their children. Steele (40) stressed the importance of the parent's closely linked identifications with a harsh, rejecting mother and with a "bad" childhood self-image, which are perpetuated in their relationship with the abused child. Abusing parents inflicted traumatic experiences on their children which were similar to those they had endured during childhood. The observation that most abusing parents have frequently experienced physical abuse, rejection, deprivation, and inadequate parenting during their own childhood is one of the few which generate widespread agreement in this field.

Steele and Pollock (40) also described the abusing parent's tendency to rely on such defense mechanisms as denial, projection, identification with the aggressor, and role reversal. The last, a manuever by which the abusing parent turns towards the child for the gratification of dependency needs, has been reported by other investigators (31) as well. Galdston (12) emphasized the importance in mothers of unresolved sexual guilt derived from unconscious oedipal conflicts, associated with the conception of the child who is subsequently abused. Feinstein et al. (10) studied the behavior of women with infanticidal impulses in group therapy. These women deeply resented their parents for failing to gratify their dependency needs, and demonstrated a hatred of men which could be linked to intense rivalry with their brothers. They also exhibited phobic and depressive symptomatology.

Green (15, 16) conducted in-depth interviews with 60 mothers or female caretakers of abused children who were compared with control groups of 30 neglectful and 30 normal mothers. Twenty percent of the abusing mothers participated in follow-up interviews or psychotherapy. The mothers of the abused children could be differentiated from the controls by a more frequent perception of their child as difficult and demanding, the greater emotional unavailability of their parents and spouses, a greater overall lack of childrearing assistance and the more frequent rejection, criticism, and punishment by their own parents. This mistreatment at the hands of their parents reinforced their feelings of having been burdensome children, and facilated their identification with a hostile, rejecting parental figure. Key personality characteristics of the abusing mothers were poor impulse control, low self-esteem, heightened narcissism, and shifting and unstable identifications dominated by hostile introjects of "bad" self- and object-identifications of early childhood. Major psychodynamic elements appeared to be role reversal, the denial and projection of their own negative attributes onto their children (scapegoating), and the displacement of aggression from extraneous sources onto the child.

Contributions of the Child

The child's role in the abuse process has become a subject of increasing interest. Usually only a single child in a family is selected for scapegoating and abuse. It is the child who is perceived as the most difficult or burdensome who is the most likely to be abused. The period of infancy and early childhood during which the child is most helpless and dependent on caretakers is a particularly stressful time for most parents, and especially for those who are "abuse-prone." In fact, the majority of reported cases of child abuse occur in the first two years of life. Infants with sustained crying and irritability may have a devastating effect upon the parent-child relationship. Moss and Robson (33) noted decreases in mother-infant attachment as a result of sustained crying and fussing. Bell and Ainsworth (2) observed maternal withdrawal in mothers who were unable to control the crying of their infants. On the other hand, infants who are relatively unresponsive, passive, lethargic, and slow in development might be equally frustrating to their mothers and would tend to provoke abuse. Both irritable and sluggish infants are readily scapegoated because their mothers perceive their unresponsiveness as a rejection reminiscent of similar experiences with their own parents. This will, in turn, reinforce their sense of inadequacy.

Physically or psychologically deviant children are also vulnerable to abuse. Children with prominent physical defects, congenital anomalies, mental retardation, or chronic physical illness are not only burdensome, but are readily viewed by narcissistic parents as symbols of their own defective self-image.

Low birth weight and premature infants seem to be over-represented in the child abuse statistics (8, 26, 37). This might be explained in several ways: These infants might be perceived as "unattractive," and are more irritable than their normal counterparts. They are also prone to medical problems and developmental retardation. They manifest more feeding disturbances and often require special feeding techniques. Their delayed social responsiveness might be especially frustrating for "abuse prone" parents with high expectations of their infants. The prolonged separation between the mother and her premature infant during the early postpartum period also interferes with normal attachment behavior or maternal "bonding" (25). Recent studies have indicated that mothers who were permitted greater physical contact with their premature babies in the intensive care nursery demonstrated more effective infant care and attachment behavior following discharge than mothers who were deprived of this contact (24).

The child also contributes to his/her own abuse through his/her aggressive and impulsive behavior which is itself a common sequel of maltreatment. Thus, as the child emulates the violent behavior of his/her parents, he/she exhibits the same type of aggressiveness and provocativeness that the abuse was designed to prevent. This, in turn, creates a vicious cycle of misbehavior and abuse. The fact that many abused children incite abuse and scapegoating in foster homes attests to their provocativeness.

Environmental Stress

Parental "abuse-proneness" and the special vulnerability of a child for scapegoating and abuse might be insufficient in themselves to result in actual abuse without the presence of a stressful situation or crisis, as a catalyst. A typical childrearing crisis occurs when the equilibrium between the parental capacity and childrearing demands is disrupted. Decreased parental capacity may be caused by a loss or diminution of support from a spouse or key family member involved with child care. Physical or emotional illness in the parent might reduce his or her parenting ability, or the sudden unavailability of childcare facilities (daycare center, babysitter) might constitute an inordinate burden for working parents. The pressures of childrearing might be increased by the birth of another child, illness or deviancy of the children, or assuming the care of children of friends or relatives.

Environmental stress has often been associated with lower socioeconomic status. Gil (13) has attributed abuse almost entirely to socioeconomic determinants. A single study (22) has shown a relationship between life change and child abuse, while economic pressures have been associated with child abuse in other investigations (21, 23). The occurrence of maltreatment has been noticed in middle- and upper-class families as well (1, 4, 5, 19, 41). The actual impact of poverty on the genesis of child abuse might be somewhat overstated due to the overrepresentation of poor families in child abuse registers throughout the country. Poor abusers served by municipal agencies are more likely to be reported than their middle- and upper-class counterparts who bring their children to private physicians. In their 1972 review, Spinetta and Rigler (38) concluded that environmental stress had not been proven to be either necessary or sufficient to cause child abuse. It may, however, interact with parental personality traits and child variables to potentiate maltreatment by widening the discrepancy between limited parental capacities and the demands for child care.

REPORTING LAWS

Since 1964, all 50 states, the District of Columbia, the Virgin Islands, and Guam have enacted child abuse reporting laws. Physicians are specifically designated as mandated reporters in most states, along with other professionals such as osteopaths, dentists, chiropractors, pharmacists, nurses, hospital administrators, religious healers, teachers, and social workers. All reporting laws provide immunity from criminal and civil liability for mandated reporters. The laws of most states include penalities for nonreporting.

Friends, relatives, and neighbors are also encouraged to report suspected cases of child abuse and neglect. These nonmandated reporters are not required to identify themselves.

The agency legally designated to receive reports bears the prime responsibility for protecting children in the state. In 23 states, the reporting laws specify a single agency to receive all reports. In more than half the states mandated reporters may choose between two or more specified agencies. In the 23 states that require reporting to a single source, 17 designate a child protective agency, 5 specify a law enforcement agency, and one reports to the juvenile court. The agency receiving reports of child abuse and neglect should be able to fulfill the following criteria: It should be able to handle reports 24 hours a day, seven days a week, and should be able to investigate reports within a day. It should also maintain, at the local or state level, a central register of reports. Several states have initiated statewide reporting systems which use one toll-free telephone number for reports from anywhere in the state. Certain states, such as Connecticut, New York, and Florida require reports to be made to the local child protective agency, which must then report to the central register.

Reporting to child protective agencies is preferable to notifying a law enforcement agency because a child protective agency is able to provide supportive and crisis-oriented social services which may prevent further abuse and strengthen family functioning. Reporting to the police, sheriff, or prosecuting attorney would be perceived as a punitive act by the parents, and would seldom lead to rehabilitative efforts. Child protective agencies are usually authorized to notify the appropriate district attorney in cases of abuse or neglect accompanied by a felony or leading to the death of the child.

The major objective of reporting laws is to increase case finding, which, in itself, does not solve the problem of child abuse. However, without legal coercion, most of the maltreating families would not voluntarily seek help. The identification of larger numbers of abused and neglected children is of dubious importance if it is not followed by immediate investigation and remedial action.

The psychiatrist or mental health professional involved in the treatment of a family in which physical abuse or neglect takes place is required by law to report such maltreatment, as any other professional. Reporting is also mandatory for any recurrence of abuse by parents who are receiving help for previous maltreatment. The reporting laws take precedence over the privileged doctor-patient relationship, and, therefore, this does not constitute a breach of confidentiality. When abuse takes place, the legal rights of the child immediately precede those of the parents. The potential negative therapeutic impact of the reporting laws can be minimized if the therapist clarifies his/her obligation to report abuse at the onset of any intervention with maltreating parents. The great strain that reporting abuse imposes on an ongoing therapeutic relationship requires the clinician to make the difficult distinction between physical abuse and physical punishment which constitutes an "acceptable" level of discipline. Reporting may not jeopardize the therapeutic relationship but, even if it does, protecting the child takes priority over preserving the relationship. Therapeutic omnipotence may prevent some therapists from recognizing both their limitations and those of their patients.

INVESTIGATION

The child protective agency, generally located in county or state departments of social services, is usually authorized by law to investigate reported cases of abuse in order to determine the validity of the allegations. The investigation includes an intake process by a protective services caseworker who tries to obtain information concerning the suspected maltreatment. The worker may contact neighbors, relatives, schools, and other agencies to obtain information about the family. He/she also checks the central register for any previous reports of maltreatment involving the child, his siblings, or the parents. All information collected about a family should be available to other agencies and professionals involved in the case.

If the investigation confirms the presence of maltreatment, the child may be protected in one of the following ways: Depending on the severity of the case, the child can be hospitalized; can remain home under supervision of the child protective agency while the family is provided with supportive services; or can be placed in a shelter or foster home on an emergency basis.

If the report of abuse or neglect cannot be verified, the case is closed and the report is expunged from the central register.

PARENTAL RIGHTS

The parent, or any person alleged to have maltreated a child, should be informed of his legal rights by the local authority. These usually include the right to receive written notice of one's record in the central register and of court orders and petitions filed, the right to consult legal counsel, the right to a court hearing prior to removal of the child, the right to refuse agency services unless mandated by a court, and the right to appeal child protective case determinations. The parents should also be protected from unauthorized disclosure of identifying information by limiting access to the records to the authorities designated in the state law.

RIGHTS OF THE CHILD

All children alleged to be abused or neglected should be entitled to representation in all legal proceedings. Many states require that the court appoint a "special" guardian, or guardian ad litem, to protect the child's interest. The guardian ad litem, usually an attorney, is responsible to the court that appointed him. As the child's advocate, he/she insures that the court receives all relevant data. He/she also acts as an investigator, gathering relevant information about the causes, nature, and extent of abuse or neglect inflicted on the child. He/she must ensure that the child's immediate and long-range interests are protected by the law, as a counterpart to the attorneys for the parents and protective service agencies who act as advocates for the parents and community, respectively.

THE JUDICIAL PROCESS IN THE JUVENILE OR FAMILIY COURT

Child protection proceedings are initiated when a petition alleging child abuse or neglect is filed. A *pretrial conference* may be held prior to any hearing in order to examine the issues and determine which reports and evidence will be admissible. The judge and the attorneys for all parties evaluate all evidence without subjecting the participants to the trauma of an adversary trial. The vast majority of cases are settled at the pretrial conference by some form of consent decree, in which the parent agrees to cooperate with the child protective agency.

If a case cannot be settled in a pretrial conference, an *adjudicatory hearing* is held. This is the "trial" stage of the proceedings in which the charges of abuse and neglect are examined and argued. At the conclusion of the trial, the judge decides whether the allegations have been proven.

A *dispositional hearing* follows the adjudication. At this hearing, the agency managing the case, usually the local child protective agency, presents a case plan to the court and the parents. The plan usually stipulates conditions and arrangements designed to guarantee the child's protection, and a time schedule within which the plan is to be carried out. The dispositional order might require counseling, psychiatric treatment, or the provision of social services for the parents. If the child is placed outside his home, a schedule for visitation should be included in the case plan. Once the plan is agreed upon, the court should insure parental compliance by periodically reviewing the participation of the parents in the rehabilitative process.

At the periodic *review hearings,* the court should determine the level of progress made by the parents in complying with the dispositional order. The case plan may be modified as needed. Parents who fail to follow through with their commitments may be threatened with termination of parental rights.

If the child's health or safety is in danger, he/she can be removed from the home on an emergency basis by the court following the filing of a petition for *temporary custody* by the child protective service agency. Temporary custody of the child is usually awarded to the local social service agency for placement of the child in a foster home, home of a relative or emergency shelter.

Termination of parental rights is a legal proceeding freeing the child from parental custody so that the child can be adopted by others without the parents' written consent. The legal grounds for termination differ from state to state, but most statutes include abandonment. Other indications are institutionalization of parents, reabuse, voluntary placement for over two years without visits by the parents, and refractoriness or repeated resistance to treatment.

RETURNING THE CHILD TO HIS NATURAL PARENTS AFTER PLACEMENT OUTSIDE OF THE HOME

Positive changes in the childrearing climate must take place before the child can be reunited with his/her parents. First of all, the parents should be able to demonstrate adequate impulse control which would allow them to utilize nonphysical forms of discipline. Other signs of improvement are a growing capacity to derive pleasure from the children and a cessation of unrealistic expectations of the children (role reversal) and some capacity for self-observation. Decreased social isolation and improved self-esteem of the parents would also reduce the likelihood of scapegoating and abuse. The capacity to utilize therapeutic intervention in a constructive manner should significantly improve parental functioning. Increased parental tolerance for the child's independence and expression of negative feelings should also be a prerequisite for the return of abused children to their parents. Final plans for the reunion should only be made after a gradually increasing schedule of parental visits outside of the home under supervision.

TESTIFYING IN COURT

Various mental health and child care professionals are called upon to testify in court on cases of child abuse and neglect as regular or expert witnesses. A regular witness testifies about factual material derived from direct case observation. An expert witness, recognized as an authority, is permitted to give his professional opinion based upon his education and experience, without firsthand knowledge of the case. Pediatricians are requested to provide medical testimony confirming the presence of abuse or neglect. Psychiatrists are frequently asked to assess the presence and degree of psychiatric disorders in maltreating parents which might seriously impair their childrearing capacities. Psychiatrists might also be able to predict the risk for abuse in a given family based upon such factors as marital conflict, parental impulsivity, external stress, and the availability of parental support systems. Child psychiatrists may be called upon to document the adverse impact of abuse and neglect on the child's development and psychological functioning, and to recommend the most suitable environment for the child's physical and emotional welfare. Social workers, nurses, psychiatrists, and other members of a multidisciplinary treatment staff may be required to describe the parents' motivation and response to therapeutic intervention, and report on the current childrearing climate in the home.

Good court testimony requires a thorough knowledge of the case, based upon careful examination, evaluations, and treatment when applicable. Complete medical, evaluation, and treatment records required by the court should be reviewed by the witness. Prior to his/her court appearance, the witness should have a definite idea about what is best for the child and family, and be prepared to recommend this opinion to the court in a clear and concise manner, avoiding the use of medical or psychiatric jargon. All reports and recommendations should be shared with the parents prior to the court appearance and they should be encouraged to attend the hearings. In cases where the testimony may be viewed by the parents as opposed to their best interest, one should avoid an accusatory or adversarial tone, which could impair the parents' relationships with the current or future treatment facility.

TREATMENT FOR CHILD ABUSE

Treatment of Abusing Parents

The major thrust of treatment with abusing parents is to protect the children from further injury and to strengthen the family and its childrearing capacity. To this end, intervention with abusing parents must be designed to modify the major components of the child abuse syndrome: the personality traits of the parents that contribute to "abuse proneness," the characteristics of the child that make him/her more difficult to manage and enhance scapegoating, and the environmental stresses which either increase the burden of child care or deplete the childrearing resources of a family. The child abuse syndrome requires a crisis-oriented, multidisciplinary approach with a capacity for providing the parents and children with a wide variety of home-based comprehensive services. Innovative techniques such as homemaking assistance, regular home visiting by nurses, social workers, and lay therapists, and a 24-hour hot-line for emergences will assist abusing families to cope with environmental pressures and provide them with childrearing support. The availability of crisis nurseries and day care facilities for infants and preschool children will relieve the child care burden and facilitate the identification of pathological or deviant traits which would increase the child's vulnerability to abuse or scapegoating. Childrearing education, based on an understanding of the child's physical and psychological development, will modify inappropriate parental expectations for precocious and premature performance. Individual and group psychotherapy and counseling attempt to resolve or attenuate parental conflicts and personality traits which contribute to abuse proneness. Family therapy and therapeutic monitoring of parent-child interaction are geared towards the exploration and modification of distorted and inappropriate interactions and communications between parents and children. Self-help groups, such as Parents Anonymous, have proven effective in providing emotional support, peer acceptance, and parent education for many abusing parents.

Intervention with abusing parents poses special difficulties beyond those usually encountered in poor, unmotivated, and psychologically unsophisticated multi-problem families. The effects of ongoing investigative and punitive procedures inhibit the establishment of a confidential and trusting therapeutic alliance. The suspiciousness and basic mistrust of authority exhibited by these parents, resulting from their long-standing experience of humiliation and criticism by their own parents and authority figures, is intensified by their contact with case investigators and court personnel. This poses a barrier to the development of a therapeutic relationship unless it is dealt with specifically. This problem may be overcome by clearly divorcing the functions of the child protective agency and the courts from those of the therapeutic team.

Staff members of these agencies must be viewed as advocates of the parents. Evaluations and progress reports required by the court or child protective agency should be fully explained and shared with the parents before they are submitted.

The fragile self-esteem of these parents makes it difficult for them to accept advice and help from the therapeutic team. Suggestions concerning childrearing and household management are frequently construed as criticism and rejected. The parents require continual reassurance and support during the initial stages of treatment. Their own dependency needs must be gratified before "demands" can be placed on them.

Another group of obstacles to treatment is determined by strong feelings of anger and revulsion elicited in the therapist by child abusers. Most individuals instinctively condemn and dislike anyone who would intentionally injure an innocent infant or child. Many therapists are additionally burdened by rescue fantasies in which they attempt to save the child from a threatening situation by overidentifying with a "good" parent. Some staff members might feel pressure to "reform" the abuser by transforming him or her into a model parent.

An additional reservoir of negative feelings, or countertransference, towards the abusing parents stems from their provocativeness and masochism. They often exhibit a strong unconscious need to sabotage all therapeutic efforts by regarding them as repetitions of previous humiliating interactions with their parents and spouses. Typical examples of such provocative behavior are arriving late or missing appointments, expressions of overt hostility towards the therapists, and an overall lack of respect or commitment to the treatment process. Needless to say, a successful therapeutic outcome will not be possible unless the treatment personnel are able to recognize and control such feelings of anger and self-righteous indignation towards the parents.

Despite the formidable difficulties encountered during intervention with abusing parents, most of them can be rehabilitated. Pollock and Steele (36) estimate that 80 percent of these parents can be treated with satisfactory results under optimal conditions. Our own treatment program at the Downstate Medical Center in Brooklyn, New York has helped the majority of families involved. Its basic goals and techniques help the parent establish a trusting and gratifying relationship with the therapist and other adults, which is facilitated by an initially noncritical need-satisfying therapeutic posture. The parent is "indulged" and permitted to experience the type of dependency gratification he or she was previously unable to obtain. "Giving" to the parent may take the form of childrearing advice, home visiting, securing medical and social services for the family as an advocate of the parent, and being available in emergencies. The parent is helped to improve his/her devalued self-image by the mobilization of his/her assets with eventual educational and vocational assistance. The therapist or visiting nurse provides the parent with a model for childrearing. Group therapy has been helpful in facilitating social involvement with peers and the community. As the parents experience gratification and support from the treatment staff, and strengthen peer relationships, they will no longer require their children to fulfill a disproportionate share of their dependency needs. The ultimate goal of intervention is to enable the parents to derive pleasure from their children and to increase their capacity for successful nurturing.

Treatment of Abused Children

Numerous studies have recently documented a wide range of cognitive, developmental, neurological and emotional deficits among abused children which tend to persist after the cessation of maltreatment (7, 17, 28, 32). Green (18) described the importance of psychiatric treatment for these children, in order to effect changes in the child's pathological inner world by modifying pathological identifications and internalized representations of their violent parents. The abused children also required assistance in improving their impulse control, using verbalization as an alternative to motor discharge, improving their poor self-image, overcoming acute anxiety states and depressive reactions, and learning to trust others. Modifications of psychoanalytically oriented play therapy and psychotherapy have been used effectively to overcome these deficits, while psychoeducational intervention has been used to reverse cognitive deficits and learning disabilities. Treatment has been successful in interrupting the vicious cycle in which the abused child recreates the original sadomasochistic relationship with his parents and others which, if unchecked, leads to further rejection and traumatization. Timely intervention with abused children can also prevent their commonly observed transformation into abusing parents in the following generation. Psychotherapy with abused children should be carried out in the context of a multidisciplinary treatment program for the family. The provision of mental health services for abused and neglected children by public mental health agencies has been recently recommended as a federal standard for child abuse and neglect treatment programs (9).

REFERENCES

1. ALLEN, H., TEN BENSEL, R., & RAILE, R. (1969). The Battered Child Syndrome. *Minnesota Medicine*, 52:1345-1349.
2. BELL, S. M. & AINSWORTH, M. D. S. (1972). Infant Crying and Maternal Responsiveness. *Child Develop.*, 43:1171-1190.
3. BESHAROV, D. (1975). Child Abuse Rate Called "Epidemic." *The New York Times*, November 30.
4. BOARDMAN, H. E. (1962). A Project to Rescue Children from Inflicted Injuries. *Social Work*, 7:43-51.
5. BRYANT, H. (1963). Physical Abuse of Children—An Agency Study. *Child Welfare*, 42:125-130.
6. COHEN, M., RAPHLING, D., & GREEN, P. (1966). Psychological Aspects of the Maltreatment Syndrome of Childhood. *J. Pediatrics*, 69:279-284, 1966.
7. ELMER, E. (1965). The Fifty Families Study: Summary of Phase I, Neglected and Abused Children and Their Families. Children's Hospital of Pittsburgh, Pa.
8. ELMER, E. & GREGG, G. S. (1967). Developmental Characteristics of Abused Children. *Pediatrics*, 40:596-602.

9. Federal Standards for Child Abuse and Neglect Prevention and Treatment Programs and Projects. U.S. Department of Health, Education, and Welfare, Washington, D.C., 1978.
10. FEINSTEIN, H., PAUL, N., & PETTISON, E. (1964). Group Therapy for Mothers with Infanticidal Impulses. *Amer. J. Psych.*, 120:882-886.
11. FONTANA, V. J.: *The Maltreatment Syndrome in Children*, 2d ed. Springfield, Ill.: Thomas.
12. GALDSTON, R. (1971). Violence Begins at Home. *J. Am. Acad. Child Psych.*, 10:336-350.
13. GIL, D. (1970). *Violence Against Children*. Cambridge: Harvard University Press.
14. GIL, D. A Holistic Perspective on Child Abuse and Its Prevention. Paper presented at the Conference on Research on Child Abuse, National Institute of Child Health and Human Development, 1974.
15. GREEN, A. H., GAINES, R., & SANDGRUND, A. (1974). Child Abuse: Pathological Syndrome of Famliy Interaction. *Amer. J. Psych.*, 131:882-886.
16. GREEN, A. H. (1976). A Psychodynamic Approach to the Study and Treatment of Abusing Parents. *J. Am. Acad. Child Psych.*, 15:414-429.
17. GREEN, A. H. (1978a). Psychopathology of Abused Children. *J. Am. Acad. Child Psych.*, 17:92-103.
18. GREEN, A. H. (1978b). Psychiatric Treatment of Abused Children. *J. Am. Acad. Child Psychiat.*, 17:356-571.
19. HELFER, R. E. (1975). The Diagnostic Process and Treatment Programs. (DHEW Publication No. (OHD) 75-69) Washington, D.C.: U.S. Department of Health, Education and Welfare, National Center for Child Abuse and Neglect.
20. HELFER, R. E. & KEMPE, C. H. (Eds.), (1968). *The Battered Child*. Chicago: University of Chicago Press.
21. JOHNSON, B. & MORSE, H. (1968). Injured Children and Their Parents. *Children*, 15:147-152, 1968.
22. JUSTICE, B. & DUNCAN, D. F. (1976). Life Crisis as a Precursor to Child Abuse. *Public Health Reports*, 91:110-115.
23. KEMPE, C. H., SILVERMAN, F., STEELE, B., DROEGENMUELLER, W., & SILVER, H. (1962). The Battered Child Syndrome. *J.A.M.A.*, 181:17-24.
24. KENNELL, J. H., JEROULD, R., WOLFE, H., CHESLER, D., KREGER, N. C., McALPINE, W., STEFFA, M., & KLAUS, M. H. (1974). Maternal Behavior One Year After Early and Extended Post-Partum Contact. *Dev. Med. Child Neurol.*, 16:172-179.
25. KLAUS, M. H. & KENNELL, J. H. (1970). Mothers Separated from Their Newborn Infants. *Pediat. Clin. North Amer.*, 17:1015-1037.
26. KLEIN, M. & STERN, L. (1971). Low Birth Weight and the Battered Child Syndrome. *Am. J. Dis. Child.*, 122:15-18.
27. LIGHT, R. J. (1973). Abused and Neglected Children in America: A Study of Alternative Policies. *Harvard Educational Review*, 43:556-598.
28. MARTIN, H. (1972). The Child and His Development. In *Helping the Battered Child and His Family*, C. H. Kempe and R. E. Helfer (Eds.). Philadelphia: J. B. Lippincott.
30. MERRILL, E. (1962). Physical Abuse of Children: An Agency Study. In *Protecting the Battered Child*, V. DeFrancis (Ed.). Denver: American Human Association.
31. MORRIS, M. & GOULD, R. (1963). Role Reversal: A Necessary Concept in Dealing with the Battered Child Syndrome. *Am. J. Orthopsych.*, 33:293-299.
32. MORSE, W., SAHLER, O. J., & FRIEDMAN, S. B. (1970). A Three-Year Follow-up Study of Abused and Neglected Children. *Am. J. Dis. Child.*, 120:439-446.
33. MOSS, H. A. & ROBSON, K. S. (1970). The Relation Between the Amount of Time

Infants Spend at Various States and the Development of Visual Behavior. *Child Development*, 41 (2):509-517.

34. New York City Central Registry for Child Abuse, 1965.

35. New York City Central Registry for Child Abuse, 1977.

36. POLLOCK, C. & STEELE, B. (1972). A Therapeutic Approach to Parents. In *Helping the Battered Child and his Family*, C. H. Kempe and R. E. Helfer (Eds.). Philadelphia: J. B. Lippincott.

37. SIMONS B., DOWNS, E., HURSTER, M., & ARCHER, M. (1966). Child Abuse. *N.Y. State J. Med.*, 66:2783-2788.

38. SPINETTA, J. & RIGLER, D. (1972). The Child Abusing Parent: A Psychological Review. *Psychol. Bull*, 77:296-304.

39. STEELE, B. (1970). Parental Abuse of Infants and Small Children. In *Parenthood: Its Psychology and Psychopathology*, E. Anthony and T. Benedek (Eds.). Boston: Little, Brown & Co.

40. STEELE, B. & POLLOCK, C. (1968). A Psychiatric Study of Parents who Abuse Infants and Small Children. In *The Battered Child*, R. E. Helfer and C. H. Kempe (Eds.). Chicago: University of Chicago Press.

41. YOUNG, L. (1964). *Wednesday's Children: A Study of Child Neglect and Abuse*. New York: McGraw-Hill, 1964.

8

SEXUAL MISUSE OF CHILDREN

CAROL C. NADELSON, M. D. and ALVIN A. ROSENFELD, M.D.

The phrase "sexual abuse of children" is widely used in the professional literature. It derives from child abuse statutes which have included sexual acts between adults and children as a form of abuse. The child, because of age, is considered the abused party, while the adult is considered the perpetrator, legally responsible for the act. Despite this apparent clarity, there is considerable confusion in the definition of "sexual abuse" (27). Cases of sexual abuse may be prosecuted under a variety of different laws, including child abuse statutes, molestation, sexual assault, rape, indecent exposure, and corrupting the morals of minor. The term "sexual misuse," defined as "exposure of a child to sexual stimulation inappropriate for the child's age and role in the family" (3), may be clearer since it allows for increased flexibility in concepts and for definition within a specific culture.

Since standards of "appropriate" or "typical" sexual behavior within a family differ between cultures, socioeconomic groups, etc., this is particularly useful. For instance, in Melanesia, parents may have intercourse in front of their children, while in other countries a father could be accused of indecent exposure if he walked around the home naked. Thus, applications of the sexual abuse standards in a country as heterogeneous as the United States are difficult unless one is rigorous in limiting prosecution to clearly socially deviant behavior. While some form of "incest taboo" exists in all cultures, the nature of the prohibitions varies with regard to who is to be considered taboo and the specifics of circumstances and relationships.

The term "sexual abuse" is also confusing with regard to the acts to

Partial support for this work was made possible by grants to Dr. Rosenfeld by the National Institute of Mental Health Training Grant MH 14449, and by the Boys Town Center for Youth Development at Stanford University.

be included, the ages of the participants, and the relationships between the participants. It refers to acts ranging from genital touching to coitus; the age of the child ranges from infancy through late adolescence; and the relationship between the child and the adult may be nonexistent, as in many cases of indecent exposure, or perhaps as intimate as parent and child, as in some cases of incest. Force may or may not be used, the child may be severely traumatized, or may show no clearly demonstrable response or injury.

PREVALENCE

Since the definition of sexual misuse is unclear, and the boundaries between appropriate and inappropriate sexual behavior within the family are not absolute, the prevalence of all forms of sexual misuse (rape, abuse by strangers, neighbors, family members, and/or parents, indecent exposure, etc.) remains unclear. However, a number of surveys indicate that childhood sexual experience with an adult is far from uncommon. Landis (18) asked 1800 college students about their experiences as children with sexually deviant adults. He found that fully one-third of both males and females had had some such personal experience. While retrospective data are subject to distortion, this study does indicate that the experience occurs with greater frequency than is generally acknowledged. In a similar study, Gagnon (8) confirmed Landis' prevalence figures for women. Furthermore, in contrast to prior suggestions that this is a lower-class phenomenon, Gagnon's work suggested that victims occurred in all classes, although it was reported somewhat more frequently among lower socioeconomic classes. Gagnon also suspected that lower-class women were subjected to "a larger proportion of the more serious offenses (e.g., father-daughter incest, assaultive coitus)." While all questionnaire studies have their limitations, in both of these studies, 75 to 90 percent of the women who had been sexually involved with an adult as children had been approached by an exhibitionist or had been fondled by a stranger on a single occasion. The remainder were involved with someone they knew, often over a prolonged period of time.

In a more recent study, Finkelhor (7) surveyed 530 female college students with regard to their early sexual activity with an adult. Nineteen percent of the women reported such an experience during childhood, and 44 percent of this group stated that it occurred with a family member. Of the one-sixth of the population from this sample who were in the lowest socioeconomic group, 33 percent had had such an experience, and an even higher percentage had sexual experiences with a family member.

While noncontrolled studies are difficult to evaluate in terms of prevalence, reports from psychiatric clinics stated that three to five percent of psychiatric patients of all ages (4, 20, 22) have had an incestuous experience. In one report, six out of 18 consecutive female patients reported this experience (22). Therefore, in contrast to earlier impressions that incest is rare (an incidence of about one per million population) (30), it seems that incest is far more common than previously suspected.

Recent attention to the prevalence of sexual abuse has encouraged more careful assessment of a variety of signs and symptoms, which had previously been ignored or not explored beyond initial questions or examination. Protective care workers have noted that a significant percentage of children coming to their attention as "abused" are being sexually misused at home. Medical personnel have also noted more sequelae of sexual molestation. Branch and Paxton (2) have reported an increased incidence of gonorrhea in children between one and nine years of age, and Brant and Tisza (3) have found a large number of children coming to emergency rooms with genital injuries, infections, or rashes which are apparently caused by sexual abuse, although they are often not initially identified as such.

Childhood rape has also been increasingly documented in the last decade. Burgess and Holmstrom (5) have reported that they see a substantial number of children coming to emergency rooms complaining of rape. Hayman and Lanza (11) reported their findings in more than 1200 rape cases, noting victims as young as 15 months of age. In their report, 12 percent of the rape victims were under 12 years of age, and 25 percent were between the ages of 13 and 17. This suggests that a substantial number of children are rape victims. These exact figures are difficult to obtain and evaluate, in part because of confused conceptual frameworks and terminology, and also because of the large number of estimated unreported cases.

INCEST AND CHILDHOOD RAPE

The major distinction between the overlapping categories of childhood rape and incest involve (a) the difference in the relatedness between the adult and child, and (b) the issue of consent. Incest is often narrowly defined as sexual intercourse, or more broadly as "grossly aberrant sexual behavior" (25) between two people who are too closely related to marry, regardless of age. Consent is not a specific factor as it is in rape, where the definition is sexual intercourse without consent. Regardless of the prior relationship, the ability of the participants to consent is the central factor.

All incest between adults and children can be considered a form of rape since the age of the child makes it impossible for him/her to give consent, regardless of the degree of alleged or observed provocation. The nature of the family relationship makes intimidation, overt or covert, a factor. Even an older adolescent, who would be considered cognitively competent to consent, cannot ordinarily be considered to be legally consenting in incestuous relationships, since the affectional and power relationships between parent and child alter the concept of "free choice." The child may perceive that there is no choice, or he/she may be fearful of reprisal or deprivation if he/she refuses. In fact, the parent generally does have the power to inflict hardship or pain on the child. Thus, even when the parent or even the child states that the child consented, this perception cannot be accepted at face value. However, there are cases where a child may secondarily aquire and use power derived through the incest relationships to control parental behavior.

While in both rape and incest the nature of the sexual act remains an important component of the definition, in both situations this narrow perspective is limiting. A spectrum of behaviors which ranges from actual sexual seduction to overstimulation exists and has specific implications for those involved (27). Thus, a parent may be sexually provocative and disturbing to a child, but he/she is not technically committing incest; and, while intercourse may not be forced, other sexual acts without the consent of the partner are still not considered rape.

In "rape," the sexual act is coital and forced, while incest is a broader category of aberrant family sexual life that includes a spectrum of behaviors ranging from rape, incest, actual sexual seduction, and "incestuous" behavior, such as overstimulation, on the one hand, to total affectional neglect on the other (24). This is not to diminish it as an offense, only to place it in perspective. There are specific implications for those involved in each form of aberrance. Thus, a parent may be overtly sexually provocative, although not engage in specific sexual acts, but may be responsible for serious behavioral or psychological problems in his/her children. This can be seen as aberrant "incestuous" behavior, although it is not technically incest.

In contrast to rape, many incestuous experiences continue over time and, in some cases, have even been reported as "enjoyable" to the child. How can one assess this without considering intimidation and betrayal based on the nature of the relationship? While the child seeks affection and attention, the parent may not be able to discriminate between tenderness, sexuality, love, and domination.

Another important issue is the nature of the sexual act, particularly in incestuous situations. Most often the act is inappropriate to the child's physical stage of development, e.g., sexual intercourse is not usual with prepubescent children. Thus, using sexual intercourse to define either incest or childhood rape does not seem appropriate; rather, a spectrum of behaviors should be considered.

PRESENTATION

While rape generally presents as an acute traumatic situation, there are a variety of ways that incest becomes apparent.

There are several patterns of incestuous activity, ranging from one-time rape by either a parent or another relative, to endogamic or repeated incest. In this latter situation, the participants and sometimes the rest of the family collude and rarely allow it to be known outside of the family. The fact of the incestuous relationship is often revealed when one partner decides that the incest should end. This is particularly likely to occur when the child becomes an adolescent. Most often a daughter, upon reaching adolescence, grows more interested in peer relationships and in heterosexual activity outside the family, and finds a way to halt the incestuous relationship. She may, at this time abruptly end the relationship herself or she may tell somebody (her mother, other siblings, or friends) so that they will act to end it. The single incestuous event may be handled by subsequent avoidance or by open confrontation and accusation. In the latter case, a child may find him/herself (a) not believed, (b) accused of perpetrating the event, or (c) having provoked the immediate incarceration of the offender by an outraged parent.

Weiss et al. (31) divided female children who were molested into two groups, "accidental" and "participant." "Accidental" victims are usually approached by an exhibitionist, fondled by a stranger, or raped on a single occasion. More likely to tell the parent of the event when it does not involve a family member, they are frequently brought to an emergency room, since there is often concern on the parents' part that genital damage or trauma has occurred. However, parents often refuse to prosecute the perpetrator because they feel that the process will increase the trauma to their child. Court procedures and the attitudes of physicians often serve to reinforce this feeling. Families often prefer to handle the problem within the family, or to seek professional help without involving legal authorities. Parents, however, cannot always be supportive. Lewis and Sarrel (19) state that the parents may try to deal with their own sense of failure in parenting by "vociferous attempts to punish or attack the offending adult . . . the child observes the reaction of rage in the parents and develops a revulsion against all future sexual feelings and experience" (p. 796), resulting in an intensification of adaptive problems for the child.

Children involved sexually over a period of time are called "participant" or "collaborative" victims (8). In this situation, it is usually most difficult to detect sexual misuse. This is because they are often involved with a person with whom they are well acquainted, even if it is not a family member. In some cases through threats, intimidation, or bribes, in others through affection, the child remains silent. Other friends or family members, e.g., the mother or siblings may also be aware of what has transpired but collude in the silence because they also feel vulnerable.

The relationship is often revealed because of a medical problem in the victim or in a younger child in the family or neighborhood. At times, genital abrasions, irritations, or other genital trauma, or repeated vaginal or vulvar infections in a child will alert medical professionals to the possibility that sexual misuse has occurred (22). Venereal disease in a child older than one year of age is almost invariably transmitted by sexual means. (Opthalmic gonorrhea can be transmitted to a newborn during passage through the birth canal (13).) Though some argue that venereal diseases can be transferred by fomites, this is an unlikely mode of transmission for this disease to children.

Some children who are raped cannot put it into words. They may be seen in clinics or emergency rooms with other symptoms, including sleep disturbances, changes in patterns of behavior, withdrawal from previously important relationships, phobias, learning problems, unexplained depression or excessive clinging, episodes of crying, enuresis, or encopresis. At times, somatic complaints are seen, e.g., headaches, stomachaches. These may be conversion phenomena. Adolescents who have been sexually abused may make it known by running away, or they may begin to use drugs, become promiscuous, contract venereal disease, or become pregnant. There is very little descriptive material in the literature on how to separate the manifestations of sexual abuse from nonsexual etiologies of the same problems in children and adolescents.

Burgess and Holmstrom (5) described a "rape trauma syndrome" in children which is similar to that experienced by adults, with differences consistent with the developmental stage of the young victim. Thus, nausea, vomiting, and enuresis are more frequent, in addition to the symptoms seen in adults. While most rape victims react to the threat to their lives, regardless of age, adolescents tend to feel more embarrassed. For children, problems at school are important. They are concerned about how the event will affect them at school, or about the reactions of their peer group. Of the 23 victims described, all but three experienced symptoms for many months. These included nightmares, phobias, fears of being left alone, panic reactions on seeing either the assailant, the crime scene, or a symbolic reminder of the assault. Sexual fears were prominent and difficult for the child to discuss, since the issue was likely to be new, unfamiliar, and embarrassing. Parallel to the adult rape victim's desiring to move, children often wished to change schools or became school phobic.

Families often respond intensely to rape of their child. While these reactions usually emanate from caring, they can, at times, be distressing for the victim. While parents may need to blame someone, the person blamed may be the assailant, the child, and/or themselves. Thus, some parents may exacerbate the situation by expressing anger for the child's "stupid" behavior, or becoming concerned about their adolescent's sexual "provocativeness," then punishing the child by restricting privileges. When the parents assume the responsibility for the event themselves, they feel that they have been inadequate parents, that they should not have allowed the child to go out, or that they should not go out themselves. This may contribute to a child's developing a "phobic" attitude subsequent to the rape.

In circumstances where a relative outside the nuclear family or a baby sitter molests a child, parents may have previously disbelieved the child until clear evidence supporting the youngster's complaint becomes available. Then, they may feel very guilty. The sexual issues which may surface later may be difficult for parents to handle, especially if there has been no prior discussion about sex with the child.

As with the adult, the child may have a silent reaction in which he/she tells no one about the rape. Burgess and Holmstrom (5) suggest that one can be alerted to the possibility of an assault when the following symptoms occur without any other evident cause: acute onset of somatic symptoms, gastrointestinal symptoms, sleep disturbances and enuresis in a child under ten; and withdrawal from one's usual activities and relationships at home and school. The physician should not overlook the fact that male children may also be victimized. While much of the literature on children focuses on whether or not a "real" rape occurred, one must not overlook the fact that, in many cases, a child will not report a rape, but will present with symptoms.

There is very little systematic, long-term data on the impact of rape or incest on a child. Katan (14), reported on her analytic work with six adult women who were raped in childhood. The common theme for all six women was "low self-esteem" and "aggression turned against the self." They felt keenly that the traumas had caused "irreparable damage." Rosenfeld et al. (27) reported finding sexual problems and depression in adults who had had early incestuous relationships; and behavior and learning disorders were reported in children. Herman and Hirschman (13), in their report on 15 victims of father-daughter incest, emphasize that "the severity of subsequent complaints was related to the degree of family disorganization and deprivation in histories rather than to the incest history per se." Furthermore, they state that the women they studied all entered therapy with a "sense of being different, and distant from ordinary people." Other problems included subsequent marital conflict and abuse within marriage. While this group may not be representative, since they were seen for psychotherapy, the issues they raise merit further, more systematic study.

FAMILY DYNAMICS

In the "accidental" situation involving a child and a stranger (31), there do not seem to be any predisposing factors. While it is not clear what particular dynamics apply to molestation by a neighbor, family friend, or relative other than a parent, it is likely that issues involving the potential for ongoing contact, intimidation, continued vulnerability, and betrayal are important factors.

In incest, particularly the endogamic variety, it is clear that the issues are complex. While the law considers the child an innocent victim of the adult perpetrator, in these families, distorted forms of family interaction often include all family members in the incestuous interaction. Both parents may play a role: The father is the active perpetrator of the incest and the one who is held legally responsible because he is the "aggressor"; the mother, who may, by virtue of her passivity, be a covert supporter of the incest, may not even be consciously aware of the events or she may be aware but not take action to stop the activity for a variety of reasons, frequently because of chronic depression (4) or because she is frightened of the repercussions for herself or one of her children. The child is unfortunately caught in a family which cannot provide an atmosphere in which social and personal intimacy can coexist in the absence of sexual involvement, and is therefore "exploited" (9).

Sexual involvement on the part of the father is not at a "genital" level, but it represents a less mature search for gratification of basic dependency needs through use of genital organs. This form of incest can be thought of as a "symptom" of defective family functioning (21). Generational boundaries which support distinction between social and psychological roles of parents and children have been obliterated in these families, although the outward manifestations of social conformity are often maintained.

In their own early histories, both parents have often experienced multiple losses, both actual and psychological, and have made an agreement, usually unspoken, to keep the marriage "intact," regardless of the circumstances. Lustig (21) has argued that, in these families, incest serves as a homeostatic, tension-reducing mechanism which keeps the family intact by permitting satisfaction of all needs within the family. Thus, no member needs to seek satisfaction outside of it. The endogamic incestuous family is seen as depriving and neglectful, and the incestuous relationship may provide the child with the only attention available. Thus, although incest is a sexual activity, its psychological meaning is not directly sexual but serves other purposes, embodying a search for safety, comfort, and nurturance for both parents and children. In other situations, incest serves as a vehicle for domination and for enforcing compliance by adults who are incapable of dealing with the uncertainties of usual human relationships.

THE "SEDUCTIVE" CHILD

In endogamic families, the child has learned that sexual behavior is a way to gain attention from grownups. The behavior of these children can seem to be "seductive" or sexually arousing to adults. The term "seductive," however, is ill defined and value laden. It can imply the attribution of blame to the child although in this situation it actually refers to behavior that stimulates sexual feelings in nonpedophilic adults, combined with an ability to make others feel extremely involved and protective. Since the child has learned to expect this response and if the sexually arousing behavior is not responded to the child may become upset or depressed, it is important to emphasize, however, that the child does not necessarily recognize the sexual meaning of the behavior in an adult way, nor can the child be seen as culpable.

This "seductiveness" represents learned behavior on the child's part. Sexuality and sexual arousal are a means to obtain nurturance, perhaps because, in these families, the child's needs cannot be satisfied through more sublimated channels. It is a desperate attempt to adapt to adults' desires to obtain affection. In the literature, many authors (1) have commented on this "charming" and "seductive" quality in children who had been molested or involved incestuously, and Weiss (private written communication) noted that some of the more than 70 molested children he evaluated in his classic study (31) of almost 30 years ago not only behaved in a "seductive" manner during the psychiatric interview but they then told their parents that the physician had tried to molest them. Krieger et al. (16) found that similar behavior can occur in therapy and that it represents an attempt to discover whether the new therapeutic situation is safe or demands the same techniques the home atmosphere had required.

The fact that the child may seem to be seductive does not make him/her less, but rather more, a victim of exploitation. In this context, the child is a victim of a distorted and depriving family situation rather than of a sexual "act" or perversion (26). Furthermore, not only is the child a victim of his/her family, but the parents are victims of their past, which is sometimes remarkably similar to their child's present. Their life histories, including incestuous relationships, seem to create a defect in their parenting abilities and make them prone to expose their children to similar experiences (27). Thus, endogamic incest seems to be a multi-generational victim-victim relationship.

REPORTING SEXUAL MISUSE

Reporting requirements for sexual abuse vary between states. Although every state has laws concerning child abuse, not all of these laws include sexual abuse. In every state, however, sexual activity between adults and children is considered a crime, but regulations and categories for prosecution differ. In some localities, these activities are prosecuted as "undermining the morals of a minor," while in others they are considered "molestation."

Furthermore, reporting procedures also vary. In certain states, cases of sexual abuse or misuse must be reported to a protective care agency, which will then conduct an investigation. In other states, reports are transmitted directly to legal authorities, with the police investigating. In the case of incest, whether the child is removed from the family under a care and protection statute varies among cases and states.

Legal clarity on sexual abuse can facilitate intervention in those severe forms of sexual misuse where the normative boundaries of affectional life in the family have been broadly transgressed. Because these boundaries may be culturally determined and hence variable, laws and requirements may also differ. Thus, while incest is universally prohibited, it is not universally a crime, e.g., it is a serious ethical and moral infraction of Japanese culture, but it is not prosecuted under the criminal law. In fact, it usually comes to the attention of authorities only when infanticide resulting from incestuous union is reported (17).

LEGAL INTERVENTION AND ROLE OF THE COURT

Once a case of sexual misuse or incest is recognized, and a decision has been made to prosecute, an important factor must be considered: the impact of the court procedure on the child and family. Some legal experts tend to favor vigorous prosecution, while others are concerned about the impact of this on those involved. In Britain, for example, Henriques (12) encourages parents to prosecute because he believes that this will remove serious sexual offenders from society, preventing similar occurrences with other children, since without prosecution there is no guarantee that the abuse will cease or that other children will not be involved. Others disagree, finding prosecution more traumatic than the occurrence itself (15).

The potential for traumatization often begins before there is contact with the law. Emergency room procedures, including the physical examination, may be perceived as a repetition of the sexual trauma. While in an acute trauma accurate evidence must be collected (obtaining information, examining the witness, and maintaining an unbroken chain of evidence), at times this concern can override respect for a child's sensitivities. In some areas, consideration has been given to the use of well-trained, same-sexed, nonuniformed officers to interview children who have been sexually molested. This may also take place in a less threatening setting than police headquarters or the hospital emergency room. When the child is brought to court because of a criminal charge against the adult, procedures generally allow for cross-examination. The potential for traumatizing the child may be minimized in these cases by holding proceedings in a more private setting, e.g., the judge's chambers, or a private interview room. If the child is forced to retell the story over and over again, often months or years after the actual occurrence, or if he/she is subjected to strenuous cross-examination, he/she may be psychologically traumatized and may even be unable to remember or accurately recount the story. The use of an audio or videotape recording may reduce the necessity for repetition if it is legally permissible. Furthermore, if the child has been raped by a stranger, he/she may be frightened at seeing the rapist again in court or in a police lineup, and may have terrifying fantasies or even develop a traumatic neurosis.

In Israel, because of the potential for emotional repercussions, counselors who are trained to take testimony from children are employed and are empowered to testify in their stead, sparing the child the need to appear. Under our adversarial legal system, however, this would not be permissible in criminal proceedings where a plea of "not guilty" has been entered, and cross-examination is a right of the accused adult. In what De Frances (6) reported were well-selected cases for prosecution, 40 percent were dismissed outright before the trial had proceeded, thus subjecting children to what emerged as confusing and unproductive examination and questioning. For the fewer than 200 prosecuted cases, over 1,000 court appearances were required for the children involved. The interpretation of this situation on the part of the child is important. It may be seen as a negation of their experience or as confirmation that they are not being truthful. On the other hand, Lenore C. Terr (personal communication) has suggested that preventing a child from testifying may be traumatic if the child sees prosecution as a way of obtaining retribution and wants to testify. Parents are often reluctant to prosecute because of these concerns as well as because of the fear that the rapist may continue to be a real danger to the child who is "pressing the case" or to the family. This is not entirely unrealistic, since threats are often made.

In incestuous situations, there may be a greater degree of flexibility regarding the charges. As Wald (29) has pointed out, it is often possible to avoid criminal proceedings by charging neglect. This protects the child from the trauma of cross-examination. Furthermore, the case is less likely to be contested if the charges are civil rather than criminal. Hearings can be held in private, and following neglect proceedings, according to Wald, authorities are more likely to look after the child's interests by tending toward therapeutic approaches rather than by focusing on seeking punitive sanctions.

Stringent, severe prohibitions against incest do encourage recommendations for punitive sanctions toward parents involved in incest in most localities. Since some jurisdictions consider that this solves the "problem," little attention is paid to the circumstances which gave rise to the incest. Thus, the adult perpetrator is often incarcerated with no further services provided for the child or family.

New types of intervention have been instituted in some communities, including an extensive program in Santa Clara County, California (10), where a child abuse treatment program in the juvenile probation department offers a wide range of therapeutic approaches together with self-help groups focusing on family issues. Families have received this program positively, although systematic and careful study of the program has not yet been reported. What the results of these more compassionate approaches will be over time remains to be seen. However, it is clear that, in incest cases, careful clinical judgments and alternative approaches seem necessary to prevent further traumatization to the child, as often occurs when punitive action alone is undertaken (26). As Kaufman (15) has pointed out, when the incestuous parent is incarcerated, the child may feel enormous guilt over the breakup of the family, rather than over the incestuous act itself. Furthermore, the entire family system may be disrupted, and support, including economic, may be withdrawn if the breadwinner is incarcerated. Thus, in some incest cases, charges may be dropped after an accusation has been made because the child is guilty, frightened, or even more deprived. The child may wish the incest to end but does not necessarily want to lose the parent or feel responsible for their incarceration.

TREATMENT APPROACHES

In discussing childhood rape, Polak, Reyes and Fish (23) reiterate the need for limiting the questioning of a child during crisis intervention, and they emphasize the importance of preparing a child for the process, including the physical examination. They caution against questioning or examining a child alone without the presence of parents or other supportive adults.

Since the strongest and most important support system the child has is his/her family, the focus of early intervention in cases of actual rape should be to facilitate communication and empathy among family members, so that they are able to support the child. There are, of course, wide variations in parents' perceptiveness, willingness, and ability to talk openly about the experience. They usually need someone available with whom to discuss the difficulties of such communications. Parents should be reassured that their child is not "ruined" and that, in the case of rape, if the experience is handled calmly, openly, and supportively, available information, though scanty, and clinical judgment suggest that later sequelae are minimized.

How one talks to a child about his/her feelings and about the details of a sexual assault depends on age, who the perpetrator is, and the relationship with other family members. All interventions must be tailored to that particular child, including the use of appropriate terminology and/or play techniques. Some children will refuse any intervention. This may represent anything, varying from pathological denial to an adaptive coping style. One should not assume one or the other without knowing the child. Children usually know and remember a great deal more than adults suspect, so there is no justification for not speaking directly with the child if the child is verbal. There is no reason to think that talking is traumatizing; rather, it may give the child permission to speak. Anger and undue pressure, however, should be avoided. Parents should be alerted to symptoms of distress in the child, so that they are aware of which kinds of responses are usual, which ones herald more complex problems. They must be aware of the need for time for the child to recover from the trauma. Again, each child is unique. Parents usually know their children better than a professional called in during a crisis. With appropriate support and guidance, they are best able to tailor interventions to their child.

In most cases, the child needs encouragement to return to her usual life-style as quickly as possible, and the counselor may need to be involved with the parents, the child, and, at times, with the school. Some children will find it difficult to return to school, and they may become more symptomatic if pressured excessively. Others may prefer to change schools or living situations. If the sexual encounter was incest, the child may or may not need to be separated from the adult until more long-term planning can occur. On occasion, family treatment is instituted immediately, and the family is able to remain together. Since incest often comes to light because the family system which maintained it is disrupted, these families often are fragmenting when they are seen.

Finally, the decision of whether or not to prosecute is particularly complex when a child is involved since, as discussed above, additional trauma may be imposed on the child. The family needs the opportunity to discuss options and consequences. In the event the family wishes to proceed in spite of the child's ambivalence or wishes not to, it is likely that prolonged counseling support will be necessary. In these cases, it might be helpful to explore the parents' motivation.

While everyone needs some help in coping with the acute phase after sexual trauma, the types of intervention required may differ. In assessing what kinds of resources to offer to children and their families, one must consider previous adjustment, family interaction, and the age of the child. Stress tolerance, adaptive resources, and environmental supports are important aspects. Since there is a danger of lowered self-esteem, the child needs reassurance about how he/she handled the experience and about his/her efforts to cope following it. The child must be offered the opportunity for constructive catharsis with a caring and empathetic person. Restitution is interfered with by lack of support, and condemnation reinforces guilt and lowers self-esteem.

An additional therapeutic goal, if possible, is to utilize the crisis experience for some further growth. The trauma may be too great for this. However, at times genuine gains may be made. In deciding upon the particular approach to be recommended, it is useful to differentiate short-term crisis goals from long-term issues which may require referral for individual psychotherapy. Most often, group therapy is not well received initially. Parents and children desire the opportunity to discuss their specific experiences and responses. Groups may be most helpful after the initial crisis stage, when sharing the continuing concerns and symptoms may be supportive and provide affirmation that the trauma does not need to be denied or negated. Those children requiring long-term therapy are more likely to have had difficulty resolving crises in the past, or the events may have been particularly traumatic for some specific reason, e.g., the person involved, the events or other life issues which have occurred such as the recent death of a close relative. They may exhibit a deterioration of relationships, phobic reactions, or sexual anxiety. Depression may be persistent, and long-term sequelae may lead to problems, especially with sexual adjustment in later life.

It is particularly difficult to make recommendations for a child as a witness in a criminal proceeding. This is so because molested children vary considerably with regard to their emotional maturity and stage of psychosexual development or cognitive development. They also vary in their ability to remember or describe the events. Prior to approximately age seven, a child is generally not cognitively capable of giving an adult form of rational recounting of a story without confusing events, times, and places. An older child who has been traumatized may also experience similar difficulties. Often, those involved in the legal proceedings are so concerned with the outcome of the case that they do not recognize the child's particular limitations.

The literature is filled with discussions about whether reports of incest are fantasy or reality. Although, as noted above, the young child may distort reality, it has been our experience that many, if not most, of these reports are true in older children. We must remember, however, that, in some younger children, an actual molestation has occurred, but the wrong person may have been accused. Also, younger children may feel guilty for some matter unconnected with sex and use such an accusation as a vehicle to express that guilt. At very early ages fantasy and reality may be difficult to separate because of the child's immature modes of expression (28).

If the report is believed to be valid, and no violence has occurred, but the decision to prosecute is made, then there would be no laboratory or emergency room findings. Thus, the child will have to be witness since he/she was, most likely, the only other person present at the time of the molestation. Under these circumstances, steps must be taken to protect the child to whatever extent possible. It has proven useful in some cases to foster the development of a relationship between one specific prosecutor and the child during the course of preparation for the trial. This may aid the child through the process. The presence of supportive and familiar adults, particularly parents, is also helpful. Some preparation, in which the child can rehearse what the courtroom will be like in a supportive play situation may also prove helpful. There is, however, no way of denying that the process of prosecution in those cases where the child is not pressing for it can be traumatic.

CONCLUSION

It is important to emphasize that, regardless of the circumstances, guilt and shame are almost always experienced, even by young children. These feelings are often related to the perception that they were in some way responsible for the sexual encounter. Often the responses of parents, peers, and professionals support this view. Rather than understanding the helplessness, powerlessness, and vulnerability of the child, he/she may actually be blamed, or covertly made to feel responsible for the events. In the case of incest, the violation of the contact with a caretaker is of primary importance. This, coupled with the resulting family dissolution, especially if the child is blamed, may be extremely traumatic. Even the child who ostensibly permitted the incestuous relationship is not able to predict the negative reaction that he/she will have at a later time. An encounter with law enforcement agencies may reinforce guilt, or even be seen as a punishment.

REFERENCES

1. BENDER, L. & BLAU, A. (1937). The Reaction of Children to Sexual Relations with Adults. *Am. J. Orthopsych.*, 7:500-518.
2. BRANCH, G. & PAXTON, R. (1965). A Study of Gonococcal Infections Among Infants and Children. *Public Health Reports*, 80:347-52.
3. BRANT, R. & TISZA, V. (1977). The Sexually Misused Child. *Am. J. Orthopsych.*, 47:80-90.
4. BROWNING, D. H. & BOATMAN, B. (1977). Incest: Child at Risk. *Am. J. Psych.*, 134: 69-72.
5. BURGESS, A. W. & HOLMSTROM, I. L. (1974). Rape trauma syndrome. *Am. J. Psych.*, 131:981-986.
6. DE FRANCIS, V. (1969). Protecting the Child Victims of Sex Crimes Committed by Adults. The American Humane Association, Denver.
7. FINKELHOR, D. (1978). Unpublished Doctoral Thesis.
8. GAGNON, J. (1965). Female Child Victims of Sex Offenses. *Soc. Probs.*, 13:176-192.
9. GALDSTON, R. (1971). Dysfunctions of Parenting, the Battered Child, the Neglected Child, the Exploited Child. In *Modern Perspectives in International Child Psychiatry*, 3:571-588, J. G. Howells (Ed.). New York: Brunner/Mazel.
10. GIARETTO, H. (1976). The Treatment of Father-Daughter Incest. *Children Today*, 5:2-35.
11. HAYMAN, C. R. & LANZA, C. (1971). Sexual Assault on Women and Girls. *Am. J. Obstet. Gynec.*, 109:480-486.
12. HENRIQUES, B. (1961). Sexual Assaults on Children: II. A Magistrate's View. *Brit. Med. J.*, 1629-1631.
13. HERMAN, J. & HIRSCHMAN, L. (1977). Father-daughter incest. *Signs: Journal of Women in Culture and Society*, June.
14. KATAN, A. (1973). Children who were raped. *The Psychoanalytic Study of the Child*, 28:208-224.
15. KAUFMAN, I., PECK, A., & TAGIURI, L. (1954). The family constellation and overt incestuous relations between father and daughter. *Am. J. Orthopsych.*, 24:266-279.
16. KRIEGER, M., ROSENFELD, A., GORDON, A., & BENNETT, J. J. (1980). Problems of Psychotherapy of Children with a History of Incest. *Am. J. Psychother.*, 34(1): 81-88.
17. KUBO, S. (1959). Researches and Studies on Incest in Japan. *Hiroshima J. Med. Sciences*, 8:99-159.
18. LANDIS, J. (1956). Experiences of 500 Children with Adult Sexual Deviation. *Psychiatric Quart. Suppl.*, 91:91-109.
19. LEWIS, M. & SARREL, J. (1969). Some Psychological Aspects of Seduction, Incest, and Rape in Childhood. *J. Am. Acad. Ch. Psych.*, 8:609-619.
20. LUKIANOWICZ, N. (1972). Incest. *Brit. J. Psych.*, 120:301-313.
21. LUSTIG, N., DRESSER, J., SPELLMAN, S., & MURRAY, T. B. (1966). Incest. *Arch. Gen. Psych.*, 14:31-40.

22. MOLNAR, G. & CAMERON, P. (1975). Incest Syndromes: Observations in a General Hospital Psychiatric Unit. *Can. Psych. Assoc. J.*, 20:373-377.

23. POLAK, P., REYES, M., & FISH, L. (1975). The Management of Family Crises. In *Emergency Psychiatric Care*, H. Resnik and H. Ruben (Eds.). Bonill, Md.: Charles Press.

24. ROSENFELD, A. A. (1977). Incest: A Clinical Spectrum. Presented at Annual Meeting of American Academy of Child Psychiatry, Houston.

25. ROSENFELD, A. A. (1979a). Incidence of a History of Incest Among 18 Female Psychiatric Patients. *Am. J. Psych.*, 136 (6):791-795.

26. ROSENFELD, A. (1979b). Endogamic Incest and the Victim-Perpetrator Model. *Am. J. Dis. Ch.*, 133:406-410.

27. ROSENFELD, A., NADELSON, C., KRIEGER, M., & BACKMAN, J. H. (1977). Incest and Sexual Abuse of Children. *J. Am. Acad. Ch. Psych.*, 16:327-339.

28. ROSENFELD, A., NADELSON, C., & KRIEGER, M. (1979). Fantasy and Reality in Patients Reports of Incest. *J. Clin. Psych.*, 40:159-164.

29. WALD, M. (1975). State Intervention on Behalf of "Neglected" Children: A Search for Realistic Standards. *Stanford Law Review*, 27:985-1040.

30. WEINBERG, S. (1955). *Incest Behavior*. New York: Citadel Press.

31. WEISS, J., ROGERS, E., DARWIN, M., & DUTTON, C. E. (1955). A Study of Girl Sex Victims. *Psych. Quart.*, 29:1-27.

9

TERMINATION OF PARENTAL RIGHTS

DIANE H. SCHETKY, M.D. and DAVID L. SLADER, J.D.

This chapter will review some of the problems associated with long-term foster care and discuss termination of parental rights as an alternative for children who are unable to be returned home.

FOSTER CARE: ITS PROMISE AND PERFORMANCE

Foster care is an institution which has survived with tenacity amidst controversy and permutations. Its origins are not known, though it is said to have been practiced among Anglo-Saxons, Welsh and Scandinavians and it was popular in ancient Ireland. In contrast to the situation today, it was then practiced primarily among the well-to-do and regarded as a means of promoting training for children and social cohesiveness (13).

Foster care first emerged in this country in the 19th century in the form of indenture. Later, Charles Loring Brace of the N.Y. Children's Aid Society viewed foster care as a means of rescuing children from city slums. With missionary zeal, he initiated a program responsible for placing 31,000 youths into homes in the West between 1853 and 1921 (3). His work was attacked because he failed to place children in homes with the same religious orientation and because it posed a threat to traditional institutional care. Not too surprisingly, states receiving partial subsidy for institutional care of children were likely to be more resistant to using foster care than those who were not (20). Foster care as an alternative to institutions was utilized in the early 20th century and Trotsky (27) was the first to do research comparing the two.

Further opposition to foster care arose when it attempted to accommodate delinquent youths. The public sympathy went out to destitute, orphaned children but did not extend to delinquents, whom many believed to be in need of authority and more punitive treatment. Healy and Bronner (11) refuted some of these notions in their work, which

107

demonstrated the successful adjustment of many delinquent children to foster care. Since the 1950s there has been a plethora of studies dealing with foster care, some of which will be referred to in this chapter.

In 1973, there were more than 300,000 children in foster care in the U.S. (28). Approximately 50 percent of all neglect hearings result in the child's being removed from home (18). In spite of the frequency with which children are removed from their homes, guidelines for when removal is indicated remain unclear (2) and standards for when the child is returned to the home are vague or introduce issues unrelated to the reasons for the child's removal.

The Child Welfare League states that "Foster Family Care offers the child, who would otherwise lack adequate parental care and who can not remain in his own home, a closer approximation to normal family life living than other types of substitute care, and is particularly adapted to meet the child's normal needs in a family centered society" (4). It defines Foster Family Care as "The Child Welfare Service which provides substitute family care for a *planned* period for a child when his own family can not care for him for a temporary or extended period and when adoption is neither desirable nor possible." It goes on to state that "long-term placement resulting from lack of adequate planning or casework with parents is not considered an acceptable practice" and further stresses the need for ongoing professional help to parents, foster parents, and child to "help in dealing with problems involved in separation and placement" (4).

In reality, many children in foster care lack ongoing relationships with caseworkers and in one study 50 to 60 percent of children had no contact with their caseworker over a two-month period. When the caseworker did make contact it was more likely to be with the foster mother than with the child (12). Continuity of caseworkers is a problem, with annual turnover running as high as 36 percent in some public child welfare agencies (26) and many foster parents complain that there are times when they do not even know who their caseworker is (14). Foster parents claim that they are not given relevant information about the children in their care and in one study only 26.1 percent were told how long they could expect the child to be with them (25). Further, a study of a well staffed child care agency revealed that less than half of the foster children served understood why they were in foster care (25).

Although foster care is designed as a *temporary* measure, studies show that a child placed in foster care has a 50 percent chance of remaining there three years or longer (29). The longer a child is in foster care, the less likely he or she is to be adopted or returned home and Maas and Engler (17) suggest that a child who has been in foster care for longer that 18 months has a remote chance of either being adopted or returned home. Fanschel, in a more recent five-year longitudinal study, found 36.4 percent of 624 children remained in foster care for five years, with 56.1 percent returned home and only 4.6 percent adopted, and the remaining 2.9 percent institutionalized (7). Older children and Caucasian children were most likely to have been returned home. One-half of children entering placement at under two years of age remained in foster care. This seems particularly tragic considering the demand for infants in adoption agencies, how readily adoptable most infants are, and how critical these early years are in terms of development. Fanschel's data, however, contradict the notion that children are doomed to remain in foster care if not discharged within two years, as he found that one-fourth of the children in his study returned home after two years in foster care. The best predictor of returning home was frequent parental visiting (7).

A study of foster children in the southeast estimated that 9.6 percent of 3000 children could benefit from termination of parental rights and adoption proceedings, yet only 220 petitions to terminate parental rights were filed in 1976. The author suggests that given conditions of optimal agency resources, probably one-third of all children in foster care could be returned to parents or relatives (25). Because of inadequate staffing, case planning, and court surveillance, many children become lost in the limbo of foster care with no plans made towards either reintegrating them into their families or freeing them for adoption. Unfortunately, only 18 states require periodic court review of the status of children in foster care (29), in spite of the fact that it has been shown to be an effective means of expediting children out of foster care (8).

For the child who is left in foster care there are multiple problems to contend with: separation from biological parents, fear of the unknown, feelings of being different, shifting agency personnel, loyalty conflicts over having to relate to two sets of parents, hesitant or ambivalent attachments, and the fear of rejection, separation, and yet another move. Given these stresses, it is difficult for the child in foster care to maximize potential for normal emotional growth. Children in foster care show a much higher incidence of emotional maladjustment and learning difficulties than do control children (5, 24) and Boehm (1) concludes that emotional difficulties in foster children "tend to increase with the passage of time" (1). The foster care system itself is unstable and, through no fault of the child, placements may fall through; if a child is experiencing problems at the time of placement, he or she remains at an even higher risk for multiple placements.

Foster and Freed noted,

> Children are persons and the law should recognize that fact, although it will take some doing. The status of minority is the last legal relic of feudalism and the arguments for and against perpetuation of that status have a familiar ring. In good measure they are the same arguments that were advanced over the issues of slavery and the emancipation of married women (9).

This section will attempt to explore the legal and philosophical standards as well as the psychological basis for the child's rights.

Defining the Rights of the Child

The maintenance of the relationship between parents and their biological child is as much the right of the child as of the parent. Just as surely, the right of the parent cannot be terminated without terminating the right of the child to the parent. However, rights of the child, due to his/her dependent status, are not one-dimensional. He/she also possesses the right, that is, the overpowering need, to have parents to call his/her own on a continuous basis and to be free of physical and sexual mistreatment. The balancing of these sometimes conflicting rights is, from the child's perspective, the issue in a proceeding to terminate the parent-child relationship.

The right of the child to the maintenance of his/her relationship with his/her biological parents is, as a general rule, the foremost guarantee of the child's interest. The family, when functioning, serves the child's primary emotional needs for continuity, consistency and identity. Tampering with the biological family is, correspondingly, usually adverse to his or her interests.

When someone other than the biological parents has provided for the child's care and custody, the interests of the child which are normally attached to the biological parent-child relationship, i.e., continuity, consistency, and identity, may have been transplanted by time and affection onto what can be called the "psychological" parent-child relationship. This most commonly exists when a child has experienced a long-term warm and stable relationship with foster parents or custodial relatives. The maintenance of that relationship, when it exists and can be perpetuated, may be the primary right of the child.

More precious, perhaps, than the right to a particular parent is the right of the child to have someone to call "parent." The child in foster care or in an institution without hope of a prompt return to his original family may find himself in the limbo of being no one's child. He/she is an orphan of the living, and his/her legal tie to his or her biological parents may be the sole obstacle to adoption, the only adequate alternative to long-term foster care or institutionalization.

Under early Roman law, a father had the power of life or death over his children on the theory that having given the child life, he had the right to take it away. Today, children are "persons" within the meaning of the Constitution of the United States, and as "persons" they have the right to be free from unwarranted assault upon their bodies and their minds, even when the assailant is their parent.

Weighing the Rights of the Child and Parent

The rights of a child to his or her psychological home, to some home, or to a home free of abuse are in obvious potential conflict with the rights of the biological parents to possess the child. That conflict is resolved as a practical matter by adherence to statutory standards for termination of the parent-child relationship. The usual criteria, which look to the fulfillment or neglect of parental duties (rather than to the quality of the relationship from the child's perspective), include desertion for a specified period of time; abandonment (i.e. parent's declaration that he/she has no intention of returning); and unfitness by reason of conduct (i.e. abuse or neglect) or condition such as mental illness or retardation which presents a risk of serious physical danger to the child.

In a conflict between the fundamental rights of a child and the fundamental rights of a parent, two underlying social considerations govern the outcome. On the one hand is a well justified apprehension whenever the coercive arm of the government enters into the private domain of the family. It is the family which, more that any other factor, deprives the state of a monopoly of unfettered power; any diminution of the prerogative of parents is a corresponding and ominous increase in the power of the state.

On the other hand, the interest of society is not served when children are grievously mistreated, grossly neglected, or allowed to languish in the limbo of foster care. Unless the chain of mistreatment is somewhere broken, abuse breeds abuse from one scarred generation to another. As recently articulated by Goldstein, Freud and Solnit, "Each time the cycle of grossly inadequate parent-child relationships is broken, society stands to gain a person capable of becoming an adequate parent for children of the future" (10, p. 7).

The balance resolves itself into the imprecise principle that parents have a general right to act toward their child as they see fit, even when it is detrimental to the child's welfare. The child's rights are, or should be, superior in these regards:

1) He or she is entitled to have some adult functioning on a permanent basis in the role of nurturing parent;

2) He or she is entitled to maintain that relationship once it has been ratified by time and affection; and

3) He or she is entitled to a minimal level of freedom from abuse and exploitation within that relationship.

When those rights are not being served by the relationship between a child and his or her biological parents and when they would be better served by severing that relationship and freeing the child for adoption, it is the child's right for that separation and reattachment to occur.

IMPLEMENTING TERMINATION OF PARENTAL RIGHTS

The Honorable Justine Wise Polier has commented "That courts have power to terminate such rights when for valid reasons it becomes necessary to remove a child from the custody of natural parents, gives few clues as to what is or should be done. . . . What is done to terminate parental rights is done in a hesitant and tragically slow fashion. The lack of clarity, the confusion and uncertainty about the termination of parental rights on the part of public agencies, private agencies, and the courts all contribute to the procrastination and ineffectiveness that mark the handling of such cases" (21).

Unfortunately, there exist no uniform standards regarding the indications for termination of parental rights though several model statutes have been proposed (19, 23, 29).* Statutes in most states are extremely vague and in others overly restrictive. For instance, some states will not

---

* Levine discusses the deficiencies of existing statutes and provides an excellent bibliography on the legal issues as well as needs of the child, and existing state laws pertaining to termination of parental rights (16).

consider terminating parental rights unless an adoptive home has been found for the child. Unfortunately, it is difficult to place a child in a potential adoptive home unless the child is legally free for adoption. Most statutes remain parent centered, focusing on parental fault rather than the child's needs, with little consideration given to the child's concept of time and the fact that he/she does not share the adult's capacity for frustration tolerance and postponement of gratification of needs.

Wald had proposed that termination be based on the length of time the child has been in foster care and suggests that it should be the norm after a specified period of time (six months for the child under three and 12 months for the older child) unless there are reasons why it would be harmful. He further advocates termination at the initial neglect hearing in cases where 1) the child has been abandoned, 2) there have been previous charges of abuse from parents with respect to this child or a sibling, and 3) the child has previously been removed from the home and now must be removed again (29).

The state of Oregon has taken the lead in aggressively pursuing termination of parental rights as a means of effecting permanent placement for children unable to return home as an alternative to indefinite foster care. Freeing Children for Permanent Placement was a three year demonstration project conducted in Oregon and funded in 1973 by the Children's Bureau of the Office of Child Development.* The project identified 509 children who seemed destined to remain in foster care indefinitely and sought to provide them with permanent homes. Permanent plans were thought of in terms of returning children home, formalizing long-term foster care arrangements or freeing them for adoption. The children in the project had been in foster care for over one year, were considered by caseworkers unlikely to be returned home, but were felt to be adoptable. The project focused on aggressive casework techniques and also contracted for legal representation for the children through the Public Defender's Office and had access to the services of a child psychologist. Returning children home had the highest priority and, where this was not possible, adoption by foster parents, new parents, or relatives was explored, leaving permanent foster placement as a last alternative.

At the onset of the project, the concept of termination of parental rights was foreign to many caseworkers and courts, and considerable reluctance was encountered from judges, state's attorneys and court work-

* The savings in foster care payment were greater than one million dollars and equaled the expenses of supporting the project in the first two years (6).

ers. Special training was given to selected social workers who were given limited case loads.

At the conclusion of the project, 66 percent of the children were in permanent placement (26 percent returned to parents, 20 percent adopted by new parents, 20 percent adopted by foster parents) with 90 percent of the permanent placements intact at follow-up two years later. Children who were doing well at time of placement were likely to continue doing so. Those returned to their parents were also doing well but not as well as those in other placements. A sense of permanence, not necessarily legal, was found to be the best predictor of a child's well being (15).

The Role of the Child Psychiatrist in Termination of Parental Rights

In view of the number of termination cases now being heard, child psychiatrists and psychologists are increasingly being called upon to make recommendations to the court with respect to which course of action is in the best interest of the child. Secondly, they are often asked about the likelihood of the parents' conduct or condition altering sufficiently to permit return of the child home within the foreseeable future. Ideally, one's evaluation should include assessment of parents, child, parent-child relationship as well as the child's relationship with surrogate parents. However, one is often forced to work under less than optimal conditions when parents are unavailable or unwilling to participate in the evaluation.

The evaluation is conducted along the lines outlined in Chapter 3, and, where possible, one observes the child with various parent figures. The reasonably intact parent will usually put his or her best foot forward and be attentive to the child at least while under observation. However, with some families these brief interactions are most revealing, particularly where there is much covert aggression which they fail to recognize, but which is readily apparent in name calling, testing, and the parent's need to put down the child or encourage his or her aggression. Commonly, one also observes role reversal or the child playing a significant role in marital dysfunction. For example, a four-year-old's mother handed him a pair of boxing gloves and suggested that he "punch Daddy out," commenting that it would be an opportune time to give his diabetic stepfather a "shiner" since he had not yet taken his insulin that day. Many parents will display age-inappropriate expectations for their child and show little appreciation of developmental norms or the child's feelings. Their behavior may also indicate their commitment to the child. For instance, a 15-year-old chronic runaway sang the following prophetic lullaby to her infant, "Rock a bye baby on the tree top, when the wind blows the cradle will rot"!

Much emphasis is placed on the parents' background with an eye towards where they are in their emotional development and what their strengths and capacity for change might be. A study of 51 parents who had their parental rights terminated found that the majority came from backgrounds of educational, social, economic and social disadvantage (22). The cyclical nature of their parenting skills was evident as one looked at their childhoods which were replete with disturbed parent-child relationships, family disruption, alcoholism, neglect, physical and sexual abuse. Many had experienced out-of-home placements as children. As adults, they functioned marginally and displayed difficulties in interpersonal relationships. Their parenting was characterized by deficiency in empathy and they tended to regard their children as existing to satisfy their own needs. Diagnostically, 35 percent of the mothers were schizophrenic and neglect of their children was the major reason for agency involvement. In contrast, the fathers were not psychotic and were likely to be diagnosed as antisocial or inadequate personalities.

Important questions to ask oneself in assessing the parent's potential are:

1) Is the parent currently able to meet the child's needs?
2) What is the parent's current level of functioning and does this represent an arrest in development or a regression?
3) Is the parent's condition treatable and, if so, is the parent motivated to change and willing to accept therapy?
4) What is the parent's past record with respect to following through with recommendations for treatment? (Almost all will profess motivation at the time of the hearing.)
5) If the parent is deemed treatable, will help improve the parent sufficiently in time to meet the child's needs within the child's time perspective?
6) What is the impact of the parent's pathology or conduct on the child and what ameliorating factors might be present such as the protection of a spouse or grandparent?
7) Does the child have special needs or problems that require exceptional parenting skills?

In weighing the pros and cons of termination of parental rights, one must give careful consideration to the strength of the child's ties to the parents. The children who maintain close emotional ties to their parents, with or without any reciprocity on their part, are not likely to be good candidates for termination of parental rights because the strength of these ties usually preclude attachment to new parents. Schetky et al. (22) studied children involved in termination proceedings and found that almost all of them had relinquished emotional ties to their parents prior to formal termination of that relationship by the court.

Some exceptions exist, however, and in instances where there is no likelihood of parents ever being able to resume custody of a child in the foreseeable future, it may be in the child's best interest to allow him or her, with the help of therapy, to mourn the unavailable parent, relinquish the intensity of the relationship, and move on to form new attachments. For example, a woman seeking to regain custody of her two children became despondent and made a serious suicide attempt which left her with irreparable brain damage necessitating a lifetime of nursing home care. Her parental rights were terminated, but her children continued to visit her while eagerly awaiting adoption by their foster parents. A similar situation arises when a father murders his wife and the children lose the surviving parent through incarceration. In one such instance, the father agreed to the adoption of his children by an aunt and uncle and was willing to assume the role of uncle to his children. In such cases, as with children who are adopted at an older age and choose to maintain some casual contact with their biological parents, the parent-child relationship is greatly attenuated but not entirely relinquished. Hopefully, the child comes to accept the fact that the father or mother is no longer available to them in the role of parent. As noted by Derdeyn in Chapter 10, the continued relationship may offer the child important links to the past and a chance to check reality with fantasy, but the risk is that it may jeopardize the relationship between child and adoptive parent.

Termination of parental rights may not be advisable when a child is living with relatives who do not want to adopt. Grandparents may not wish to alienate a child by seeking permanent custody of grandchildren, and identity and continuity may be less of an issue for the child living with relatives. The dangers remain, however, in that the parent may choose to interfere or abruptly uproot the child and that the child may be subjected to the same adverse influences and conditions that contributed to the parent's pathology.

One must also determine whether the child is adoptable in the event that parental rights are terminated. Age, sex, physical appearance, disabilities, intelligence, race, and behavior problems all affect a child's chances for being adopted. However, who is adoptable is often a function of who will have the child and how diligently agencies are willing to search for homes for hard-to-place children. From the child psychiatrist's standpoint the most crucial issue with respect to adoptability is the child's capacity to develop relationships. Some children who have been bounced around a lot, particularly in the critical early years, are only capable of shallow, self-serving, interpersonal relationships which are often the precursors to serious character disorders in adult life. The alternatives for these children are return home, permanent foster care, or in some instances residential care or a group home.

In summary, there is no absolute formula for determining when to recommend termination of parental rights. One must weigh a variety of factors including severity and duration of parent's condition or conduct, likelihood of change and reintegration of the child into the home within a reasonable time, who the child views as the psychological parent, what options are available to the child in the event that the parent-child relationship is severed, and what course of action will be least detrimental to the child.

REFERENCES

1. BOEHM, B. (1958). *Deterrents to Adoption of Children in Foster Care*. New York: Child Welfare League of America, 22:28.
2. BOEHM, B. (1962). An Assessment of Family Adequacy in Protective Care. *Child Welfare*, 41:10.
3. BRACE, E. (1894). *The Life of Charles Loring Brace*. New York: Charles Scribner's Sons.
4. *Child Welfare League of America Standards for Foster Family Care Service*. (1959). New York: Child Welfare League of America, Inc., 3-5.
5. EISENBERG, L. (1962). The Sins of the Fathers and Urban Decay and Social Pathology. *Am. J. Orthopsych.*, 32:5-7.
6. EMLEN, A., LAHTI, J., DOWNS, G., McKAY, A., & DOWNS, S. (1977). *Overcoming Barriers to Planning for Children in Foster Care*, Vol. 2. A Report on Freeing Children for Permanent Placement. Washington, D.C.: U.S. Department of Health Education and Welfare.
7. FANSCHEL, D. (1976). Status Changes of Children in Foster Care. Final Results of the Columbia University Longitudinal Study. *Child Welfare*, 55:143-171.
8. FASTINGER, J. (1976). The Impact of New York Court Review on Children in Foster Care: A Follow Up Report. *Child Welfare*, 55:515-544.
9. FOSTER, H. & FREED, D. (1974). A Bill of Rights for Children. In *The Youngest Minority*, S. Katz. ABA Press, 318.
10. GOLDSTEIN, J., FREUD, A., & SOLNIT, A. (1973). *Beyond the Best Interests of the Child*. New York: Free Press.
11. HEALY, W. & BRONNER, A. (1936). *Reconstructing Behavior in Youth*. New York: Knopf.
12. JETER, H. R. (1963). *Children, Problems, and Services in Child Welfare Programs*. Washington, D.C.: U.S. Department of Health, Education and Welfare, 155-158.

13. JOYCE, P. (1913). *A Social History of Ancient Ireland*, 14. London: Longmans, Green & Co.

14. KADUSHIN, A. (1967). *Child Welfare Services*. New York: Macmillan Co., 420.

15. LAHTI, J., GREEN, K., EMLEN, A., ZADNY, J., CLARKSON, O. D., KUEHNEL, M., & CASCIATO, J. (1978). A Follow-up Study of the Oregon Project: A Summary. Portland: Regional Research Institute for Human Studies.

16. LEVINE, R. (1975). Foundations for Drafting a Model Statute to Terminate Parental Rights: A Select Bibliography. *Juvenile Justice*, August, 1975, 42-56.

17. MAAS, H. & ENGLER, R. (1959). *Children in Need of Parents*. New York: Columbia University Press, 390.

18. MNOOKIN, R. (1973). Foster Care in Whose Best Interest? 43 *Harvard Ed. Review*, 599:606-638.

19. NATIONAL COUNCIL OF JUVENILE COURT JUDGES. (1976). Model Statute for Termination of Parental Rights. *Juvenile Justice*, Nov. 3-8.

20. POLIER, J. (1941). *Everyone's Children. Nobody's Child*. New York: Charles Scribner's Sons.

21. POLIER, J. (1958). *Parental Rights. The Need for Law and Social Action*. New York: Child Welfare League Assoc., 4-11.

22. SCHETKY, D., ANGELL, R., MORRISON, C. V., & SACK, W. H. (1979). Parents who Fail: A Study of 51 Cases of Termination of Parental Rights. *J. Am. Acad Ch. Psych.*, 18:366-383.

23. SLADER, D. & ROBART, N. (1976). *Model Dissolution of Parent-Child Relationship Act*. Portland: Project to Free Children for Permanent Placement.

24. SWIRE, M. & KAVALER, F. (1977). Health Status of Foster Children. *Child Welfare*, 56:635-653.

25. THOMAS, G., POLLANE, L., BRANSFORD, R., & PARCHURE, S. (1977). *Supply and Demand for Foster Care in the Southeast*. Athens, Ga.: Regional Inst. and Soc. Welfare Research Institute, 46, 78.

26. TOLLEN, W. (1960). *Study of Staff Losses in Child Welfare and Family Services Agencies*. Washington: U.S. Department of Health, Education and Welfare, 12-13.

27. TROTSKY, E. (1930). *Institutional Care and Placing Out*. Chicago: Marks Nathan Jewish Orphan Home.

28. U.S. DEPARTMENT HEW (1973). Child Welfare Statistics, Pub. No. (SRS) 73-03258, NLSS Report E 9.

29. WALD, M. (1976). State Intervention on Behalf of Neglected Children: Standards for Removal of Children from their Homes, Monitoring the Children in Foster Care and Termination of Parental Rights. *Stanford Law Review*, Vol. 28, No. 4, 623-705.

30. WEINSTEIN, E. (1960). *The Self Image of the Foster Child*. New York: Russell Sage Foundation.

10

ADOPTION

ANDRE P. DERDEYN, M.D.

Adoption, like many of our social institutions, continues to be in a process of change. Spanish immigrants brought to the United States the influence of Roman adoption, which almost exclusively served the needs of the adopter (35, 69). In the United States, the basic purpose of adoption changed to primarily benefiting children in need of homes. It is of note, however, that institutionalization was thought to be beneficial for children, and orphanages continued to be built in great numbers until the early part of the 19th century, when placing-out began to replace both institutionalization and indenture as the major modes of finding homes for children.

Until the mid-1800s, adoption, like divorce, was accomplished in this country by individual legislative acts on behalf of specific individuals (98). The first general adoption act was passed in Massachusetts in 1851, followed by similar acts in other states (96). This interest in adoption was part of a growing concern for children which was associated also with the establishment of public schools and child labor laws.

This chapter will broadly review changes in the population of children available for extra-familial adoption and the legal framework of adoption, including the controversy regarding the sealed birth record. In addition, some psychodynamics of adoption affecting the adoptive parent-child relationship will be explored, as will questions regarding continuing contact with birth parents.

CHILDREN AVAILABLE FOR ADOPTION

Until very recently adoption has primarily served infants, and there has been a reasonably clear attempt to recreate for the adoptive family the image of a biological one. There are, however, recent and significant changes in the composition of the group of children available for adop-

119

tion and in the total number of children. The pattern of adoptive placements in recent years has been one of progressively slower growth, finally dropping in 1971 (85). Changes in attitudes toward illegitimacy, greater availability of abortion with adequate medical and legal safeguards, better methods of contraception, and wider dissemination of birth control information are all having an impact upon the supply of children available for adoption. There has been a great decline in the availability of young white babies, and the decrease in overall numbers of children available for adoption would be even more dramatic were it not for the recent expansion of the pool of potential adoptees to include many children who were formerly not considered for adoption. These are the children who tended to remain in the foster care system.

The Increasing Significance of the Foster Care System to Adoption

Public concern has risen regarding children in foster care because of the increase in total numbers of children within the foster care system, and because of an increasing realization that in a great proportion of instances, foster care is by no means temporary. In Maas and Engler's classic 1959 study involving over 4,000 children, the authors predicted that over half would remain in foster care for most of their childhoods (59). In a 1973 study in the state of Massachusetts, it was found that 60 percent of children in foster care at the time of the study had been in care between four and eight years, with the average stay in excess of five years (34). The Columbia Longitudinal Study of Children in Foster Care in New York City has provided information regarding 467 families with one or more children entering foster care. The children were under 12 years of age and were entering foster care for the first time. Of the original study of 624 children, 36 percent remained in foster care at the end of five years (27). As a result of the greater awareness about the problems faced by children in foster care, new initiatives are being sought to meet their need for parenting persons.

Efforts to decrease the utilization of foster care thrust in two different directions: 1) limiting the utilization of foster care, and 2) facilitating adoption (16). The first goal, that of limiting removal of children from parental homes, is being addressed by refining the criteria by which a child can be removed from his/her home for temporary or other purposes, and by focusing more effort of welfare departments and other agencies on enhancing the parents' abilities to care for their children at home (63, 71, 93, 94). The effort to find adoptive placements focuses on the new population of children who are older, handicapped, or from minority groups.

The preceding chapter on termination of parental rights details some of the new types of efforts being made in facilitating adoption. Subsidized adoption programs comprise another such effort.

Subsidized adoption. Model subsidized adoption legislation being disseminated by the U.S. Children's Bureau has been made law in the majority of states (14, 29). Although there is considerable variation among the various states, excerpts from the Virginia law will help illuminate the focus of such legislation. An eligible child is defined as "any child who has special needs because of a handicap to placement for adoption by reason of his physical, mental, or emotional condition, race, age, or membership in a sibling group" (92, p. 62). The Virginia law lists a variety of special needs which include medical care, legal services in effecting adoption, and educational and mental health services. Eligible parents are defined as those who "are capable of providing the permanent family relationships needed by the child in all respects except financial" (92, p. 62). The objective of such legislation is to diminish the financial bar to caring for such children. It is evident that the framers of the legislation assumed that foster parents with a long-standing relationship with the child would make up the great majority of persons receiving adoption subsidies (45). At the federal level, legislation to facilitate development of programs for adoption of children with special needs has been proposed by Senator Alan Cranston (Dem. Calif.) (70). Another approach some states are taking to provide for stability and continuity of relationships for older children is that of permanent foster placement (20) which will be addressed later in this chapter.

THE LEGAL FRAMEWORK OF ADOPTION

It must be kept in mind that in spite of the rapid evolution of adoption, there continue to be influences from the past which impinge upon adoption. The most important influence from the past, when children were viewed largely as the property of their parents, is the extent to which biologic parents continue to possess a legal right to their children (17, 19).

Adoption, as we are accustomed to it, has been a recent development. Adoption was not initially a part of the child welfare system, and was arranged quite casually. The following newspaper advertisements from the 1920s give a little of the flavor: "Mother wants to give up baby boy two weeks old"; "Wanted to adopt baby girl up to four years. Will furnish ideal home and best refs" (9, p. 139). Adoption remained largely a private matter until the mid-20th century. Adoption by deed without court proceedings of any kind persisted well into this century in a few jurisdictions. Until 1931 in Texas, a child could be adopted by filing with the county clerk a written statement of adoption. If the natural parents were living, this statement was accompanied by a written transfer of parental authority (39, 89). It was after World War II that the present system of agency adoption with screening and preparation of parents and counseling with the biological parent (s) was established (43).

Availability for Adoption

Children usually become available for adoption in one of two ways: 1) through voluntary consent of their parents, or 2) through a judicial termination of parental rights, most often on the basis of unfitness or abandonment (12). Usually, one of these two events has occurred before any adoptive placement will be made, particularly placement by an agency.

1) *Parental consent.* The most critical problem in the area of voluntary parental consent arises when a biological parent seeks the child's return after placement has occurred but before an adoption decree has been rendered. The period elapsing between placement and final decree varies typically from six to 12 months. Sometimes the legal process after placement involves two judicial decrees, the first of which is referred to as interlocutory. Some states have enacted provisions greatly restricting the right of a parent to revoke consent while others have left considerable discretion with the courts. In some states there is less likelihood that the biological parents' attempts to revoke consent will be successful if the child was surrendered to a licensed placement agency rather than to the adoptive couple in a private placement (1, 68).

2) *Involuntary termination of parental rights.* Unlike the situation in which a parent who has voluntarily consented to adoption may retain some rights until the final adoption decree, a judicial termination of parental rights effects a total and irrevocable loss. Generally, younger children are the ones given up by voluntary consent. The presumption in favor of custody in the biological parent is so great, and the movement of the judiciary so slow, that years have often elapsed by the time a child becomes available for adoption by termination of parental rights.

Whether parental rights are voluntarily or forcibly terminated, there remains an interval between placement and completion of the legal adoption. Goldstein, Freud, and Solnit in their book, *Beyond the Best Interests of the Child,* take exception to there being any delay in adoption, emphasizing that to facilitate emotional commitment and bonding, adoption should be immediate and final (33).

PSYCHODYNAMIC ISSUES IN ADOPTION

Although studies on incidence of psychiatric disturbance in adopted children have inherent methodological weaknesses (49), they do indicate that child psychiatric consultation is sought more frequently by adoptive families than by the general population (41, 61, 77, 80). Surely there are a number of factors besides severity of disturbance that influence whether or not a child comes to a child guidance clinic. However, if one views adopted children's overrepresentation at child psychiatric facilities as a sign of family system disturbance, it can be surmised that adoption poses a greater challenge to parents than does the raising of biologic children. A discussion of the emotional tasks and challenges of adoption follows.

Adoptive Parenthood

Infertility. In most cases, infertility has not been suspected by either of the adults and a major coming to grips with an altered view of body-image and self-concept is required of the prospective adoptive parent. Parents' unresolved feelings about infertility are thought to be a major contributor to family problems (4, 53, 88). Recognized and unrecognized hostility towards the partner held responsible for the inability to have children may continue to contaminate family relationships and the child may become the target of some of this hostility, representing the parent's inability to affirm the parental biologic roles and reminding the parent of what is not possible (81).

Loss of the hoped-for biologic child. Somewhat analogous to Solnit and Stark's findings regarding parents of impaired children (82), adoptive parents must acknowledge emotionally that the adopted child is a replacement for the child that they cannot have. The danger here is that if the parents are not able to adequately grieve the wished-for biologic child, the extent of their attachment to the adopted child may be attenuated.

The absence of pregnancy as a developmental phase. Most couples are graced with many months of increasingly concrete evidence that they are going to become parents. Whatever limitation of activity or mobility pregnancy requires of the woman serves as a focus for helping both partners to work through some of the changes occurring in the marital relationship (5, 7, 8). The presence of the new child can be increasingly anticipated and the pending loss of freedom and of being able to attend to each other's needs will unavoidably be faced due to various aspects of the pregnancy. In adoption, the working through process of whatever is most crucial to that particular couple is made more difficult because there is no pregnancy, and because it can never be predicted when a child will become available for adoption. There may be an analogy here to a problem which affects biological families when a child is born prematurely. When the child must be kept in an incubator for an appreciable period after birth, there is a measurable decrease in parental attachment behaviors, perhaps indicating some impairment of bonding (46, 50).

Rescue fantasies. Deutsch and Schechter have called attention to the liability in the parent-child relationship when the adopting parent suffers from an excess of rescue fantasy regarding the adopted child (22, 76). When in the course of normal conflict inherent in child raising there is frustration of these saviour fantasies, a very angry response from the adoptive parents too often results. Problems in this area may be closely connected to the issue of failure to work through the loss of the child one cannot have, as described above. When the child has had significant deprivation in the past and exhibits the characteristic sequelae of emotional withdrawal, indiscriminate friendliness, or provocative behavior (55, 57), however, even the most mature adoptive parents will feel rejected and will require support.

Entitlement. Adoptive parents who bring their children to child psychiatric clinics have commonly been observed to feel they have only a tenuous right to their adopted child (90). Unconscious oedipal determinants of this phenomenon have been well described by Schechter (75). These feelings of adoptive parents are usually expressed in terms of a lack of "entitlement" to the child (6, 26, 53, 95). The author has on a number of occasions heard adoptive mothers of nonpatient children remark that they wished the biologic mother could see what a good job they had done of raising the child. Again, this attitude which may afflict the adoptive parent is in major part the result of insufficient resolution of the losses and issues inherent to the developmental process of adoptive parenthood (47).

The role of the agency. Most people in the field agree that the potential for adoption is greatly enhanced with adequate parental resolution of the issues presented above. The goal of such resolution is not to deny differences between adoptive and biological parenthood; rather, the goal is to acknowledge and to accept comfortably the differences (48). Agency adoptions are thought to be preferred because of the caseworker's facilitating the accomplishment of the psychological tasks of adoptive parenthood. One of the difficult problems in this area, however, is the dual function of the agency social worker, who is supposed to screen the parents for adoption as well as to prepare them. It has been observed that parents do not always look upon the agency as a benign helper (72, 76), and it has been the observation of the author that even in group meetings of parents of nonpatient adoptive children, there is a high degree of resentment regarding intrusion or scrutiny by agency caseworkers. This impediment, in addition to the fact that the human psyche has a great resistance to accepting losses of any sort, would suggest that even under the best of circumstances preparation for adoptive parenthood must remain quite incomplete. There are data indicating a high degree of success for private adoptions (98), and a 1976 Danish study indicated no superiority of agency over private adoptions regarding scores for psychopathology or for the parent-child relationship (25). A decided advantage of agency adoption is the sounder legal foundation achieved by the agency's counseling the biologic parent(s) regarding giving up the child, as mentioned previously.

Another issue which agencies will be called upon to address in their preparatory work with parents relates to adoption of deprived children of any age (13). Either agency personnel should have skills in working in this area, or the agency should arrange for consultation or continuing psychotherapy for parents adopting children with this type of problem.

Adoption for the Child

Adoption most basically offers children the opportunity to be raised by people who desire to have a child and who have generally made difficult conscious decisions and gone to efforts which most biological parents do not even approach on their route to parenthood (48). When writing or reading a chapter such as this which focuses on difficulties and differences in adoption, one can easily overlook the simple and charming fact that adoption allows infertile adults and children in need of parents to come together as a family.

In spite of the data indicating an overrepresentation of adoptive families seeking child psychiatric services, other data indicate that the majority of adoptions go well indeed. In a study of 500 adoptions ten years after placement, Witmer et al. found little difference between adoptees and controls in ratings of social and emotional functioning (98). In a study regarding adoption of older children, Kadushin found that about 85 percent of a series of 91 adoptions were successful. These children were between five and 11 years of age at adoption (42).

One could surmise that, on the surface, adoption should not make much difference to a child adopted early in life, for the child can have no perspective on the identity of the caretaking adults. Later, however, when a child is told of adoption, he or she must deal with the incomprehensible questions of who are the other parents and why did they leave him or her. The almost universal agency practice of advising parents to start telling their child about adoption early has been objected to on theoretical grounds because the confusion engendered could lead to problems in the development of conscience and the ego ideal (24, 67). The psychological separation process of adolescence does appear to be complicated by the fact of adoption, an issue which will be taken up later in a discussion of identity.

For some adopted children the developmental process may be impeded by parental deprivation or disruption of relationships prior to the adoptive placement. Following placement, the adoptive status may predispose to destructive parent-child patterns of relating.

Maternal (parental) deprivation. This has two important components. The first has to do with the child's knowledge of having been given up for adoption. Without going into primitive aspects of childhood thinking regarding causality (18), suffice it to say that many children "solve" this unfathomable mystery by assuming that they were unlovable, dirty, or otherwise unrewarding to their biologic parents. Probably of even more significance to the adoptive child is his or her assumption that abandonment could well happen again, often leading to a high and continuing level of separation anxiety. The other aspect of maternal deprivation has to do with measurable developmental effects upon the child, irrespective of the child's memory, thought content, or even conscious knowledge of the issue of adoption or of loss of parenting persons (99). This is, of course, made worse if the child goes to a succession of foster homes or experiences adoptive failures before entering his/her final adoptive placement (69.

Interactional issues. When things do not go well in adoption, there is often a combination of some of the issues discussed above: a deprived child who may not respond optimally to his adoptive parents' attention, and parents with excessive amounts of rescue fantasy and insufficient feelings of entitlement. This soon leads to increasing frustration and hostility on the part of the adoptive parent(s), and increasing separation anxiety and, often, aggressive behavior on the part of the child (86). In some instances, parental knowledge about the child's biologic parents' behavior leads the adopted parent to expect undesirable behavior of the child.

Antisocial behavior. In those adopted children who are brought to psychiatric facilities, there is a notable incidence of complaints of sexual behavior in girls and of aggressive behavior in boys (62, 64). In spite of the actual behavior being exhibited by the child, there is also a high degree of parental concern regarding antisocial behavior, often far out of proportion to the actual behavior the child is exhibiting. There are at least two major sources for this type of parental concern. The first has to do with guilt on the part of the adoptive parents, but primarily the mother, for having another woman's child (95). Another aspect is the adoptive parents' knowledge of or fantasies about the behavior of the natural parents, whose union produced the child and whose weakness or immorality (in the adoptive parents' view) led to the child's being put up for adoption (24, 48, 76). Both of these issues—their fantasy of the biological parents' immorality and their guilt and fear that they might not deserve the child—stimulate in the adoptive parents anxieties of conscience. Their concerns about the child's becoming antisocial and their guilt about not having a right to the child may lead them to expect from the child excessive reassurance and affirmation of their parental role. When this is not forthcoming and the parents cannot change, then the relationship predictably deteriorates (56).

The remaining major issue faced by adopted children has to do with questions of identity, which commonly arise primarily in adolescence (83).

Identity issues in adoption. One of the central dynamic theories explaining the identity problems of adolescent adopted children is based upon concepts initially postulated by Freud. Because these ideas have been focused upon by many writers (30, 54, 97) and because Freud's discussion is so lucid, excerpts of his paper, *Family Romances,* will be presented here (28).

Freud noted that as the child's intellectual growth increases, he "gets to know other parents and compares them with his own, and so comes to doubt the incomparable and unique quality which he has attributed to them" (28, p. 74). In normal development, there are times when a child "feels he is not receiving the whole of his parents' love. . . . His sense that his own affection is not being fully reciprocated then finds a vent in the idea . . . of being a stepchild or an adopted child" (p. 75). Then, "the child's imagination becomes engaged in the task of getting free from the parents of whom he now has such a low opinion and of replacing them by others, occupying, as a result, a higher social station" (p. 76). He noted, however, that "these works of fiction . . . still preserved, under a slight disguise, the child's original affection for his parents. The faithlessness and ingratitude are only apparent. If we examine in detail the commonest of these imaginative romances, the replacement of both parents or of the father alone by grander people, we find that these new and aristocratic parents are equipped with attributes that are derived entirely from real recollections from the actual and humble ones; so that in fact the child is not getting rid of his father but exalting him" (p. 76).

Freud then focuses upon the central function of the family romance at adolescence: facilitating dealing with loss of the primary relationship with parents which is necessitated by or even defines adolescence. "Indeed the whole effort at replacing the real father by a superior one is only an expression of the child's longing for the happy, vanished days when his father seemed to him the noblest and strongest of men and his mother the dearest and loveliest of women. He is turning away from the father whom he knows today to the father in whom he believed in the early years of his childhood; and his fantasy is no more than the expression of regret that those happy days have gone" (p. 78). In this way the adolescent is helped in accomplishing psychological separation from parents in two ways: he or she may devalue his or her parents, which appears to be one of the requisites by which adolescent children can separate from their parents, if it is not indeed inevitably due to their being able to view their parents in greater perspective than previously; but also, the family romance allows the adolescent a final identification with parents, in essence taking a somewhat idealized part of them along as one is in the process of leaving them.

The family romance for most people is adaptive. The images of the exalted fantasy parents and the lowly real ones, as pointed out by Freud, are not very distinct from each other. In the case of adopted persons, due to their awareness of two sets of parents, these images may be much more disparate, and the family romance may not facilitate psychological development and separation from the adoptive parents. The adopted person may find that he or she cannot in the process of psychologically separating simultaneously devalue and identify with parents who are not known. At this time, curiosity about biologic parents increases, and the person may develop a determination to locate the biologic parents.

Kornitzer emphasizes that the adolescent knows that an essential part of him or herself has been lost through adoption (52). Sants introduced the term "genealogical bewilderment" to describe the confusion and uncertainty of a developing person who has vague or vanishingly little knowledge regarding biologic parents (73). Many adult adoptees continually search faces for resemblances and wonder if a person they talked with or observed might be a relative. Sants described adoptees' developing a fear of committing incest, and this has indeed frequently been an issue in the author's clinical experience with adult adoptees. The legal system generally follows societal concerns about incest and consanguinity. In a recent case in a state with no statutory prohibition against marriage of brother and sister related by adoption, a court disallowed marriage because of its duty to protect the integrity of the family (38). However, a provision forbidding such marriage in another state was found to be unconstitutional because freedom to marry is a fundamental right (37). The issue of genealogical bewilderment brings us to the often published search of adult adoptees for their biologic parents.

ADOPTEES AND THEIR BIOLOGIC PARENTS

Adoptees have been participants in the broad social movement to increase individual civil rights. Their concerns about identity (their own and that of their biologic parents) have led to interest in open adoption and to legal attacks upon the sealed adoption record.

The Search for Biological Parents

In recent years adopted adults have become more vocal in their search for biologic parents. Triseliotis studied 70 adults requesting copies of their birth certificates in Scotland, with the goal of seeking information or actual reunion with birth parents (91). The author felt that most of these were unhappy and lonely people, particularly those who sought reunion with, rather than simply more information regarding, biologic parents. The great majority found they had achieved considerable satisfaction from gaining additional information.

In 1976 Sorosky, Baran, and Pannor reported on 50 American adult adoptees who had reunions with their birth parents (84). Forty of these people found the experience satisfying, and only 10 percent of the birth parents reacted adversely to the reunion. The data do not indicate that a poor relationship with the adoptive parents was a primary reason for making contact with the birth parents. Their results led these authors to suggest opening original birth records to adult adoptees and to advocate open adoption, as well as suggesting that agencies accept the charge of working with all three components of the adoption triangle (2). How some of these issues currently stand in the law will follow a brief discussion of open adoption.

Open Adoption

Open adoption has been advocated most vocally by Baran, Pannor, and Sorosky (3) who made the study of reunions of adoptees with birth parents cited above. In open adoption, the child and his or her biologic parents continue to have contact with each other. Currently, this type of adoption takes place in some European countries (23). This type of adoption would allow a child of any age to temper fantasy with reality regarding biologic parents and the reasons they gave him or her up for adoption. For an older child, open adoption might permit the continuation of important links to the past, as would foster care with tenure (32) or permanent foster placement (15).

There are a number of important potential problems for the adoptee inherent to continuing contact between child and biologic parents: attenuation of the adoptive parent-child bond; possibly even greater predisposition to identity confusion; and great opportunities for the development of loyalty conflicts. Further, contact with birth parents would likely make adoption much less attractive to potential adoptive parents.

The Sealed Adoption Record

In response to a rise in queries from adoptive parents, agencies have been providing an increased amount of information regarding biologic parents to adoptive parents both at the time of adoption and subsequently. Generally speaking, an adult adoptee must have a court order to have access to his or her birth certificate in all but three states (51). Although the right of the adult adoptee to petition the court to unseal the adoption record is gaining increasing recognition, the courts are conservative, tending to respond only to such practical issues as health and property (65). Courts are, however, beginning to take into account the adoptee's psychological needs. In a New Jersey case (58), the court held that an adoptee's psychological need to know the identity of biologic parents may constitute "good cause" under the statutes of that state.

In this case, as in others like it (36), the court required a procedure to protect the interest of the biologic parent. In these cases the sealed record statutes have not been overthrown. Instead, "good cause" has been defined in each case and the principle has been laid down that neither the adoptee nor the biologic parent has absolute rights (51). There are a number of pressing and conflicting interests at stake in such cases. These interests include: 1) the psychological needs of the adoptee; 2) the need to protect the privacy of the biologic mother from intrusion by the adoptee; 3) and the privacy of the adoptive family from the intrusion by the biologic parent; 4) and, in the public interest, there is the need to maintain the integrity of the adoption process, which depends upon confidentiality. Stephenson aptly points out that an Adoption Reunion Registry such as one proposed in British Columbia would kindle adoptive parents' anxieties regarding entitlement and loss of their children back to the biologic parents (87). It does not appear that there will be an overthrow of sealed record statutes, in spite of arguments that secrecy in adoption abridges the adoptee's constitutional rights (11, 78).

ADOPTION AND THE OLDER CHILD

A recent opinion aptly expressed the accepted view regarding the effect of adoption upon former relationships: "public policy demands that an adoption carry with it a complete breaking of all ties" (10, p. 1135). In view of this policy, adoption for an older child with a memory of and even some degree of continuing contact with biologic parents poses somewhat of a dilemma. For a child who, for example, has been in foster care several years and is occasionally visited by parents, the prospect of a "complete breaking of all ties" may be very upsetting because of real emotional ties, unrealistic hopes for reunion with biologic family, and the threat to identity posed by the break with the past. Such a child may refuse to be adopted, and he or she may suffer painful conflicts if adoption takes place (31, 44, 66).

In a case discussed in detail elsewhere (21), siblings 10 and 12 years of age were adopted by the foster parents who had cared for them during the previous two years. The children were seen in a court consultation prior to a hearing regarding termination of rights of their biologic parents. Both children appreciated the reciprocal warm ties of affection with their adoptive parents, but both felt they *should* be taking care of their biologic parents. The older child was able to make the distinction that in order for her to go back home, her father would have to stop drinking; the younger child simply wanted to return to the home of his biologic parents. The children's anxieties regarding termination of the right of their parents were considerably allayed by their foster parents' agreeing to facilitate their visiting their biologic parents. The children both agreed to be adopted by their foster parents, in spite of concerns about their biologic parents' anger. The younger of the two was the more dubious about adoption and did not wish to change his name; the older changed her name quite eagerly. They have continued to visit their biologic parents infrequently and the older sister corresponds quite regularly with them.

For the children described above, and for many of the older children not available for adoption, some of the old policies do not quite fit. It is the task of judges, attorneys, and consultants to fashion dispositions which correspond to these children's emotional needs, to the extent that their needs can be ascertained. In spite of the inflexibility of the law in this matter, it has been common agency practice to encourage the maintenance of past ties when placing older children (79).

For an older child the adoption decision cannot be a unilateral one: as Bernard has stated it, "instead of older children *being adopted,* they and their parents really need to *adopt each other"* (6, p. 526). For some older children, permanent foster care might be less threatening with regard to their identities and to their continuing contact with aspects of their past lives than adoption might be, and might still adequately facilitate the development of the foster parent-foster child bond.

COMMENT

For young children and their adoptive parents, the process, the joys, and the problems of adoption do not appear to be changing appreciably. What is changing, however, is that as time goes on, relatively fewer young children are becoming available, and quantitatively as well as relatively, more older children will become available for adoption due to increasingly aggressive efforts to terminate the rights of abusing, neglectful, or abandoning parents (40). Perhaps eventually these recent initiatives in terminating parental rights will lead to increased numbers of younger children becoming available for adoption as well.

REFERENCES

1. ALDRICH, C. K. (1965). Hazards of Adoption. *Abbottempo,* 3:14-15.
2. BARAN, A., PANNOR, R., & SOROSKY, A. D. (1974). Adoptive Parents and the Sealed Record Controversy. *Soc. Casework,* 55:531-536.

3. BARAN, A., PANNOR, R., & SOROSKY, A. D. (1976). Open Adoption. *Soc. Work*, 21:97-100.

4. BARNES, M. J. (1953). The Working-Through Process in Dealing with Anxiety Around Adoption. *Am. J. Orthopsych.*, 23:605-615.

5. BENEDEK, T. (1959). Parenthood as a Developmental Phase. *J. Am. Psychoanal. Assoc.*, 7:389-417.

6. BERNARD, V. W. (1974). Adoption. In *American Handbook of Psychiatry*, Vol. 1, S. Arieti (Ed.). New York: Basic Books, Inc., pp. 514-534, 2nd. ed.

7. BIBRING, G. (1959). Some Considerations of the Psychological Processes in Pregnancy. *The Psychoanalytic Study of the Child*, 14:113-121.

8. BIBRING, G., DWYER, T., HUNTINGTON, D., & VALENSTEIN, A. (1961). A Study of the Psychological Processes in Pregnancy and of the Earliest Mother-Child Relationship. *The Psychoanalytic Study of the Child*, 16:9-72.

9. BREMNER, R. H. (1971). *Children and Youth in America*, Vol. II. Cambridge, Mass.: Harvard University Press.

10. *Browning* v. *Tarwater* (1974), Kan., 524 P.2d 1135.

11. BURKE, C. (1975). The Adult Adoptee's Constitutional Right to Know His Origins. *South. Calif. Law Rev.*, 48:1196-1220.

12. CLARK, H. H. (1968). *The Law of Domestic Relations in the United States*. St. Paul, Minn.: West Publishing Co.

13. CLIFTON, P. M. & RANSOM, J. W. (1975). An Approach to Working with the "Placed Child." *Child Psych. Hum. Developm.*, 6:107-117.

14. COMMENT (1976-7). The Implementation of Subsidized Adoption Programs: A Preliminary Survey. *J. Fam. Law*, 15:732-769.

15. DERDEYN, A. P. (1977a). A Case for Permanent Foster Placement of Dependent, Neglected, and Abused Children. *Am. J. Orthopsych.*, 47:604-614.

16. DERDEYN, A. P. (1977b). Adoption in Evolution: Recent Influences on Adoption in Virginia. *South. Med. J.*, 70:168-171.

17. DERDEYN, A. P. (1977c). Child Abuse and Neglect: The Rights of Parents and the Needs of Their Children. *Am. J. Orthopsych.*, 47:377-387.

18. DERDEYN, A. P. (1977d). Children in Divorce: Intervention in the Phase of Separation. *Pediatrics*, 60:20-27.

19. DERDEYN, A. P. & WADLINGTON, W. J. (1977). Adoption: The Rights of Parents Versus the Best Interests of their Children. *J. Am. Acad. Ch. Psych.*, 16:238-255.

20. DERDEYN, A. P. (1978). Virginia's Legislators Address the Needs of Children. *Va. Med.*, 105:32-35.

21. DERDEYN, A. P., ROGOFF, A. R., & WILLIAMS, S. W. (1978). Alternatives to Absolute Termination of Parental Rights After Long-Term Foster Care. *Vanderbilt Law Rev.*, Vol. 31:1165-1192.

22. DEUTSCH, H. (1945). A Study of Adoptive Mothers in a Child Guidance Clinic. *Soc. Casework*, 26:587-594.

23. EHRENZWEIG, A. A. & JAYME, E. (1973). *Private International Law; A Comparative Treatise on American International Conflicts Law, Including the Law of Admirality*, Vol. 2, Special Part, Jurisdiction, Judgments, Persons (Family). Dobbs Ferry, N.Y.: Oceana Publications, Inc., pp. 212-259.

24. EIDUSON, B. T. & LIVERMORE, J. B. (1953). Complications in Therapy with Adopted Children. *Am. J. Orthopsych.*, 23:795-802.

25. ELDRED, C. A., ROSENTHAL, D., WENDER, P. H., KETY, S. S., SCHULSINGER, F., WELNER, J., & JACOBSON, B. (1976). Some Aspects of Adoption in Selected Samples of Adult Adoptees. *Am. J. Orthopsych.*, 46:279-290.

26. FANSHEL, D. (1962). Approaches to Measuring Adjustment in Adoptive Parents. In

Quantitative Approaches to Parent Selection. New York: Child Welfare League of America.

27. FANSHEL, D. (1976). Status Changes of Children in Foster Care: Final Results of the Columbia University Longitudinal Study. *Child Welf.*, 55:143-171.

28. FREUD, S. (1959). Family Romances (1909). In Sigmund Freud's *Collected Papers, Vol. 5*, J. Strachey (Ed.). New York: Basic Books, Inc., pp. 74-78.

29. GALLAGHER, U. M. & KATZ, S. N. (1975). The Model State Subsidized Adoption Act. *Child. Today*, 4:8-10.

30. GEDIMAN, H. K. (1974-5). Narcissistic Trauma, Object Loss, and the Family Romance. *Psychoanal. Rev.*, 61:203-215.

31. GILL, M. M. (1978). Adoption of Older Children: The Problems Faced. *Soc. Casewk.*, 59:272-278.

32. GOLDSTEIN, J. (1975). Why Foster Care—For Whom For How Long? *The Psychoanalytic Study of the Child*, 30:647-662.

33. GOLDSTEIN, J., FREUD, A., & SOLNIT, A. J. (1973). *Beyond the Best Interests of the Child.* New York: Free Press.

34. GRUBER, A. (1973). *Foster Home Care in Massachusetts.* Commonwealth of Massachusetts Governor's Commission on Adoption and Foster Care.

35. HUARD, L. A. (1956). The Law of Adoption: Ancient and Modern. *Vanderbilt Law Rev.*, 9:743-763.

36. *In re Anonymous* (1977). *Fam. Law Reporter*, 4:2105-2106.

37. *In re MEW and MLB* (1977). *Fam. Law Reporter*, 3:2601-2602.

38. *Israel v. Allen* (1978). *Fam. Law Reporter*, 4:2396-2397.

39. JACOBS, A. C. & GOEBEL, J. (1952). *Cases and Other Materials on Domestic Relations.* Brooklyn: Foundation Press, 3rd ed.

40. JONES, M. L. (1977). Aggressive Adoption: A Program's Effect on a Child Welfare Agency. *Child Welf.*, 56:401-407.

41. KADUSHIN, A. (1966). Adoptive Parenthood: A Hazardous Adventure? *Soc. Wk.*, 11:30-39.

42. KADUSHIN, A. (1970). *Adopting Older Children.* New York: Columbia University Press.

43. KADUSHIN, A. (1976). Child Welfare Services—Past and Present. *Child. Today*, 5:16-23.

44. KATZ, L. (1977). Older Child Adoptive Placement: A Time of Family Crisis. *Child Welf.*, 56:165-171.

45. KATZ, S. N. & GALLAGHER, U. M. (1976). Overview: Subsidized Adoption in America. *Fam. Law Quart.*, 10:3-54.

46. KENNELL, J. H., JERAULD, R., WOLFE, H., CHESLER, D., KREGER, N. C., McALPINE, W., STEFFA, M., & KLAUS, M. H. (1974). Maternal Behavior One Year After Early and Extended Post-Partum Contact. *Develpm. Med. Child Neurol.*, 16:172-179.

47. KENT, K. G. & RITCHIE, J. L. (1976). Adoption as an Issue in Casework with Adoptive Parents. *J. Amer. Acad. Child Psych.*, 15:510-522.

48. KIRK, H. D. (1964). *Shared Fate.* New York: Free Press.

49. KIRK, D., JONASSOHN, K., & FISH, A. D. (1966). Are Adopted Children Especially Vulnerable to Stress? *Arch. Gen. Psych.*, 14:291-298.

50. KLAUS, M. H., JERAULD, R., KREGER, N. C., McALPINE, W., STEFFA, M., & KENNELL, J. H. (1972). Maternal Attachment: Importance of the First Post-Partum Days. *New Eng. J. Med.*, 286:460-463.

51. KLIBANOFF, E. B. (1977). Genealogical Information in Adoption: The Adoptee's Quest and the Law. *Fam. Law Quart.*, 11:185-198.

52. KORNITZER, M. (1971). The Adopted Adolescent and the Sense of Identity. *Child Adoption*, 66:43-48.

53. KRUGMAN, D. C. (1964). Reality in Adoption. *Child. Welf.*, 43:349-358.
54. LAWTON, J. J. & GROSS, S. Z. (1964). Review of Psychiatric Literature on Adopted Children. *Arch. Gen. Psych.*, 11:635-644.
55. LEADING ARTICLE. (1977). Adoption of Deprived Children. *Brit. Med. J.*, 2:280-281.
56. LEWIS, D. O., BALLA, D., LEWIS, M., & GORE, R. (1975). The Treatment of Adopted Versus Neglected Delinquent Children in the Court: A Problem of Reciprocal Attachment. *Am. J. Psych.*, 132:142-145.
57. LOADMAN, A. E. & McRAE, K. N. (1977). The Deprived Child in Adoption. *Develpm. Neurol.*, 19:213-223.
58. *Lovallo* v. *New Jersey State Registrar* (1977), New Jersey Superior Court, Chancery Division.
59. MASS, H. & ENGLER, R. (1959). *Children in Need of Parents.* New York: Columbia University Press.
60. McEWAN, M. T. (1973). Readoption with a Minimum of Pain. *Soc. Casewk.*, 54:350-353.
61. McWHINNIE, A. M. (1967). *Adopted Children—How They Grow Up.* London: Routledge & Kegan Paul.
62. MENLOVE, R. L. (1965). Aggressive Symptoms in Emotionally Disturbed Adopted Children. *Child. Develpm.*, 36:519-532.
63. MNOOKIN, R. (1973). Foster Care—in Whose Best Interest? *Harvard Educ. Rev.*, 43:599-638.
64. OFFORD, D. R., APONTE, J. F., & CROSS, L. A. (1969). Presenting Symptomatology of Adopted Children. *Arch. Gen. Psych.*, 20:110-116.
65. PANNOR, R., BARAN, A., & SOROSKY, A. D. (1976). Attitudes of Birth Parents, and Adoptees Toward the Sealed Adoption Record. *J. Ontario Assn. Children's Aid Societies*, 19:1-7.
66. PANNOR, R. & NERLOV, E. A. (1977). Fostering Understanding Between Adolescents and Adoptive Parents Through Group Experiences. *Child. Welf.*, 56:537-545.
67. PELLER, L. (1963). Comments on Adoption and Child Development. *Bull. Phila. Assoc. Psychoanal.*, 13:1-14.
68. PODOLSKI, A. L. (1975). Abolishing Baby Buying: Limiting Independent Adoption Placement. *Fam. Law Quart.*, 9:547-554.
69. PRESSER, S. B. (1971). The Historical Background of the American Law of Adoption. *J. Fam. Law*, 11:443-516.
70. Public Law 95-266, 95th Congress, April 24, 1978, 92 Stat. 205-211.
71. RODHAM, H. (1973). Children Under the Law. *Harvard Educ. Rev.*, 43:487-514.
72. ROTHENBERG, E. W., GOLDEY, H., & SANDS, R. M. (1971). The Vicissitudes of the Adoption Process. *Am. J. Psych.*, 128:590-595.
73. SANTS, H. J. (1964). Genealogical Bewilderment in Children with Substitute Parents. *Brit. J. Psychol.*, 37:133-141.
74. SCHECHTER, M. D. (1960). Observations on Adopted Children. *Arch. Gen. Psych.*, 3:21-32.
75. SCHECHTER, M. D. (1967). Psychoanalytic Theory as it Relates to Adoption. *J. Am. Psychoanal. Assoc.*, 15:695-708.
76. SCHECHTER, M. D. (1970). About Adoptive Parents. In *Parenthood: Its Psychology and Psychopathology*, E. J. Anthony and T. Benedek, (Eds.). Boston: Little, Brown, & Co., pp. 353-371.
77. SCHECHTER, M. D., CARLSON, P. V., SIMMONS, J. Q., & WORK, H. H. (1964). Emotional Problems in the Adoptee. *Arch. Gen. Psych.*, 10:109-118.
78. SCHEPPERS, R. C. (1975). Discovery Rights of the Adoptee—Privacy Rights of the Natural Parent: A Constitutional Dilemma. *Univ. San Fernando Valley Law Rev.*, 4:65-83.

79. SHAPIRO, M. (1957). *A Study of Adoption Practice, Vol. III, Adoption of Children with Special Needs*. New York: Child Welfare League of America, Inc.
80. SILVER, L. B. (1970). Frequency of Adoption in Children with the Neurological Learning Disability Syndrome. *J. Learn. Dis.*, 3:11-14.
81. SIMON, N. M. & SENTURIA, A. G. (1966). Adoption and Psychiatric Illness. *Am. J. Psych.*, 122:858-868.
82. SOLNIT, A. & STARK, M. (1961). Mourning and the Birth of a Defective Child. *The Psychoanalytic Study of the Child*, 16:523-537.
83. SOROSKY, A. D., BARAN, A., & PANNOR, R. (1975). Identity Conflicts in Adoptees. *Amer. J. Orthopsych.*, 45:18-27.
84. SOROSKY, A. D., BARAN, A., & PANNOR, R. (1976). The Effects of the Sealed Record in Adoption. *Am. J. Psych.*, 133:900-904.
85. STATISTICAL ABSTRACT OF THE UNITED STATES (1974). U.S. Bureau of the Census, U.S. Department of Commerce. New York: Grosset & Dunlap.
86. STEIN, J. M. & DERDEYN, A. P. (1980). The Child in Group Foster Care: Issues of Separation and Loss. *J. Am. Acad. Ch. Psych*, 19:90-100.
87. STEPHENSON, P. S. (1975). The Emotional Implications of Adoption Policy. *Compr. Psych.*, 16:363-367.
88. TAYLOR, A. D. & STARR, P. (1972). The Use of Clinical Services by Adoptive Parents. *J. Am. Acad. Ch. Psych.*, 11:384-399.
89. Texas Revised Civil Statutes (1925), Articles 42, 44.
90. TOUSSIENG, P. (1968). Principles, Convictions and Values Underlying Current Adoption Practices with Consideration of Problems Relative to Natural Parents, Infertility and Identity. In *The New Face of Social Work*. New York: Spence-Chapin Adoption Service, pp. 75-78.
91. TRISELIOTIS, J. (1973). *In Search of Origins: The Experiences of Adopted People*. London: Routledge & Kegan Paul.
92. Va. Code Ann. 63.1-255 (1975), Charlottesville, Va.: The Michie Company, Law Publishers, Vol. 9A, p. 68.
93. WALD, M. (1975). State Intervention on Behalf of "Neglected" Children: A Search for Realistic Standards. *Stanford Law Rev.*, 27:985-1040.
94. WALD, M. (1976). State Intervention on the Behalf of "Neglected" Children: Standards for removal of Children from their Homes, Monitoring the Status of Children in Foster Care and Termination of Parental Rights. *Stanford Law Rev.*, 28:623-706.
95. WALSH, E. D. & LEWIS, F. S. (1969). A Study of Adoptive Mothers in a Child Guidance Clinic. *Soc. Casewk.*, 50:587-594.
96. WHITMORE, W. H. (1876). *The Law of Adoption in the United States, and Especially in Massachusetts*. Albany, N.Y.: J. Munsell.
97. WIEDER, H. (1977). The Family Romance Fantasies of Adopted Children. *Psychoanal. Quart.*, 46:185-200.
98. WITMER, H. L., HERZOG, E., WEINSTEIN, E. A., & SULLIVAN, M. E. (1963). *Independent Adoptions: A Follow Up Study*. New York: Russell Sage Foundation.
99. YARROW, L. (1964). Separation from Parents During Early Childhood. In *Review of Child Development Research*, Vol. 1, M. Hoffman and L. Hoffman (Eds.). New York: Russell Sage Foundation, pp. 89-136.

Part III

THE JUVENILE OFFENDER

11

DIAGNOSTIC EVALUATION OF THE DELINQUENT CHILD: PSYCHIATRIC, PSYCHOLOGICAL, NEUROLOGICAL AND EDUCATIONAL COMPONENTS

DOROTHY OTNOW LEWIS, M.D., F.A.C.P.

The diagnostic evaluation of the juvenile offender is not a search for simple causes. It is, rather, an exploration of vulnerabilities. Behaviors are rarely singly determined. Biological, psychodynamic, and environmental or social factors in combination affect what we do. Therefore, no evaluation is complete that fails to take into account the multiple determinants of a child's antisocial behavior.

Delinquent behaviors occur, for the most part, under conditions of socioeconomic deprivation (4, 21, 31). There are those who have suggested that antisocial behaviors are as common in the middle class as in the lower socioeconomic classes (32), but are handled differently by police and parents. Whether or not such is the case is hard to determine. Juvenile delinquency, however, by definition refers to officially recognized antisocial acts and, as such, occurs more often in the more deprived sectors of our society. Violent acts by juveniles are of greatest concern and have been well documented to be more prevalent in the lower socioeconomic and minority populations of our country (37).

It has also been well established that juvenile delinquency and chaotic home situations are associated with each other (5, 7, 27, 35). Disrupted homes and households in which there are friction and violence are often characteristic of the backgrounds of delinquent youth, and those kinds of factors have been used to explain juvenile deviance (7, 15, 23). Psy-

chodynamic factors, particularly the sociopathic inclinations of parents
and their transmission to children, have also been used to explain away
juvenile antisocial behavior (11).

Unfortunately, the social and psychodynamic factors contributing to
the delinquent behaviors of children are often so flamboyant and so
easily recognized that there is a tendency for psychiatrists, psychologists,
and neurologists to overlook or minimize the importance of other kinds
of vulnerabilities that contribute to the development of antisocial
behaviors.

The Psychiatric Evaluation

The psychiatrist requested to evaluate a delinquent child has a special
responsibility, greater even than the responsibility of the child guidance
clinic psychiatrist or the private practitioner. His/her report may be used
to determine the child's capacity to stand trial, the child's culpability,
the treatment or lack of treatment afforded the child, and whether or
not the child will be sent home or incarcerated. The increasingly punitive developments in the handling of children (i.e., lowering the age at
which a child can be tried and punished as an adult) increase the psychiatrist's responsibility. It is, therefore, with fear and trembling—or
at least with appropriate humility and caution—that the psychiatrist
evaluating a delinquent minor approaches his task.

The usual 20- to 60-minute psychiatric interviews with delinquent
children, particularly in the absence of other psychiatric, medical, and
social information, almost invariably afford inadequate opportunities to
make accurate psychiatric diagnoses. Although the inadequacy of a single
short interview is as true of the evaluation of the truant or runaway as
it is of the violent juvenile, in the latter situation the consequences of
venturing a psychiatric opinion on the basis of a single brief interview
can be disastrous. Rather than capitulate to unreasonable time limitations (based usually on limitations of funds to pay for evaluations), the
psychiatrist must insist on adequate time in which to perform his/her
evaluation. If forced to make a statement after a single brief interview,
unless the child is flamboyantly disturbed and the requirements for treatment obvious, the psychiatrist is well advised to use the brief contact with
the child to assess what further diagnostic measures are required before
an accurate psychiatric assessment can be furnished and to indicate this
in his/her report. This report should be entitled "Preliminary Psychiatric
Impression" or a synonym for this title in order to document the inadequacy of the report.

Psychiatric Interview with a Parent or Relative

It is extremely desirable that, in addition to interviewing the child, a parent or relative also be interviewed. A parent can furnish information about perinatal factors, early life experiences, and medical events about which a child has no information. Furthermore, a parent can provide information regarding the mental health of other family members than can shed light on the psychiatric status of the child.

Naturally, if the child has been raised in a household with a psychotic relative, his/her experiences can be expected to have influenced the child's thinking and behavior in particular ways. A paranoid mother may convey to the child a sense of pervasive danger and even teach him/her to be wary and to carry weapons at all times. A brain-damaged, violent father may not only set an example of impulsiveness, but may also batter the child and inflict central nervous system damage which will contribute further to the child's antisocial adaptation (12, 16, 18, 19, 30).

At this time, psychiatrists are beginning to appreciate more and more the hereditary predisposition to certain kinds of psychiatric disorders. Family members can furnish invaluable clues to the understanding of certain aberrant childhood behaviors. Schizophrenia (8, 9, 10, 28), manic-depressive illness (29, 36), and even minimal brain dysfunction (3) are now thought to be influenced in part by hereditary factors. The discovery that a child has a paranoid schizophrenic parent may shed light on the physiological underpinnings of his inordinately suspicious, sometimes violent and bizarre behaviors. Similarly, the knowledge that an adolescent who is periodically out of control, destructive, and verbally and physically abusive has a manic-depressive parent should encourage the psychiatrist to explore the possibility that such a disorder contributes to the behavior that called the child to the attention of the police. Most important, knowledge of heritable psychiatric disorders in family members has implications for possible effective treatment for the child. Behaviors previously dismissed by the psychiatrist as simply characterologic may, with the benefit of an accurate family history, be recognized as manifestations of other kinds of effectively treatable psychopathology.

An example of the usefulness of a family history is the case of a youngster incarcerated for reported arson and vandalism. While incarcerated, the child tore at his flesh and frequently banged his head against the wall, behaviors interpreted by the correctional staff as simply attention-getting devices. When an attempt was made to reach the boy's mother, it was learned that she had been psychiatrically hospitalized on different occasions, had been diagnosed schizophrenic, and that between hospitalizations was nomadic and unreachable. Although the boy was usually coherent and responsive, he tended to keep to himself and seemed inordinately suspicious of others. He also had marks on his arms where he had deliberately burned himself. Because of the boy's extreme discomfort, suspiciousness, and self-mutilation, and in light of his family history of psychosis, he was treated with low therapeutic doses of an antipsychotic agent. Although the boy's self-mutilation decreased, he complained of sleepiness and he continued to be withdrawn. During an interview, the child reported having once been treated by a psychiatrist at a clinic with a blue pill that really helped him. He was able to identify the medication from pictures in the Physician's Desk Reference (P.D.R.). When his medication was changed to the alerting phenothiazine the boy had identified, within a short period of time he was able to function well in the correctional institution, to handle himself in an open setting, and eventually to gain admission to a boarding school. We learned subsequently of a sibling who had been placed in a residential setting who also responded well to the identified medication. Had our initial family history been more detailed, had it included previous medications that had been useful to the boy and to his first-degree relatives, we would probably have been able to provide effective treatment more rapidly.

It is common practice in child guidance clinics and juvenile courts to have parents interviewed by probation officers and to have only the child seen by a psychiatrist. Many of the children who come to juvenile court have parents who suffer from serious psychopathology (14, 15). In addition to furnishing information regarding relatives, interviews with parents by skilled clinicians permit an assessment of parental medical and psychiatric status. It is, therefore, advisable that the individual who interviews the parents have expertise in psychiatric interviewing and diagnostic evaluation. Otherwise, there is the real danger that the seriously disturbed parent who, for example, has been incarcerated, will be dismissed as merely sociopathic, or that the extremely depressed parent who frequently drinks to excess will be dismissed as simply alcoholic. On the other hand, the recognition of the nature of parental psychopathology has implications not only for understanding and treating the child, but also for arranging for effective treatment for the parent to enable the parent to function more appropriately and provide a supportive environment for the child.

The Medical History

Many delinquent children, particularly those who have committed numerous and serious antisocial acts, have extremely poor medical histories (16, 17). In the case of violent juveniles, medical problems are often characteristic of their entire lives, beginning with perinatal problems (19) and continuing throughout childhood. Head and face injuries and child abuse are particularly common in the histories of violent delinquents. Because of the multiplicity of biopsychosocial factors affecting the lives of delinquent children, it is often impossible to determine the contribution of particular medical events. Sometimes, however, it is possible to document the onset of deviant behaviors following particular trauma to the central nervous system. For example, one boy who had remained out of trouble with the law became extremely violent and paranoid and actually raped and assaulted several women following a car accident in which he sustained severe head injury. Another boy became assaultive and unmanageable following an episode of encephalitis at age five. Yet another youngster, a teenage girl who had been considered her "mother's angel," became involved in a multiplicity of antisocial acts and began to experience episodes of violent behaviors for which she had no memory following an episode of meningitis.

All of the children described above came from multi-problem families. Prior to central nervous system trauma, however, they had been able to cope adequately with their environments. Following the central nervous system trauma, the first child became overtly psychotic and violent, the second hyperactive and destructive, and the third developed episodic violence with memory impairment for the violent acts. In each case, discovery of the medical factors preceding the antisocial behaviors led to further diagnostic assessments and eventually to trials of specific therapeutic interventions. Of note, the child who had suffered encephalitis at age five and who continued to be unmanageable throughout childhood was found to respond well to low-dosage amphetamine and barbiturate medication and to function well in a therapeutic setting where, without medication, he had previously been unwelcome. The teenaged girl, who was found to have an epileptiform electroencephalogram, responded well to Dilantin and, on antiepileptic medication, suffered no further violent episodes. The paranoid youngster who raped and assaulted women was able to function well in an open setting at a correctional school for approximately a year, during which time he was provided with weekly psychotherapy and minimal dosages of phenothiazine medication. Unfortunately, he ran away from the school while on a home visit and subsequently raped and attempted to murder another woman. In all of these cases, careful histories enabled staff to understand important medical contributions to the children's behavior and plan individualized therapeutic interventions.

Of note, in two cases, medical histories were obtained not only from children and relatives, but also from hospital records. Optimally, medical histories should be obtained from children, parents, and hospital or clinic records. Hospital records frequently contain vital information that children and parents are either unaware of or are reluctant to disclose. Similarly, children and their parents may recount symptoms and medical events that have not been recorded in medical charts.

Psychiatric Interview with the Child

One might anticipate that children interviewed in the context of a juvenile court or correctional setting, many from ethnic minorities, would be reluctant to talk with white, middle-class professionals. Psychiatrists might be especially suspect. Over the course of several years of interviewing within a court clinic and within a correctional setting, we have not found social and ethnic differences to impede communication, except, of course, in cases in which serious language obstacles exist. In fact, we found that children and their families were usually pleased to have the lengthy undivided attention of a trained diagnostician.

It was hard to assess the importance of confidentiality in establishing rapport since, in most of our cases, children could be assured of confidentiality and that nothing they disclosed that they did not want others to know would be placed in a report or record. Occasionally this kind of confidentiality could not be guaranteed because of legal considerations, and in such cases the child was so informed and encouraged to consult with his lawyer and/or parents regarding psychiatric evaluation. In a few instances, children preferred either not to be interviewed or to discuss issues unrelated to the act of which they were accused. In several cases, when the child was of limited intelligence or was obviously psychotic and unable to make a responsible decision regarding evaluation, interviews were not performed or were postponed until either a responsible adult could make the decision for the child, or until the child was legally committed to the state and psychiatric evaluation was ordered for purposes of disposition. In such cases the child was informed of his status, counseled about the use to be made of the information he gave, and told with whom it would be shared. In all but a handful of cases, children and families welcomed the opportunity to participate in the evaluation. This fact may be more a reflection of the sparse attention given most delinquent children and their hunger for communication with caring adults than a reflection of motivation for treatment. In any case, interviews usually flowed freely, and in many instances it was a struggle for the interviewer to terminate the session after an hour and a half or two hours. Suffice it to say that our concerns about possible communication barriers and confidentiality were greater than the children's or their parents'.

Most delinquent children are in their teens, and expect to talk rather than play with a psychiatrist. We did not, therefore, make use of games or play materials other than pencils and paper or colored markers. However, even older children accepted and took pleasure in drawing when verbal communication became difficult.

It almost goes without saying that a major aspect of the psychiatric interview concerned psychodynamic issues. Anger and its expression obviously are major themes, particularly for violent adolescents. Of note, although the majority of violent incarcerated children have come from families in which they have witnessed and been the victims of violence, many abused children are not conscious of their rage toward parents or siblings. Even the most psychotic and abusive mother may consciously be revered by the child she has injured. It is important that the psychiatrist whose function is only to evaluate and who does not have responsibility for treatment appreciate the strength of the child's denial of anger and refrain from premature interpretations, the consequences of which he will not be available to discuss and work through with the child. Children in detention and correctional schools are more aware of their loneliness and sadness than of their rage at the parents who, often, have abandoned them.

Children can furnish surprisingly useful historical information about their upbringing and medical histories. Just as parents or hospital records must usually furnish information about pregnancy, delivery, and developmental milestones, so only the child can describe lapses of consciousness, hallucinatory episodes, and a wide variety of subjective experiences of which parents are totally unaware. Frequently parents have forgotten or have been unaware of important events affecting a child's functioning, including serious falls from high places, loss of consciousness, and car accidents (not to mention drug usage and alcohol usage and their effects). For example, one girl whose mother had died had been drinking heavily for years and suffering blackouts, facts of which her father, her guardian, was totally ignorant. Another family knew that one of their children had fallen downstairs and lost consciousness, but did not recall which child it was. In the course of the evaluation, it became clear that the injured child was the only child in the family who was truant, could not concentrate, and ran away sporadically, only to be found living in squalor in neighboring communities.

Years of work interviewing delinquent children, their parents, and reviewing hospital records have clarified the usefulness of multiple sources of information about a child.

The Mental Status Examination

No matter how obvious the social and psychodynamic forces influencing a child's antisocial behaviors, the psychiatrist who focuses exclusively on these kinds of issues will often fail to uncover other equally important factors affecting behavior. It is as important that the psychiatrist perform a meticulous mental status evaluation as it is for him/her to explore family relationships. Even the most astute clinician cannot be expected to discern whether or not a child is well oriented, has experienced hallucinations, is delusional, or has an impaired short-term memory unless he focuses deliberately on these issues. Appearances are often deceiving. The fact that a child appears to be socially appropriate does not mean necessarily that he/she is of normal intelligence, that he/he does not hallucinate or suffer from perceptual motor problems that are not evident in the course of ordinary conversation.

The sensitive clinician can ask, in a context that is nonthreatening, the kinds of questions that might ordinarily be anxiety-provoking. For example, assessing the presence or absence of hallucinatory experiences can be accomplished in the course of taking a medical history. After discussing family, friends, school, sports, and, perhaps, some of the difficulties surrounding the behaviors that brought the child to court, the interviewer can introduce an ostensibly different set of questions. We might say, "Now I'd like to ask you some medical questions. How is your health? Have you ever been in the hospital? Any accidents?" After inquiring about loss of consciousness, headaches, and dizziness, we will ask, "How are your eyes? Do you wear glasses? Have your eyes ever played tricks on you? What was that like?" We will go on to ask about things looking far away or very near, objects becoming blurry or changing shapes. We have found that the invitation to discuss visual experiences often enables a child to describe episodes that have puzzled or frightened him/her but about which he/she had never spoken. Several children reported episodes when they were reading and the print seemed to disappear and the pages seemed blank. One child described watching television and experiencing the sensation that the screen was getting smaller and smaller. These kinds of symptoms, along with multiple episodes of déjà vu, falling spells, or acts for which memory was impaired or absent, were sometimes clues to the existence of psychomotor epilepsy.

The medical interview can continue with such questions as, "How are your ears? Do you ever get earaches? Have your ears ever played tricks on you? What was that like? Have you ever had the experience of thinking someone said something to you and you were mistaken? What was that like?" We have found that many paranoid children will recount episodes in which they thought a person called them an obscenity (or, worse, called their mother a bad name), and they have wheeled around and attacked perfectly innocent bystanders. One such incident was actually observed to occur on a secure unit for violent children. A small boy leaving an interview room turned suddenly and, out of the blue, punched another youngster standing in the hall. When asked by staff members why he had done this, the boy responded in anger, "He just called me a motherfucker!" Not a word had been said to or about the assaultive child.

The same technique described for visual and auditory assessments can be used for olfactory ("Do you get colds much? Do you get nosebleeds? Do you ever have the experience of smelling something and no one else smells it?"), gustatory, and tactile experiences.

The assessment of paranoid thinking is among the most difficult tasks that confront the psychiatrist evaluating delinquent children. A wariness of the interviewer is certainly to be expected in light of the possible consequences of the interview. When wariness moves into inordinate suspiciousness is a clinical judgment that must be made, and the reasons for making such a judgment must be well documented in any report. It is, however, a mistake for the interviewer to assume that carrying dangerous weapons or being ready at all times to be attacked is a normal concomitant of lower socioeconomic class existence. A child can be from a tough part of town and still not feel the need to carry multiple knives, crowbars, or loaded guns. One youngster who lived in a "tough" part of town was, nevertheless, unlike his peers in that he kept to his room, had a gun in the top drawer of his dresser, and carried knives and a gun when he did venture downtown. The mother of another extremely violent youngster reported that he stole knives from the kitchen and secreted them throughout his room, placing one over the molding of the door to his room. Several other youngsters complained of always being followed or sensing people were in the bushes waiting to hurt them. They carried weapons at all times. These kinds of children taught us the usefulness of asking in detail about feelings of endangerment or persecution. We considered paranoid symptomatology to be present if a child not only reported feelings of endangerment and persecution by a wide variety of different persons, but also either acted in response to these feelings (e.g., attacking another individual out of the blue, secreting multiple weapons) or felt seriously troubled by them.

We found that for most delinquents the most threatening part of the mental status evaluation was not the assessment of hallucinations, delusions, or paranoia, but rather the testing of the child's ability to work with numbers and to remember digits forward and backward. These aspects of the mental status examination were probably threatening both because of their association with schoolwork and because they tended to reveal impairments of which the child was vaguely aware. We found, for example, in a comparison of more and less violent children (20) that 69.5 percent of the more violent children were unable to subtract serial 7s, compared with 33.3 percent of the less violent group $(\chi^2_y = 6.138, p = .014)$. Similarly, 60.8 percent of the more violent group could not remember even four digits backward compared with 13.3 percent of the less violent group $(\chi^2_y = 8.627, p = .004)$. Difficulties with these kinds of tasks, while not pathognomonic of any particular disorders, may suggest to the clinician possible short-term memory deficits, impulse disorders, attentional disorders, and learning disabilities, all of which can then be explored further in psychological, educational, and neurological assessments.

Suffice it to say that the psychiatrist who fails to perform a detailed mental status evaluation will miss discovering a variety of potentially treatable disorders. Many of these disorders, left untreated, contribute to a delinquent child's social maladaptation.

Psychological Testing

It is erroneous to assume that even the most meticulous and sophisticated psychiatric assessment can bring to light all of the problems of personality and cognitive functioning tapped by psychological testing. In fact, psychotic thought processes and intellectual retardation, aspects of functioning that one might expect to be most easily recognized by means of psychiatric interviewing, unless the psychosis or retardation is flamboyant, are often far from obvious and among the most difficult aspects of functioning to assess. The wary, paranoid youngster may reveal disorders of thinking on a Rorschach protocol which he had concealed easily during psychiatric interviews. Even extremely intellectually limited youngsters are often able to conduct themselves in socially appropriate ways, giving the psychiatric interviewer little indication that serious intellectual deficits, elucidated through testing, do exist. And, of course, psychological testing can often reveal perceptual motor disturbances rarely elicited during psychiatric interviews.

The choice of psychological tests, their administration, and the interpretation of results are topics of greater scope than can be encompassed in this chapter. Some investigators and clinicians have found the Halstead-Reitan battery of tests particularly useful in the diagnosis of delinquent children (1). Such detailed examinations are undoubtedly useful.

Budgets, considerations of time, and limitations in professional proficiency and experience often make the use of tests such as the Halstead-Reitan battery impracticable. Much, however, can be learned about the functioning of a delinquent child by means of more usual measures such as the Wechsler Intelligence Scale for Children and the Rorschach test. The WISC is useful not only for assessing intelligence, but also for assessing many different aspects of thinking, behavior, perception, and attention. In addition to providing clues to perceptual problems and cognitive difficulties, the WISC is a valuable tool for documenting fluctuating states of attention. A number of children whom we evaluated were observed to vary markedly in their performance within individual subtests, answering difficult questions with ease and being totally unable from time to time to respond to much easier questions. Moreover, at one moment some children would be able to repeat six digits backward, while at the next moment they would be unable to recall three digits in reverse. This quality of performance, while sometimes evident during testing, often came to light only at the time the test was scored. We found that many children with this kind of intra-subtest pattern also had other symptoms suggestive of attentional disorders and/or epilepsy. Thus, differences among individual subtest scores did not always convey adequately the quality of a child's difficulties. In other words, final scores did not reflect the ways in which tasks were approached and accomplished.

Responses on the Rorschach test, in addition to contributing to the understanding of psychodynamic issues, were found to be most useful as indicators of a child's internal controls and ability to organize his thoughts coherently. Perseveration, bizarre percepts, impulsivity, or marked disorganization on the Rorschach often suggested the existence of central nervous system dysfunction or latent psychosis that had previously been overlooked. On the other hand, hardly a single Rorschach report failed to comment on latent anger, unconscious rage, and violent fantasies, most of which could be deduced from the situation of the population being tested and from psychiatric interviews.

Psychological testing is most useful when it brings to light hitherto overlooked disorders. When, however, a child's performance on psychological testing fails to reveal any evidence of emotional or cognitive disturbance, it is imperative that the psychologist indicate in his/her report the limitations of psychological test results and that testing is not a substitute for complete psychiatric, neurological, educational, and social evaluations.

For the child's well-being, it is important that the psychologist make explicit the fact that psychological tests (like other kinds of brief evaluations) reflect only the functioning of a given child at a given point in time. We learned this lesson painfully when two children, found on testing to demonstrate no abnormalities, were sent to correctional schools without benefit of further evaluations. There they subsequently developed flamboyant psychotic symptomatology and required psychiatric hospitalization. Our impression, on reviewing the cases, was that their latent serious psychopathology might have been revealed had more complete evaluations been performed prior to institutionalization.

Educational Assessments

It is well established that many delinquent children have learning disabilities (1, 3, 22, 25). Our own work indicates that especially violent delinquents have even more serious learning disorders than do less violent delinquents (20).

Neither standard psychiatric nor standard psychological evaluations assess the kinds of skills that educational testing is designed to measure. Again, which tests to use and the interpretation of specific tests are topics beyond the scope of this chapter.

Obviously, reading and mathematical abilities should be evaluated. But more information than scores on reading or mathematical tests is required if programs are to be designed to meet the specific needs of individual delinquent children. Problems in auditory discrimination and/or comprehension, visual discrimination and/or comprehension, and sequencing may exist separately or may coexist. Programs to remedy one kind of learning disorder may be completely inappropriate for another.

At this point, it should be noted that discrete learning disabilities may exist concurrently with serious emotional problems or in the presence of identifiable neurological disorders. The psychiatrist cannot assume that a borderline psychotic delinquent child's poor school performance is necessarily a reflection of his psychotic disorder alone. Nor can he/she be certain that, for example, the poor school performance of an epileptic child is necessarily a function of his epilepsy. In other words, treatment of a neurotic, psychotic, or neurological disorder, while of benefit to aspects of a given child's functioning, may not improve his reading or mathematical performance and his functioning in other areas of social adaptation.

An example of the simultaneous but ostensibly independent existence of psychosis and specific learning disabilities is the case of a violent paranoid psychotic youngster evaluated on a unit for especially violent delinquent children. This boy, seemingly as a result of his psychotic thought processes, inordinate suspiciousness, and discomfort with peers, had been truant from school for years. It would have been easy to dismiss his extremely poor reading scores as the consequence of failure to attend class. After several weeks on a secure unit, the youngster developed enough trust in the clinical staff to agree to a trial of antipsychotic medication. Medication was instituted slowly to avoid side effects as much as possible. The results of this treatment were gratifying, and after several weeks the boy was able to interact with peers and staff with relative comfort. One day, several weeks after medication was instituted, this child approached the learning disabilities specialist on the clinical team and asked, "Could you teach me to read?" She thereupon explained to him that she could try to do this, but that certain kinds of educational tests would be required to discover exactly what kinds of difficulties he was having. Detailed educational testing (in this instance including the Woodcock Reading Mastery Tests, the Keymah Diagnostic Arithmetic Test, and the Slingerland tests) revealed extreme difficulties in visual discrimination and sequencing. In fact, this child, of low normal intelligence, could not even sequence sounds sufficiently to read the words "rat" and "bat" after having been taught the words "mat" and "cat." A special program was devised, making use of colors and sounds, to improve this child's visual discrimination and ability to sequence. Needless to say, there was great rejoicing on the unit when this child, Joe, learned to read, "Joe is a cool cat."

This kind of experience demonstrates the fact that psychiatric disorders and learning disabilities can exist independently. It also illustrates the need for psychiatric and educational evaluations, and underlines the necessity for institutions caring for delinquent children to be prepared to treat psychiatric and educational disorders. Our work with extremely violent incarcerated delinquent children suggests that it is especially common for seriously delinquent children to suffer from both psychiatric and learning disorders.

The Neurological Evaluation

Obvious neurological deficits such as grand mal epilepsy or hemiparesis are unlikely to be seen often in the delinquent population (although a history of grand mal seizures is not uncommon). This may be because flamboyantly impaired antisocial children, like flamboyantly psychotic delinquents, are likely to be recognized as "sick" and channeled to therapeutic facilities during early childhood. A meticulous neurological assessment, however, is likely in many instances to reveal subtle neurological impairment, particularly in seriously delinquent, violent youngsters. For example, in a recent study major neurological abnormalities (i.e., a history of grand mal epilepsy, a grossly abnormal encephalogram, a positive Babinski sign, or a head circumference two or more standard deviations from the mean for age) were found in 46.3 percent of extremely violent delinquents, compared with 6.7 percent of less violent delinquents (χ^2_y = 6.499, p = .011) (20). Moreover, 98.6 percent of extremely violent children had one or more minor neurological signs (e.g., choreiform movements, poor coordination, inability to skip), compared with 66.7 percent of less violent delinquents (χ^2_y = 16.275, p = .001) (20). Choreiform movements, psychomotor epileptic symptoms, inability to skip, and a greater than 10 percent discrepancy between right and left palm strikes were especially characteristic of the very violent delinquent children studied (20).

As important as the actual neurological physical findings are the findings obtained from detailed neurological histories. The neurologist would do well to assume that he/she may be the only clinician who will take an adequate history, an assumption that in most cases is probably legitimate. Questions about illnesses, accidents, injuries, headaches, dizziness, blackouts, reactions to alcohol and drug abuse, déjà vu, macropsia, micropsia, and visual, auditory, olfactory, gustatory, and tactile misperceptions or hallucinations should be an integral part of the neurological assessment. In the case of violent delinquents, questions regarding precipitants of violence, memory for violent and nonviolent behaviors, ability to cease fighting, lapses of fully conscious contact with reality, and whether or not fatigue or sleep follow these kinds of experiences should be ascertained.

The same kinds of questions to be asked by the psychiatrist should also be covered by the neurologist. Even questions related to inordinate suspiciousness are essential to the neurological evaluation. It has been reported in a number of publications that paranoid ideation is often associated with psychomotor epilepsy (6, 15, 24, 26, 33, 34).

Methods for approaching these kinds of questions have already been discussed in the section on the psychiatric evaluation. They are as applicable to the neurological as to the psychiatric interview. The neurologist must remember (as must the psychiatrist) that his certification is in both neurology and psychiatry.

Although an electroencephalogram is an obvious component of the neurological evaluation, the results of these tests at this time are more often confusing than helpful. Even sleep encephalograms in children add little to a diagnosis such as psychomotor epilepsy. Diagnosis of psychomotor epilepsy is clinical and does not depend on the results of an encephalogram. Frequently the neurologist, testifying in court, is faced with the insurmountable task of convincing a judge and jury that a normal EEG does not preclude the existence of epilepsy. Whether or not sleep EEGs in children are more revealing of psychopathology than waking EEGs remains a question. Often a trial of antiepileptic medication in delinquent children with psychomotor epileptic symptoms is more useful than an electroencephalogram.

A problem in evaluating the juvenile delinquent with neurological signs of impairment arises from the fact that the majority of delinquents come from families in which psychiatric and social problems abound and could, in and of themselves, explain deviance. The neurologist must therefore try to make sure that his/her knowledge of the psychosocial factors affecting the child not blind him to the possible contribution of neurological impairment.

CONCLUSION

When a delinquent child receives a thorough evaluation, including psychiatric, psychological, educational, and neurological assessments, it is the rule rather than the exception to be faced with a multiplicity of more or less contradictory findings. Usually a seriously delinquent child suffers from several different kinds of vulnerabilities which combine to influence his/her antisocial behavior. A judicious approach might be to think long and hard before attributing a child's delinquent behaviors to social and psychodynamic factors exclusively. Although social and psychodynamic factors are almost invariably part of the picture, they often fail to reflect a child's specific, often treatable, vulnerabilities. These kinds of vulnerabilities may make him/her less capable than his peers to cope with his emotionally stressful environment and therefore to behave in socially appropriate ways.

REFERENCES

1. BERMAN, A. & SIEGAL, A. (1976). A Neuropsychological Approach to the Etiology, Prevention, and Treatment of Juvenile Delinquency. In *Child Personality and Psychopathology: Current Topics*, Vol. 3, Anthony Davis (Ed.). New York: John Wiley & Sons, pp. 259-294.
2. CANTWELL, D. P. (1976). Genetic Factors in the Hyperkinetic Syndrome. *J. Am. Acad. Ch. Psych.*, 15:214-223.
3. CANTWELL, D. P. (1978). Hyperactivity and Antisocial Behavior. *J. Am. Acad. Ch. Psych.*, 17:252-262.
4. CLOWARD, R. A. & OHLIN, L. E. (Eds.), (1960). *Delinquency and Opportunity: A Theory of Delinquent Gangs.* New York: Free Press.
5. COHEN, A. K. (1955). *Delinquent Boys: The Culture of the Gang.* New York: Free Press.
6. GLASER, G. H., NEWMAN, R. J., & SHAFER, R. (1963). Interictal Psychosis in Psychomotor Temporal Lobe Epilepsy: An EGG-Psychological Study. In *EEG and Behavior*, G. H. Glaser (Ed.). New York: Basic Books, pp. 345-365.
7. GLUECK, S. & GLUECK, E. (1950). *Unraveling Juvenile Delinquency.* New York: Commonwealth Fund.
8. HESTON, L. L. (1966). Psychiatric Disorders in Foster Home Reared Children of Schizophrenic Mothers. *Brit. J. Psych.*, 112:819-825.
9. HESTON, L. L. (1970). The Genetics of Schizophrenia and Schizoid Disease. *Science*, 167:249-256.
10. HESTON, L. L. (1977). Schizophrenia. *Hosp. Pract.*, 12:43-49.
11. JOHNSON, A. M. & SZUREK, S. A. (1952). The Genesis of Antisocial Acting Out in Children and Adults. *Psychoanal. Quart.*, 21:323.
12. KOENIGSBERG, D., BALLA, D. A., & LEWIS, D. O. (1977). Juvenile Delinquency, Adult Criminality, and Adult Psychaitric Treatment: An Epidemiological Study. *Child Psych. Human Develpm.*, 7:141-146.
13. LEWIS, D. O. (1976). Delinquency, Psychomotor Epileptic Symptoms, and Paranoid Ideation: A Triad. *Am. J. Psych.*, 133:1395-1398.
14. LEWIS, D. O. & BALLA, D. A. (1976). *Delinquency and Psychopathology.* New York: Grune & Stratton.
15. LEWIS, D. O., BALLA, D. A., SHANOK, S. S., & SNELL, L. (1976). Delinquency, parental Psychopathology and Parental Criminality. *J. Am. Acad. Ch. Psych.*, 15:665-678.
16. LEWIS, D. O. & SHANOK, S. S. (1977). Medical Histories of Delinquent and Non-Delinquent Children. *Am. J. Psych.*, 134:1020-1025.

17. LEWIS, D. O. & SHANOK, S. S. (in press). A Comparison of the Medical Histories of Incarcerated Delinquent Children and a Matched Sample of Nondelinquent Children. *Child Psych. Human Developm.,* 1979.

18. LEWIS, D. O., SHANOK, S. S., & BALLA, D. A. (1979a). Parental Criminality and Medical Histories of Delinquents. *Am. J. Psych.,* 136:288-292.

19. LEWIS, D. O., SHANOK, S. S., & BALLA, D. A. (1979b). Perinatal Difficulties, Head and Face Trauma, and Child Abuse in the Medical Histories of Serious Juvenile Offenders. *Am. J. Psych.,* 36:419-423.

20. LEWIS, D. O., SHANOK, S. S., PINCUS, J. H., & GLASER, G. H. (1979). Violent Juvenile Delinquents: Psychiatric, Neurological, Psychological and Abuse Factors. *J. Am. Acad. Child Psych.,* 18:307-319.

21. MATZA, D. (1969). *Becoming Deviant.* Englewood Cliffs, N.J.: Prentice-Hall.

22. MURRAY, C. (1976). The Link Between Learning Disabilities and Juvenile Delinquency. Prepared for the National Institute for Juvenile Justice and Delinquency Prevention, OJJDP, LEAA, Washington, D.C.

23. OFFORD, D. R., ALLEN, N., & ABRAMS, N. (1978). Parental Psychiatric Illness, Broken Homes, and Delinquency. *J. Am. Acad. Ch. Psych.,* 17:224-238.

24. POND, D. G. (1957). Psychiatric Aspects of Epilepsy. *J. Indian Med. Assoc.,* 3:1441-1451.

25. POREMBA, C. D. (1975). Learning Disabilities, Youth and Delinquency: Programs for Intervention. In *Progress in Learning Disabilities,* Vol. III, H. R. Myklebust (Ed.). New York: Grune & Stratton, pp. 123-149.

26. PRESTON, D. N. & ATACK, E. A. (1964). Temporal Lobe Epilepsy: A Clinical Study of 47 Cases. *Canad. Med. Assoc. J.,* 91:1256-1259.

27. ROBINS, L. N., WEST, P. A., & HERJANIC, B. L. (1975). Arrests and Delinquency in Two Generations: A Study of Black Urban Families and Their Children. *J. Child Psychol. Psych.,* 16:125-140.

28. ROSENTHAL, D., WENDER, P. H., KETY, S. S., SCHULSINGER, F., WELNER, J., & OSTER-GAARD, L. (1968). Schizophrenics' Offspring Reared in Adoptive Homes. In *Transmission of Schizophrenia,* D. Rosenthal and S. S. Kety (Eds.). Oxford: Pergamon Press, pp. 377-391.

29. ROSENTHAL, D. (1971). *Genetics of Psychopathology.* New York: McGraw-Hill.

30. SHANOK, S. S. & LEWIS, D. O. Medical Histories of Abused Delinquents. Unpublished.

31. SHAW, C. R. & McKAY, H. D. (1942). *Juvenile Delinquency and Urban Areas.* Chicago: University of Chicago Press.

32. SHORT, J. F., JR. & NYE, F. I. (1958). Extent of Unrecorded Delinquency. In *Society: Delinquency and Delinquent Behavior,* H. L. Voss (Ed.). Boston: Little, Brown, pp. 52-59.

33. SMALL, J. G., SMALL, I. F., & HAYDEN, M. P. (1966). Further Psychiatric Investigations of Patients with Temporal Lobe and Nontemporal Lobe Epilepsy. *Am. J. Psych.,* 123:303-310.

34. TREFFERT, D. A. (1964). The Psychiatric Patient with an EEG Temporal Lobe Focus. *Am. J. Psych.,* 120:765-771.

35. WEST, D. J. & FARRINGTON, D. P. (1973). *Who Becomes Delinquent?* London: Heinemann Educational Books.

36. WINOKUR, G., CLAYTON, P., & REICH, T. (1969). *Manic-Depressive Illness.* St. Louis: C. V. Mosby.

37. WOLFGANG, M. E., FIGLIO, R. M., & THORSTEN, S. (1972). *Delinquency in a Birth Cohort.* Chicago: University of Chicago Press.

12

STATUS OFFENDERS: EMERGING ISSUES AND NEW APPROACHES

HERBERT S. SACKS, M.D. and HELEN L. SACKS, M.S.W.

INTRODUCTION

We feel bound to identify and summarize the key arguments for elimination or retention of the status offense jurisdiction in the juvenile court for an audience largely made up of child psychiatrists and allied mental health professionals before presenting our own viewpoint. The countervailing positions firmed up by developments of the past 15 years will illuminate the central questions for colleagues who have not been engaged in this debate in their daily work.

The chapter will show the relationship between the *parens patriae* doctrine and the early state juvenile justice acts, and will illustrate how evolving court decisions have reshaped the definitions of status offenders and their rights. We then examine the divided opinions of compassionate experts based on legal philosophic considerations and sociologic study unfettered by the contributions of clinicians or child development professionals. After looking at demographic aspects of the treatment of this group of youngsters, we move ahead to study some specific status offenses including sexual misconduct, truancy, disobedience to school authorities, running away and features of ungovernable behavior. Federal and state actions over the past five years on behalf of status offenders are critically reviewed with specific references to progress made in one advanced state—Connecticut. The *Noncriminal Misbehavior Standards* of the Institute of Judicial Administration/American Bar Association Juvenile Justice Standards Project are then explored together with the critique of the Council on Children, Adolescents and Their Families of the American Psychiatric Association. Our perspective in this broad controversy is prefaced by a look at the implications of the shift from a rehabilitation to a punishment model in the juvenile justice system. The major questions of state intervention, family autonomy and the individual's interests are integrated into our concluding position.

CHILD PSYCHIATRY'S ROLE IN THE PROBLEM OF THE STATUS OFFENDER

A colleague who has distinguished himself in psychiatry and the law spoke for some others in this field when he asserted, "I don't see what status offenders have to do with psychiatry."

Status offenses are those acts by children and adolescents which would not be considered crimes if committed by adults. They generally include unruly behavior, truancy, drinking alcoholic beverages, running away from home and immoral conduct. The unique developmental qualities of children and youth which distinguish them from adults warrant a separate juvenile justice system with a continuing emphasis on treatment and rehabilitation. We believe that the concepts, research findings and clinical experience of child and adolescent psychiatry are salient to the court's goals in dealing with status offenders.

Psychiatrists and allied professionals, with specific training in child and adolescent development and collaborative clinical work, are sometimes deterred from serving a critical societal need in the juvenile courts by state underfunding, overwhelming caseloads rife with severe psychosocial problems, difficulties in relating to varying levels of expertise of court personnel, and the need to master legal concepts and procedural matters. Many colleagues are limited by experience and training in approaching the clinical problems of court-connected youngsters, especially from the lower socioeconomic classes. Court clinical work is frequently beset by the demands of speedy diagnostic judgment in an atmosphere of urgency; the work calls for a professional temperament that can accommodate the pace and pressures. However, there are, in the nation, fine examples of psychiatric clinic operations with youngsters under court jurisdiction, which produce service, undertake research and train fellows in child psychiatry, psychologists and social workers for future efforts in this field.

A good number of these *youngsters in need* are emotionally disturbed and have not yielded to the services of community clinics and agencies. Each identifying label—status offender, delinquent, dependent and neglected child, emotionally disturbed child—is a legal/social/psychiatric term. The label attached to a particular child is consequent to how that child comes to the attention of the public, agency, clinic and family.

That process flows from a mélange of factors: unconscious, accidental, social class, school casefinding, police action, family concerns, medical referrals and welfare assessments. If the court is the last resort for children and families where community services have been insufficient or unobtainable, should we not have in-house clinical expertise available to judges and court personnel to provide better understanding and enable more reflective dispositions?

In some circumstances, the social history of a status offender persuades the probation officer to seek psychiatric consultation. The emerging clinical findings might suggest to the court staff that a youngster requires commitment to a psychiatric hospital for a more thorough evaluation. At the ensuing commitment hearing, the judge would require the recommendations of the psychiatric consultant to help to determine what course to follow.

The involvement of court-affiliated psychiatrists with status offenders has inspired some colleagues to attempt to translate their understanding of psychoanalytic developmental psychology into social policy. A small but growing group of child and adolescent psychiatrists in the states have influenced the writing of new legislation and the design of progressive treatment programs shaped to the developmental needs of troubled youngsters.

EARLY HISTORY AND PARENS PATRIAE

The first juvenile court was established in 1899 in Chicago and by the late 1920s all but two states, Maine and Wyoming, had enacted laws founded on the Illinois model. In 1951 Wyoming followed suit with Maine joining the nation in 1959.

The authority of the juvenile courts implied in the state statutes has its origins in the ancient common law doctrine of *parens patriae*, derived from the English constitutional system. Traditionally, *parens patriae* refers to the king's guardianship of people legally unable to act for themselves (1). In 1889, in Mormon Church v. United States, the court held that *parens patriae* "is inherent in the supreme power of every state . . . a most beneficient function . . . for the prevention of injury to those who cannot protect themselves" (2, pp. 57-58). Thus in the early twentieth century, the American courts with legislative support emphasized their right to protect children from parental neglect, and from their own lack of diligence and virtue, in keeping with a fusion of legal history and colonial antecedents (3).

With the establishment of juvenile courts in the first two decades of this century, the legislatures delegated the *parens patriae* role to these new legal structures which for a while successfully masked the grave differences in Puritan and reformer expectations for families and children. For the reformers, resort to tradition, with its sense of social order, was a useful strategy for minimizing the pervasiveness of state intervention that masked the "child-saving" programs (4). For the most part the "child-savers" were not interested or knowledgeable in the law but were philanthropists, expounders of the Protestant ethic, and social Darwinists abhoring the traditional methods of punishment of errant children and pleading for the rehabilitation model. Their writings do not reflect concern for rights of appeal or the overreach of the juvenile justice statutes drafted at the turn of the century (5). Judge Frank Orlando has demonstrated how the original statutes have been expanded to include offenses applicable only to children claiming that such inclusions are unconstitutional so that the whole fabric of a child's life—not a specific act—is on trial in some courtrooms (6).

A FURTHER DEFINITION OF STATUS OFFENSES

Our media shrilly remind us that the juvenile justice system cannot deal with violent young offenders; other critics complain that it has amazing efficiency in locking up troubled children and youth who have been charged with committing offenses that apply only to juveniles. The obverse of the protections given by the *parens patriae* doctrine is a special group of obligations youngsters have as a consequence of their status as minors. They must obey their parents; not skip school; not run away from home; avoid getting caught in immoral behavior; refrain from drinking intoxicating beverages.

Every American juvenile court has grounds for extending its intervention to cases involving anti-social but noncriminal behavior. Since the laws typically address the child's condition rather than the commission of specific acts, cases brought under such statutes are referred to as "status offenses." The status offense jurisdiction encompasses a broad spectrum of behaviors such as truancy, disobedience to parent or school authorities or guardian, running away from home, being sexually promiscuous or acting in a manner injurious to self or others. Most of the states include status offenders in the category of delinquents. The remainder, 41 percent, have created a special category beyond the usual groupings inclusive of neglect and delinquency. Status offenders comprise, according to some guesses, close to one-half of the work load of the nation's juvenile courts (7). With the attempts to dejudicialize status offenders during this decade, these figures have markedly declined so that in Connecticut, in 1976, the 2,269 status offenders represented only 12 percent of all delinquency dispositions (8). Status offenders have exhausted the creativity of acronym makers, wearing labels that vary from state to state—Person/Child/Minor/Juvenile in Need of Supervision (abbreviated PINS, CHINS, MINS, JINS); Families with Service Needs (FWSN); Incorrigible Child; Wayward Child; Miscreant Child; Ungovernable Child—but in all cases the jurisdictional target is the same—encouraging judicial intervention for noncriminal misbehavior.

LEGAL HISTORY AND MAJOR COURT DECISIONS

To return to the original juvenile court acts, the sole function of the system was to identity those children who required the special intervention of the state parent, suggesting that courts, administrative agencies and volunteers were literally thought to be parent surrogates (9). The process centered on identifying deviant children and then providing them with a better place to live while in custody. Due process did not play a role since the child was entitled to care and custody, not freedom (10). However, it turned out that under the guise of giving help and treatment, little was done to accomplish these goals and the institution's philosophies were perceived as punitive (11).

Children had practically no constitutional rights until 1966, when the Supreme Court in Kent v. United States held that children transferred to adult courts had to be managed by the basic requirements of due process and fairness. "There may be grounds for concern that the child receives the worst of both worlds: that he neither gets the protection accorded to adults nor the solicitous care and regenerative treatment postulated for children" (12). The court thus warned that identification of children for treatment without treatment provision was inequitable.

In 1967, the Supreme Court heard the case of Gerald Gault, a 15-year-old Arizonian boy, who was committed to six years in a state industrial school for making an obscene telephone call. Gault was not informed of the charges against him, of his right to a lawyer, of his privilege against self-incrimination, of his right to cross-examine the complainant or of his right to testify on his own behalf. Were the boy an adult charged with using obscene language in the presence of a woman, the maximum punishment in Arizona was a fine of fifty dollars or imprisonment in jail for not more than two months. The court ruled that the doctrine of *parens patriae* had been unconstitutionally used to deny Gault due process, that a child accused of a delinquent act had the same due process rights as an adult in criminal court (13). This decision established children's right to counsel only in the adjudication stage and the court has yet to address itself directly to the question of rights of status offenders (7, pp. 33, 39-44).

In Gault, the court implied the failure of the treatment and rehabilitation model of the juvenile justice system in its indifference to due process through the judges, practice of reading the defendant's "social history" before adjudication. Such histories often contain hearsay evidence and speculations which would be inadmissable at trial (14).

The emphasis on due process rights had the effect of forcing the state to prove its right to intervene in the life of the child (15). But the risk of such interventions before or after Gault is underscored in the comments of Goldstein, Freud and Solnit who wrote, "The law is incapable of managing, except in a very gross sense, so delicate and complex a relationship as that between a parent and child" (16, p. 8).

ACRONYMS AND LABELING THEORY

The Gault decision catalyzed the development of new acronymic categories (CHINS, PINS, etc.) since it required procedural safeguards and more precise notice of charges than appeared in the loosely drawn definitions of delinquency in the state juvenile court acts. Further, state legislatures sought to limit the stigmatizing label "delinquent" to violations of the criminal law alone. Labeling theory suggested that a stigmatized youth labeled and treated as a delinquent finds the path to antisocial offenses inviting, living up to the expectations of the label (17). This theory has come under attack recently (18, 19), but there seems to be some general agreement among the opposing factions, which include lawyers and sociologists, that incarceration leads to the internalization of delinquent values and a debased self-concept.

A more recent study of the results of juvenile court intervention affirms its negative impact on self-regard and the internalization of delinquent values, but cautions that the magnitude of the noted effects "is nowhere as strong as labeling theorists would have us believe" (20, p. 136). Instead of focusing on the impact of the court's labeling on the youngster's self-regard and its contribution to a delinquent career, the emphasis should be on the effects on labeling agents—probation officers and the police (21). Those youngsters who are labeled are more likely to appear in recidivism statistics, perhaps because of heightened awareness of them by authorities rather than the effects of a debased self-concept (22).

Since Gault, an intense and often confusing polemic has developed between those who wish to preserve court jurisdiction in cases of non-criminal misbehavior and those who believe in the elimination of court-sanctioned intervention in status offenses. Lawyers who seek constitutional grounds for elimination cite vagueness, overbreadth,* lack of due process and unequal protection of the laws. Sociologists have pointed to labeling and interference with family autonomy. Court administrators allege overloaded court dockets and failure to stimulate the development of voluntary social and psychiatric agencies (24).

COURT CHALLENGES AND LEGAL ISSUESS

There have been relatively few cases of juvenile status offense statutes brought before the courts on the grounds of vagueness, and the federal courts have usually ruled the statutes void, depriving minors of due process rights. The upper courts have implied that reformation of status offense statutes must be legislative—not judicial—since the volume of cases would overwhelm the court dockets (25). In Gesicki v. Oswald in 1971 (26), the court ruled that part of New York's "Wayward Minor" statute which dealt with children who were "morally depraved" or "in danger of becoming 'morally depraved' " was "impermissibly vague." The Federal Court rejected the argument that the state's power to deal with children was justified as *parens patriae* and ruled that the use of this doctrine to justify confinement was unconstitutional. The Supreme Court, in 1972, affirmed the Federal Court opinion without comment.

In Maillard v. Gonzalez (27), the Supreme Court, in 1974, struck

---

* Absence of specificity which permits a minor to determine whether his or her behavior falls within or without the boundaries of the law. The clarification of definitions of "status offenses" has become another area for conflict for the advocates of retention as opposed to elimination from the juvenile court jurisdiction. There is general agreement that the usual categories are definable except for children deemed "unruly," "ungovernable," "disobedient" and the like. The retention advocates cite the improved definition of the latter category by the National Conference of Commissioners on Uniform State Laws (23), and then moved beyond the legal question of the child's deeds and have fostered the concept of "families with service needs." This notion, now increasingly widespread, reduces the labeling argument, provides a jurisdictional tie with the parents and opens the court to the prospect of deploying its diagnostic and treatment services and due process protections to cope with the family unit. These developments have led to the replacement of juvenile courts with family courts in some states and have broadened court resources to include psychiatric clinics in advanced communities.

down a California law (Section 601 of the welfare code) which classified children under twenty-one who were "in danger of leading an idle, dissolute, lewd or immoral life" as wards of the court. The Supreme Court concluded that the statute was too vague and the child could not formulate a defense to a charge which included "the entire moral dimension of one's life."

Professor Aidan Gough writes that status offender statutes over ungovernable youth are infringements of the Equal Protection Clause since the defined class—children—is underinclusive because the child is subject to sanction and the parent who shares responsibility for the child's behavior is untouched by the law (25, pp. 276, 277; 28). The Supreme Court held that in the case of an adult, sanctions could not be imposed on a status offense (29) so it appears that our society applies stricter standards to children than to adults. A legal counterargument mounted by Juvenile Court Judge Arthur points out that classifications need only be rationally related to the legislative goal and that the treatment of troubled youth is certainly rational. Arthur takes a developmental point of view asserting that Americans insist that children have *unequal* protection, by citing governmental, religious and volunteer programs subsidized exclusively for children's needs. "Children have special needs to cope with in infancy and adolescence" (30). He argues that society has a crucial interest in protecting the development of the young, thus legislatures should not restrict juvenile court intervention to the same standard of restraint that is mandated for adults. However, Goldstein comments that laws are justified more on a legislative, judicial and administrative perception of an incapacity of persons [minors] to act for themselves rather than meeting societal needs (31).

DIVIDED OPINIONS ON JUVENILE COURT JURISDICTION OF STATUS OFFENDERS

Increasing pressure for the termination of the juvenile court's jurisdiction over status offenders took flight after Gault. The President's Commission on Law Enforcement and Administration of Justice, in 1967, asked that serious consideration be given to completely eliminating the juvenile court's power over children's noncriminal misbehavior (32). A policy advocating separation of status offenders from the juvenile court jurisdiction was adopted by the National Council on Crime and Delinquency (NCCD) in October, 1974 (33). The policy claims that subjecting a child to judicial sanctions for such offenses harms the child and society. Imprisonment of a status offender is disproportionate to the misbehavior; it is unwarranted punishment, and is not treatment. The NCCD pleaded for noncoercive community services (family counseling and youth service bureaus), and increasing educational and employment opportunities since "the court cannot deliver or regulate rehabilitative services" (33). The basis of the policy is the recognition that rebelliousness and resistance to authority are characteristic of the vicissitudes of adolescence and that the intrapsychic conflicts, the conflicts between the child and parents and child and school, demand available community clinical resources for help. A citation by Erik Erikson which appears and reappears in the literature opposed to retention follows:

> Youth after youth, bewildered by the incapacity to assume a role forced on him by the inexorable standardization of American adolescence, runs away in one form or another, dropping out of school, leaving jobs, staying out all night, or withdrawing into bizarre and inaccessible moods. Once "delinquent," his greatest need and often his only salvation is the refusal on the part of older friends, advisors and judiciary personnel to type him further by pat diagnoses and social judgment which ignore the special dynamic conditions of adolescence (34, p. 132).

Judge David Bazelon of the United States District Court of Appeals for the District of Columbia insists that the juvenile court jurisdiction over status offenders impedes the growth and development of community, social and psychiatric services. He postulates that schools and public agencies refer their problems to the court because "the courts have jurisdiction, exercise it and hold out promises of solutions" (35). The courts have failed in preventing delinquency (35). There is evidence that some diversion programs may have been responsible for an increase in community resources (36), but characteristic of much data collection and research methodology in this realm of intense feeling, the information is blurred and insufficient to come to sound conclusions.

Concern has been expressed by those who serve the existing court system that a proliferation of nongovernmental community agencies, which are used for diversion without a court referral, may not respect the constitutional due process established by Gault for intervention by the government. Their point is that if coercion is necessary, it should be imposed by the family and if the family cannot or will not, then only the courts can adequately protect the child (37). This argument is deemed irrelevant by those who oppose retention, since any parent or child who feels his or her rights are not being respected by a voluntary agency or clinic can discontinue the association without penalty (36, p. 653). When multiple repetitions of a child's misbehavior occur in states where the juvenile court jurisdiction is retained in one form or the other, the child will ultimately be assured his rights in court if the community agency or clinic continues to be unsuccessful in treating him and his family.

In 1971 and 1974, two California Assembly committees studying juvenile procedure and juvenile violence concluded that the juvenile court's options are limited by its history, by statute, by the training of its personnel and implied that the nature of adolescent turmoil—poorly understood, changing, ambivalent in its unconscious targets—leaves the court unable to cope with its symptoms (38, 39).

On the other hand, in 1975, the Women's Crusade Against Crime in St. Louis surveyed juvenile court judges and found that 89 percent did not believe that status offenders should be removed from the court's jurisdiction and 65 percent felt that if they were removed no community or public agency existed to cope with those youngsters who now come to court. Seventy-seven percent claimed that status offenders being detained are held since no other resource was available (40).

Judge Justine Wise Polier, a distinguished and reflective commentator, believes in not abandoning or restricting the court's jurisdiction in cases of noncriminal misbehavior but enabling it to achieve its purpose through mandating of beneficial services by the court and the public. She says, "The problems of PINS are *not* [italics added] merely normal adolescent problems" and she has found more emotional disturbance among them than among delinquents. She believes the argument specious that court intervention is unconstitutional; the PINS jurisdiction "is over conduct, not a status" (41). In her dissent to the IJA/ABA *Standards Relating to Noncriminal Misbehavior* she charges the authors of the *Standards* with "romantic and unrealistic" expectations that communities would provide appropriate care and services to children once such needs were made known. Such expectations were attributed by the *Standards* to the *fin de siècle* pioneers of the juvenile court movement. The "dejudicalization of status offenders" is not matched by "plans or requirements for creating alternative, accessible and appropriate services. The *Standards* fail to confront who is to be responsible for the development of alternative services, for their funding, for setting standards, for monitoring, and for protecting the rights of children who are either excluded or denied appropriate services" (28, p. 67).

Roy Wilkins, retired Executive Director of the NAACP, believes that the existent court system could provide rehabilitative service for status offenders only if the law and the public require it. But in no case, he avers, should the courts be empowered "to punish children for status offenses or to incarcerate them in 'training schools'" (24, pp. 19, 20). He is in essential agreement with Judge Polier's position.

RACIAL/ETHNIC/ECONOMIC DISCRIMINATION AND STATUS OFFENDERS

Roy Wilkins obviously had a special interest in the relationship between the existence of the status offender jurisdiction in the juvenile courts and racial/ethnic and economic discrimination. At this writing, for whatever reason, national information on race/ethnicity and social class is sketchy and it may be easy for advocates of either side to rush to judgment.

Paulsen stressed, in 1966, that upper- and middle-class families could keep their children out of the court's jurisdiction by providing restitution to people injured by the child's misbehavior or arrange for private psychiatric treatment, special tutoring, counseling and boarding schools (42). Indeed, one of the authors in a part-time private practice of child psychiatry has seen 15 minors in the past five years in consultation and treatment who were referred for so-called status offenses by parents, without court intervention. These youngsters were white and upper-middle-class, from homes which value educational and cultural attainments. While most of the group came from broken families, the separations of parents were only contributory to their complaints. Family life in these youngsters appeared to be less dysfunctional than a random sampling of cases seen in the New Haven court clinic. In this skewed small sample of private practice cases, within the confidentiality of the treatment relationship, more than half of the patients confessed to undiscovered delinquent acts. All but three suffered emotional disturbances of moderate severity, outside of the bounds of adolescent turmoil, which merited psychotherapeutic interventions.

Burkhart claims that the actions of children from poor, black or Chicano families are more likely to trigger police arrest or referral to juvenile court than the same actions of children from white or affluent homes (24, pp. 3, 4). In Connecticut in 1976 (43), the ethnic/racial breakdown of 2,269 status offenders was: Hispanic—35 percent, black —35 percent, white—30 percent. Blacks, making up six percent of the population in Connecticut, are overrepresented, which may be related to research findings that blacks are more likely than whites to request official intervention in problem behavior (44). Fifty percent of the youngsters were from welfare families, 10 percent from families below poverty level and 30 percent were from middle-income families.

Juvenile Judge John Collins of the Pima County Juvenile Court, Tucson, Arizona identifies status offenders in Pima County in the exact proportions as the ethnic/racial percentages of the general population: 28.6 percent Hispanics, 3.4 percent black and 68 percent white (45). The sociocultural factors making for this finding are elusive at the present and provide an interesting heuristic opportunity since it's the only reported instance in the country.

GENDER DISCRIMINATION

Those eager for elimination of the status offender jurisdiction call attention to the issue of sex discrimination. Certainly, there is agreement that the percentage of girls appearing in court far exceeds the percentage of boys (28, p. 40). In 1976, in Connecticut, 70 percent of the status offenders were girls; 30 percent boys. The percentage of girls charged for status offenses far exceeds the very low percentages of girls charged for criminal offenses (46). Three to four times as many girls as boys across the nation are detained for status offenses (47). Most runaways nationally, and in Connecticut, are girls. In Connecticut, runaways charged by the court are described as 14- and 15-year-old white girls from middle and low income families (48). The courts are always concerned about allegations of immoral conduct on the part of girls, a reflection of society's double standard and the judges' recognition that boys do not become pregnant. Thus, court observers in metropolitan areas note that almost 100 percent of immoral conduct cases are girls (49).

In the conflict over sexual misconduct, the retention advocates have made an unpersuasive case in that the sexual activity of adolescents, while of community and parental concern and requiring, at times, psychotherapeutic interventions, cannot be effectively managed by judicial intervention. There is some agreement that sexual behavior, if harmful to others, can be treated under criminal statutes, and if it reflects abuse and neglect, can be treated under those statutes (25, p. 286). Emergency removal of the youngster for brief periods of time may be helpful in self-destructive, hazardous situations which may bring the court's jurisdiction into play—a last resort maneuver. However, intervention by the state to protect the "best interests of the child" by the supervision of the child's morals is a statement that the child's interests are also the interests of the community and intrudes into the parent-child relationship (16, pp. 3-8). Goldstein, Freud and Solnit's general position has been further applied by Juvenile Judge Oram Ketcham to matters of truancy and drug and alcohol use (36, p. 648).

Contrary to the Goldstein, Freud and Solnit view are the convictions of those who believe that the state has a legitimate interest in what happens to the young. This grouping includes the National Council of Juvenile Court Judges, police departments and many youth services bureaus. They believe that part of the success of community agencies and clinics comes from the recognition that if noncriminal behavior persists, a referral to the court can ultimately be made (50).

As has been noted, virtually all status offense laws embrace a wide range of behavior, so it is useful to consider the jurisdiction with respect to some specific kinds of behavior, other than those discussed earlier in this chapter.

TRUANCY

Across the nation, school absenteeism has been on the rise in the past decade. Absenteeism may be excused or unexcused, and when unexcused for varying time periods according to different state laws, is deemed truancy. There are approximately 600,000 students in Connecticut's public schools. On an average day, 40,000 students or six to eight percent of enrolled students are absent from school. Nationwide studies reflect a higher absentee rate of 10 percent. For most Connecticut school districts truancy is defined as five to 10 days of unexcused absence. About 5,000 to 6,000 of the 40,000 Connecticut absentees, or 0.5 to 1.0 percent of enrolled students, might be considered truant, constituting a loss of about one million school days each year. The absenteeism rates are higher in the urban areas, especially in the ghetto communities where they run as much as 50 percent in contrast to five to 15 percent in the suburbs. The incidence of absenteeism is directly proportional to the incidence of truancy. The three major cities of Connecticut—New Haven, Hartford and Bridgeport—comprise only 11 percent of the school enrollment but they account for more than 20 percent of the absenteeism and more than 25 percent of the truancy (51). Apart from social class factors as seen in urban-suburban differences, truancy is also associated with frequent changes of residence (52) and primary school (53), and the increased number of second working parents in our society.

In the age group 12 to 14 years, about 15 to 20 percent of the students have been identified in Connecticut as unmotivated and unresponsive to the current methods of teaching. Truancy is a major symptom of these unmotivated early adolescents, many of whom turn up in court.*

Actions are infrequently brought against parents, and then usually under the umbrella of educational neglect petitions. As the investigation proceeds, other problems emerge such as familial alcoholism or abuse.

The Connecticut Commissioner of Education avers that the schools are insufficiently responsive to the learning needs of the young and are only modestly successful in motivating children and adolescents. In times of elevated unemployment rates and recession, the schools have failed to develop appropriate job training curricula. In general, secondary school students suffer from the lack of vocational schools and programs, industrial art facilities to teach salable skills and night school combined with daytime compensable work. The demanding entrance requirements to vocational schools often exceed the students' level of educational achievement, shutting off access to well-motivated aspirants. Unions and state labor departments are reluctant to waive minimum age requirements for 14- and 15-year-olds. The growing number of students whose primary language is Spanish adds another dimension of planning difficulty for state administrators (55).

It is commonly stated that the failure of a child to attend school may stem from emotional disturbance or physical disability, parental neglect, embarrassment about families, inadequate clothing and hunger, a fear of violence, and from the failures of educational programing. There is a literature claiming that many youths who are referred to the courts as truant engage in delinquent acts, suffer with complex family problems, have peer difficulties and exhibit severe behavioral and academic problems (56, 57). Later in adolescence some will experience emotional disorders, may engage in unlawful activity and become controlled substance and alcohol abusers (58, 59). These latter studies are fraught with methodologic problems and are largely based on questionnaire research.

An interview study of 33 sixth to eighth grade truants from three middle schools in New Haven has shown that students who are truant (truancy defined here as school absence, unexcused by parents) were likely to be experiencing substantial psychosocial difficulties. Many of these students were involved in fighting, disrupting classes, stealing, running away, firesetting and vandalism (in and out of school). Drug

---

* Of 2,109 Connecticut status offenders charged in 1975, 34 percent were truants (54).

use was frequent. Their families were subject to divorce and separation, serious illness, unemployment, parental discord and alcoholism. At least three-quarters of the families had one other truant child and half of them a child who repeated a grade (60). So it appears that no matter what the level of sophistication of research on truancy, the favored current explanation that truancy is only an adaptive response to adversity is flawed; for the most part it is a complex maladaptive response to multiple stresses, dysfunctions and social deprivations which finds expression in emotional disturbance and antisocial behavior. Indeed, the plight of the truant, his anguish and alienation are seen in its Celtic *(truan)* and Gaelic *(truaghn)* derivations, both meaning *wretched* (61).

For most of the truant population, the courts are uninvolved. The schools agree, however quietly, that attendance is the educators' responsibility. Once a truant is identified in Connecticut, parents are notified, the school guidance department becomes engaged and community agency or psychiatric clinic referral is often recommended. Most school districts employ a planning and placement team to alter educational planning in accord with the truant's needs. On another level, a variety of disciplinary measures are used, including demerits or detention, losing credit or school privileges, probation or, in some districts, suspension. If these measures fail, referrals are sometimes made to the police, juvenile courts or the State Department of Children's and Youth Services. These approaches have fallen short of the needs of these adolescents. In the last decade approximately 20 percent of Connecticut students enrolled in the ninth grade do not enroll in the 12th grade, a loss of less than 10,000 (when corrected for estimates of death or emigration out-of-state) (62). Large numbers of drop-outs make the transition from truancy, but no reliable data base is available.

When the juvenile court is involved in truancy referrals, those opposed to retention of status offense jurisdiction argue that the schools are not pushed to assume their own responsibilities or to upgrade their programs. If the court mandates a return to school without other supports and clinical interventions, damage to the whole system of education accrues. The court's efforts, no more than other well-designed therapeutic interventions in the most advanced states, have been less than effective in these situations. Those who favor retention see the court as an instrument of last resort for children and families besieged by multiple problems, where the best efforts of well-staffed schools, community clinics and agencies have not been able to address the needs. The coercive authority of the court, in the service of the child's ego, may initiate a comprehensive diagnostic evaluation. With these diagnostic findings, the court can compel targeted treatment programs for child and family which may have been resisted under voluntary conditions earlier or not have been previously considered.

In the arguments marshalled on both sides of the court jurisdiction issue, the question of compulsory education requirements is at the center. Those opposed to removal of the jurisdiction claim that if it is eliminated, students will be ill prepared to survive in the economic marketplace and the importance of education will be denigrated. On the other side, advocates cite the national disgrace of social promotions and the illiteracy commonplace in high school graduates, especially from metropolitan regions. Enforcing school attendance in disaffected and educationally disadvantaged young people without providing them with adequate programs of educational counseling, special education, alternative curricula, and vocational training, turns schools into custodial institutions and deprives motivated and talented students of the teaching and services they merit.

The states have approached the problem in different ways. Hawaii, Nevada, Ohio, Oklahoma and Utah have insisted that their students stay in school until they are 18 but have statutory provisions permitting pupils to drop out at the end of 10th grade if their parents and principals agree. In Florida and California, students can take proficiency tests before they reach the present legal ages of 16 and 18 respectively; if they pass and their parents consent, they may leave school with a certificate of achievement which will enable them to continue their education at a later time, if they so desire (63). Most educators welcome the debate on compulsory education since it delineates the schools' roles and responsibilities in a democratic society and clarifies the schools' relationship to the juvenile justice system in the context of status offense statutes. The schools and the courts both are frustrated by the failures of state legislatures and governors to call for improved programs with attendant funding.

DISOBEDIENCE TO SCHOOL AUTHORITIES

Students referred to court for disruptive behavior often are found to have an underlying history of truancy. Again those who favor eliminating the court jurisdiction claim that disobedience statutes diminish the school's responsibility and resources and encourage court referrals. In practice, the schools intervene in such situations without court referrals and do not invoke the statutes unless the behavior exceeds a tolerable degree of severity. Many schools, after exhausting their therapeutic armamentarium, will finally suspend the disruptive student. In Connecticut, it is estimated that five percent of the school enrollment of 600,000 children were suspended at least once, or close to 30,000 students in the 1977-1978 school year. One-third of the suspended students were suspended repeatedly, averaging a total of two and a half times. The patterns of suspension parallel the patterns of attendance, thus the three major cities and their ghetto areas have higher suspension rates. The suspension rates vary dramatically with 1.0 percent for elementary school students, 9.1 percent for middle and junior high school students and 14.0 percent for senior high school students (62).

The Connecticut state law requires that all expulsions be reported to the State Board of Education and that an alternative program be provided for the expelled student. The great majority of schools who expel students use homebound instruction; however, most districts do not employ expulsion. In 1977-1978, only 80 students were expelled in Connecticut, and of these half were in Hartford, where almost all of them were transferred to other public schools in town.

Suspensions and expulsions for disruption often become the means for young people to accomplish what they unconsciously want for themselves —to be free of schooling. Many are economically and educationally disadvantaged to start with, are caught up in family chaos and internal conflict and have struggled with the fatigued and unyielding local educational systems. To be released from school carries with it freedom from the demands of learning, from the acceptance of the authority of school personnel and/or parents, from the need to socialize with peers and from the need to master the expectable surging impulses of normal adolescent development (64).

The behavioral contagion from peers struggling with these same issues finds a rich medium in the most vulnerable—those whose controls are marginal. The pulsating ambience of the public high schools provides resonant background music lowering the threshold for conflict expression through disruptive behavior. A measure of the experience was defined by a class that was reading the *Odyssey* (studying epic similes, among other clever devices) and put together a poem called "Break Time at HSC" (High School in the Community—an alternative school)

Breaktime at HSC is like rush hour in New
York, like Grand Central Station on fire,
like letting wild horses out of a paddock

like a Japanese air raid
    like World War II broke out, and we lost
like a football game when the running back
    has fumbled
like having a high time.
Breaktime at HSC is like a dream come true (65).

Connecticut and New York are the only northeastern states that provide for in-school suspension in their statutes. While other northeastern states have no statutory or formal policy on the subject of in-school supervision, most states have a local option. Under Connecticut General Statutes (Sec. 10-233b), local and regional school boards may authorize teachers to remove disruptive students and send them to a designated school area, with the school principal being notified. In the event of a removal from class more than six times in a year, or more than twice in one week, then the student must be given an informal hearing (66). A revision of that statute is underway in the Connecticut General Assembly (67), which provides for an informal hearing with *each* imposition of an in-school suspension and limits suspensions to no more than 15 times or a total of 50 days in one school year.

In those Connecticut school districts using in-school suspensions, detention was employed by 80 percent, counseling by 68 percent and instruction by 65 percent. Those schools using in-school suspensions with a few students apparently resort to detention, while those using it with many students are making greater use of instructional programs.

The Connecticut educators claim that the present system of in-school suspension does not automatically contribute to a decrease of students on the streets. Police and probation officers from every section of the state are less impressed by the effectiveness of the program and are not satisfied with its implementation. They state that suspended adolescents are prime candidates for status offender and delinquent behavior. Of the estimated 6,000 students on the street daily, 400-600 are suspended with the remainder being truants. So a major quixotic argument presented by those who wish to eliminate status offenders from the court jurisdiction is blunted by one state's experience: The schools in Connecticut have seemingly behaved responsibly in dealing with those guilty of disruptive behavior and have developed limited resources. Nonetheless, when that behavior has not yielded to an in-school suspension system or rises to a level of gravity short of being juvenile crime, the juvenile court's authority is brought to bear—but only after the community agencies and clinics have exhausted their competencies.

RUNAWAYS

Everyone everywhere wants to run away from something.

> For some, the thought of running away is nothing more than an escapist fantasy; for others it can be dispelled with a change of pace or routine. But for some, there is no alternative but to take physical leave of an unbearable situation. They run away, usually in secret and in warm weather, to cut the ties that hurt. They run to hide, to escape, to forget, to follow a dream . . . to begin. Taking such leave can be a cry of pain or a sign of health seeking surface (68).

The problem of runaways is epidemic and increasing. Current estimates total over one million youngsters a year living out a universal childhood fantasy and threat to parents (69). The U.S. Congress in its Runaway Youth Act established a Federal grant program to fund locally controlled nonsecure facilities providing temporary shelter and counseling services to juveniles who have left home without permission of their parents or guardians. These facilities operate outside the juvenile justice system (70). They serve about 33,000 youths or 3.3 percent of the known runaways (69). The remaining young people receive local community services from walk-in crisis centers, clergy or others. Some may be picked up by the police, processed through the juvenile court or released to families with no support services or follow-up.

In 1976, the FBI arrested 75,000 runaways which most authorities believe represent less than 50 percent of the youth living on the streets (71). The National Health Survey (U.S. Public Health Service) claims that one of every 10 non-institutionalized youth ages 12-17 years of age has run away from home at least once. Many students of this problem believe these estimates too low. The vast majority of runaways seldom leave the general area of home, community or their state. In most states they make up the largest body of status offenders. The profile of status offenders in Connecticut at risk of detention indicated that 70 percent were female, 14 to 15 years old, white, charged with running away. One-third were known to protective services and/or the juvenile court (72). The major reasons cited for running away are family conflicts, authority struggles, money problems, physical and sexual abuse and neglect (73). Often the runaway's behavior is adaptive and rational when the youth flees to avoid unhealthy emotional and physical conditions at home. Female runaways make up the majority of youth fleeing families, stay away longer and find the experience more stressful and dangerous. There is a high correlation between runaway behavior and low involvement and achievement in school (74) and in the runaway typology study, 70 percent reported having serious school difficulties with nearly one-half dropping out of school prior to running away (73). In general, school systems are not involved in the provision of services or preventive work with runaway youth in 20 cities identified as high density runaway areas (75).

Upon running away, the youths are preoccupied with survival but most do not seek help from the traditional community agencies—the youngsters need a place to stay, food, clothing and medical care (76). Further, a high proportion of youth who are runaways for more than a few days report being exposed to exploitation in the streets through robbery, sexual molestation, physical abuse, and drugs. For the most part, when they seek help they turn to friends or parents and relatives of friends. Community based services are unknown to more than half of the runaways in studies noted above and others who sought these services complained of fears of being turned in to authorities, problems of waiting lists, identification and establishing eligibility.

Runaways suffer from varying statutes and court decisions in all the states so that in one locality an act may be regarded as legal but in others a youth may be apprehended as a status offender or delinquent. These statutes tend to isolate the young from institutions and services important to them during a runaway episode. They can't attend school outside of the communities of parents or guardians. Most cannot get medical attention without parental permission. They cannot secure employment, which leads them to "hustle" in order to survive. Finally, the helpers available—employers, runaway house staff and physicians—may be in legal jeopardy if they assist them without parental permission (77).

Short runaways occur frequently and commonly result in parental referrals to the court. They made up 51 percent of New York PINS cases in one study (49, pp. 1383, 1408); another survey indicated that 35 percent were away from home less than five days and 52.8 percent had been away less than 10 days (78). Those who support the court jurisdiction agree that interventions should be limited to cases where the youngster runs repeatedly, where his/her health and welfare are at risk and when community based services have been exhausted. Those opposed to the court jurisdiction cite the adaptive response to adversity that running away often represents. They call for noncoercive shelters* and counseling.

---

* For a discussion of shelters, see the next section *Federal Actions and State Responses On Behalf of Status Offenders.*

If the plight of the runaways leads them into repeated flight where they commit crimes, then the delinquent jurisdiction can be applied.

FEDERAL ACTIONS AND STATE RESPONSES ON BEHALF
OF STATUS OFFENDERS

In 1974, the DHEW Office of Youth Development issued a series of model acts for courts with jurisdiction over children and youth (79). A major recommendation was for the elimination of juvenile court jurisdiction over status offenders. In the same year, the Congress passed the Juvenile Justice and Delinquency Prevention Act, assigning responsibility to the Law Enforcement Assistance Administration (LEAA), a section of the Department of Justice. The Act, in part, provided that, within two years from the submission of a funding plan by the states, juveniles who are charged or who have committed offenses which would not be criminal if committed by an adult be treated in shelter facilities and not placed in juvenile detention or correction facilities (80). The Congressional intent was to minimize contact between law enforcement personnel and those charged with noncriminal misbehavior, especially runaways (81). Within the LEAA, the Office of Juvenile Justice and Delinquency Prevention was established (OJJDP) and within that bureaucratic structure, the National Institute for Juvenile Justice and Delinquency Prevention (NIJJDP) was set up. A task group of the NIJJDP identified four areas for immediate attention:

1) the deinstitutionalization of status offenders;
2) the diversion of youth from the juvenile justice system;
3) the prevention of delinquency;
4) the reduction of serious juvenile crime.

In March 1975, the task group asked state and local agencies to submit innovative proposals to remove incarcerated status offenders from institutions and to prevent future institutionalization of this group. While deinstitutionalization was the goal of the enabling Act and the LEAA, *separation* was central to the legislative intent, and *not* removal from the juvenile court system altogether (82). But the natural extension of the philosophy of deinstitutionalization was to call for the complete *decriminalization* of status offenders (which was not the position of the Act or the LEAA). *Decriminalization* has meant in the literature the complete removal of status offenders from court jurisdiction. The LEAA approached the problem ambiguously vis-à-vis the deinstitutionalization-decriminalization issue; its strategy was based upon the desire to achieve separation and thus expose the status offender population to community based treatment, avoiding and diverting youngsters from judicial processing. There was the underlying conviction that labeling leads to a delinquent career, detention in institutions achieves the same result, and since the juvenile court has failed its treatment mission, it should be replaced with a punishment model. By providing Federal funds, community programs were to be established which would better treat the young and reduce recidivism.

In 1977, amendments to the Act extended the deadline for state compliance to three years after submission of the state's original plan. A continuation of state participation will be admissible if "substantial compliance," meaning 75 percent deinstitutionalization, has been achieved and if there is an "unequivocal commitment to achieving full compliance within a reasonable time." "Reasonable time" for full compliance is no longer than two years beyond the three-year deadline (83).

The problems of implementation, of reaching precise definitions of status offenders, of facilities for detention and correction, of cost and service led to a 10-state study commissioned by the OJJDP (LEAA) and the Office of Youth Development (now Youth Development Bureau) of DHEW (84). The case studies in 1977 covered the following states: Arkansas, California, Connecticut, Florida, Iowa, Maryland, New York, Oregon, Utah and Wisconsin. In summary, the studies found that clear progress had been made in all of the states towards deinstitutionalization of status offenders, especially in removing them from correctional facilities as opposed to detention.*

All the state strategies have been different. They include clusters of action aimed at a) removal or limitation of the court's jurisdiction over status offenders, b) limitations on possible dispositions and c) the development of community based youth services. The major unsettled problem is pre-adjudicated detention, not longer-term commitment, since the states studied don't send large numbers to correctional institutions. As alternatives to detention, emergency structured shelter care, foster care, group homes and runaway houses are being used. Court and law enforcement officers need assurances for purposes of child protection and court ap-

---

* In 1976, California, Connecticut and Iowa sent no status offenders to correctional settings. However, in Connecticut a status offender can become a delinquent if he is in violation of court orders. If the same statutes exist in California and Iowa, and are utilized by the court, then the findings of the case studies in this area may be misleading.

pearances of the child in states where there is some sort of court juris-diction extant, that structured shelter care is available, especially for runaways. There are available, but only *weakly represented* in many states, services for residential psychiatric care, family counseling, psychiatric outpatient services for adolescents, alternative education programs, job-finding services and independent living arrangements. Highly structured intensive day programs—programs which can offer educational super-vision, recreation, drug and alcohol counseling, individual and family counseling and psychotherapy—while the child lives at home are lacking. Whatever services exist in a given state, they are scarcest in the rural areas. With small numbers of status offenders spread over wide areas, incarceration overutilization may occur as a solution. Those who favor retention point out that in rural areas, the probation officers carry out, as well as they can, the treatment functions of the court, many of which are catalogued above as the work of community-based services.

The 10-state study further speaks to the problem of structured shelter care for accused or adjudicated status offenders with serious behavioral problems who cannot be placed in detention or correctional institutions because of statutory prohibitions. In most cases, these nonsecure facilities are publicly operated; many are operated by the volunteer sector under contract such as the YMCA. Recently, the authors were called out during a wintry night to assist a Y facility in locating and helping a runaway 15-year-old adolescent who initially ran from his home and was ap-prehended by the local police. Referred to the court clinic, a full assess-ment revealed a diagnosis of a borderline schizophrenic state. His father was a chronic mentally ill patient at a nearby VA hospital, his mother had a long history of outpatient psychiatric treatment and his brother was in a prison ward in a Western state charged with murder and await-ing psychiatric evaluation. After adjudication, the adolescent was sent to the structured shelter awaiting a group home placement. He fled the Y across a dangerous rainswept roof four floors above ground and was picked up by the police a day later trying to cross a major bridge in New York City. This youngster is part of the status offender population which is at risk even if placed in a structured shelter. These shelters, staffed by people of goodwill but with little training, often cannot assure the child's safety.

As previously noted, the federally inspired move towards deinstitu-tionalization in 1974 has led to considerable debate about removal of status offenses from court jurisdiction around the nation. Two of the states studied, Florida and Utah, have taken steps. Florida redefined its

CIN's as dependent children, shunting them into the child welfare system and thus the court lost a caseload of 18,000 cases. For a child who is adjudicated ungovernable a second time, there is retained the option to treat him as a delinquent. In Utah, the Division of Family Services (DFS) has jurisdiction now over ungovernables and runaways but if the DFS fails, then the child can reenter the court's jurisdiction (84, p. 47).

The Connecticut situation, as an example of an advanced state, merits an overview. Clearly, the 1974 Act represented part of the impetus for changing state law. In Connecticut since 1976, most status offenders have been removed from correctional and detention facilities. But the issue of Federal compliance has been raised since there is some commingling of delinquents and status offenders in secure and nonsecure facilities. The view of Connecticut is that the needs of the child, not his label, are what is central. The commingling criteria of the OJJDP assure clear delineation between status offenders and delinquents and as noted in the introductory section of this chapter, the label identifying a child in need depends upon how he comes to public attention—delinquent, status offender, emotionally disturbed, dependent, and abused and neglected child. The service needs of each of these groups tend to be similar and have to be defined by careful assessment. Under Federal guidelines, there is risk that one set of group homes will be utilized for status offenders, another for delinquents and the problem of stigmatization comes to the fore—a problem which the 1974 Act is supposed to address.

Since many status offenders are difficult to manage, service providers may resist taking on labeled youngsters who may cause more management problems than delinquents. Thus in Connecticut, a facility serving children, other than detention or a correctional setting, may service both delinquents and status offenders if the services provided are specific to the child's needs. But this progressive, cost-effective policy flies in the face of Federal requirements even if one delinquent is present in a nonsecure facility with 40 beds. In addition, there are a few cases where children must be held involuntarily to provide treatment no matter what label they bear as a consequence of how they came to the public attention. The conflict with the Act of 1974 has led Connecticut among many other states to seek an alteration of the OJJDP guidelines or an amendment of the statute.

The Connecticut Justice Commission, Juvenile Justice Commission and the Department of Children and Youth Services (DCYS) have agreed on means of integrating the state's treatment of status offenders (85). The broad philosophic outlines suggest that the status offenders require services or environmental changes. Their behavior indicates broader problems involving the child, his family, peers and school. Since status offenses do not constitute criminal behavior, sanctions for criminal behavior should not be imposed on them. A rational integrated delivery system should be available to all children in need and not purely defined for status offenders. There continues to be a need for Superior Court jurisdiction, much as the court is involved in neglect and abuse matters. The treatment needs of some children require services in a location which the child may not voluntarily leave. Finally, where a child's needs require a restraint on his or her liberty, such a decision for restraint should be reached after notice, a hearing, the presentation of independent professional evidence subject to cross-examination, and a finding that restraint is required and will help the child.

A new Connecticut statute which incorporates these principles and modifies existent law was introduced into the General Assembly in January 1979, signed into law by the summer, with an implementation date of July 1, 1980 (86). However, in all likelihood, several bills pending before the 1980 Connecticut General Assembly will effectively delay the implementation date. It calls for the new designation of "Families with Service Needs." Only repeated behavior by status offenders can come under court jurisdiction. The court may reclassify its jurisdiction over a child to abused, neglected or uncared for when indicated. For example, a runaway for "just cause" may be treated as a neglected child. The present system of detention will continue until August 1980, the Federal compliance deadline, and in the interim the state will develop an adequate system of nonsecure facilities to serve the court and the child's needs. In the pre-adjudication phase, the court can continue the proceedings for six months, during which time a voluntary referral to community-based services may be made. If the problem is settled, then the petition may be dismissed—the court will have the power to direct orders against the parent, guardian or child's custodian. The role of the DCYS as custodian will be defined in legislative hearings, since the present statutes bar the court from directing the DCYS to adopt a specific treatment plan. The court would not usurp the role of the school but, since the court's role is to protect the child, it is available for the appeal of special education decisions. Hearing procedures for restraint of liberty of a child by DCYS were established—violation of a court order would no longer be a delinquent act or a status offense but would be judged as contempt. (The problem at this writing is still unresolved, since punishment for contempt may be worse than for a status offense or a minor delinquent act.) Police diversion appears to be effective in many areas of the state but, if both parent and child consent, the police and other state agencies may refer a child to a nonsecure setting. If parents are unavailable and the child protests such a placement, and if the police believe that to release the child is unwise or dangerous, they can hold the child long enough for court referral. If no court referral is indicated, they can hold a child for no more than six hours* until a parent or guardian is found.

CONNECTICUT PROGRESS TOWARDS DEINSTITUTIONALIZATION

The number of status offenders has declined by 80 percent from 1975 to 1977. And by 1977, 65 percent of the status offender population at risk was provided with an alternative to detention through the De-institutionalization of Status Offenders Project (87). The alternatives include group and foster homes, residential treatment centers, long-term programs, family crisis counseling, psychiatric treatment, and structured shelter care.

In 1976 the Connecticut court disposed of 2,269 status offenses, which were 11.4 percent of all delinquency dispositions. Note that status offenses are not a separate jurisdictional category in Connecticut and thus are included in delinquency data collections. Of 100 percent of the delinquent acts, the following is the distribution of status offenses:

        5.1 percent - runaways
        3.7 percent - truants
        2.0 percent - beyond control
        0.5 percent - school misconduct
        0.1 percent - indecent or immoral conduct (88).

As of May, 1977 there were no status offenders committed to the correctional setting at Long Lane but 165 status offenders were in detention (87).** The State of Connecticut has made much progress towards deinstitutionalization since 1972, and only a relatively small number of status offenders appear in court. Connecticut has already developed, though meagerly, the major service categories permitting treatment in the community and outside the court system. Although it is assumed

---

* Much like the IJA/ABA *Standards* 2.1. Child case workers agree that six hours is too short a time period and that 24 hours is a more pragmatic time limit.

** Again, these data may be misleading, since if a status offender violates a court order by his conduct on probation, he becomes a delinquent by present Connecticut law.

that the principal start-up costs of deinstitutionalization have been already borne, the state is attempting, along with other states, to get the OJJDP to change its guidelines addressed to commingling in order to avoid losing Federal funds. While the Act of 1974 and its amendments are not mandatory, Connecticut's failure to comply would jeopardize a Federal award of just less than one million dollars a year.

THE INSTITUTE OF JUDICIAL ADMINISTRATION/AMERICAN BAR
ASSOCIATION IJA/ABA JUVENILE JUSTICE STANDARDS PROJECT:
STANDARDS RELATING TO NONCRIMINAL MISBEHAVIOR

In 1971, the New York University Institute of Judicial Administration initiated the Juvenile Justice Standards Project. The American Bar Association joined as cosponsor in 1973 and a Joint Commission was created to serve as the project's governing body. That Commission, chaired by Chief Judge Irving Kaufman of the U.S. Court of Appeals for the Second Circuit, consisted of 29 members, half judges and lawyers and the balance representing other nonlegal disciplines such as sociology and psychology. But behavioral scientists were in the minority and clinicians with training in child and adolescent work were minimally represented. More than 160 experts in law and behavioral sciences participated in the drafting of 23 volumes and one summary volume, all designed "to cover the spectrum of problems pertaining to laws affecting children. They examined the juvenile justice system and its relationship to the rights and responsibilities of children" (28, p. v). The *Standards* are important because of their possible adoption by the American Bar Association as guidelines for judges, legislators, administrators, public and private agencies.

Each of the 23 volumes addresses different aspects of the juvenile justice system such as *Juvenile Delinquency and Sanctions, Schools and Education, Noncriminal Misbehavior, Youth Service Agencies, Records and Information Systems* and so on. Their interrelationship is founded on the basic principles which reappear in every volume. These include the rejection of the treatment, medical, or rehabilitation model of the court as being a failure, and the avowal of the principle of family autonomy as opposed to state intervention except where the juvenile's interests are inadequately protected without court involvement.

The *Standards Relating to Noncriminal Misbehavior* recommend the elimination of juvenile court jurisdiction over status offenses and noncriminal misbehavior and ask for a system of voluntary referral to community-based agencies in its stead (28, p. 2). The *Standards* permit limited coercive intervention where the child or adolescent is in immediate jeopardy as in certain cases of runaways, in provisions for short-term custody, for emergency medical services, and for court approval of residential placement. But the overriding principle is to opt for the least detrimental alternative consonant with the needs of the young (25, p. 279). The *Standards* insist that removal of the status offense jurisdiction will encourage people to get more effective voluntary help which may be more successful than court mandated referrals. The authors of the *Standards* believe that new and extended community services will flow from dejudicalization. Further, the evil impact of treating a non-criminal as a delinquent will be eliminated. Finally, the courts may be freed up to deal with delinquency and abuse and neglect cases which overload the docket.

Response to the IJA/ABA Juvenile Justice Standards Project, Standards Project, Standards Relating to Noncriminal Misbehavior by the American Psychiatric Association Ad Hoc Task Force of the Council on Children, Adolescents and Their Families. Many organizations concerned with the clinical care of children and adolescents were invited by the IJA/ABA to critique the work product of the Project but only the American Psychiatric Association, through the leadership of Dr. Edward Futterman, Chair of the Council on Children, Adolescents and Their Families, responded to the call. Within less than a 10-week period, 12 colleagues, including a distinguished lawyer-psychiatric social worker consultant, met as an Ad Hoc Task Force to review the volumes where a clinical outlook could contribute to a grasp of the urgent issues involving children and their families. Among the volumes reviewed was *Standards Relating to Noncriminal Misbehavior,* assigned to two independent critics** for specific assessment and as in the case of all the reviewed volumes, to the Task Force as a whole.

The Ad Hoc Task Force recommended retention of jurisdiction over acts of juvenile misbehavior but with qualifiers. In the *Standards* rewritten by the Task Force, jurisdiction of the juvenile court over noncriminal misbehavior shall be separate from delinquency and abuse and neglect matters in organization, staffing, calendars, budgeting, work-load

---

* Frank Rafferty, M.D., Chair, Paul Adams, M.D., Viola Bernard, M.D., Elissa Benedek, M.D., David Cline, M.D., Andre Derdeyn, M.D., Edward Futterman, M.D., Leonard Lawrence, M.D., Carl Malmquist, M.D., Herbert Sacks, M.D., Jeanne Spurlock, M.D., Sandra Nye, M.S.W., J.D.

** Drs. Elissa Benedek and Herbert Sacks.

and staff training. The definition of noncriminal misbehavior is widened to include juveniles between the ages of 10 through 17, whose behavior does not violate criminal law statutes but does "represent serious unreconciled conflict between the juvenile and his/her family, school or community. Such overt and public acts may include:

A. Truancy that is severe and unresolved by the school procedures described in the *Standards on Schools and Education.*

B. Runaway behavior that is prolonged in duration or repeated and endangers the safety and security of the juvenile and has not responded to voluntary reconciliation services.

C. Overt acts of aggression with the family, school or community that do not violate criminal statutes but do seriously endanger persons or property.

D. Overt acts of serious substance abuse, including but not limited to drugs and alcohol.

E. Sexual behavior that results in exploitation or endangerment of the individual juvenile (89).

The Task Force asked that records or files of youngsters under this jurisdiction follow guidelines for access and confidentiality prescribed under the *Standards on Records and Information Systems.* It requested that the limited custody associated with an endangered youngster and instituted by a law enforcement officer be extended from six hours to 24 hours in a nonsecure temporary residential setting, which is more realistic given the routine problems of informing parents, custodians or guardians and attempting to mobilize community agencies. The Task Force called for appropriate staff training prior to and during employment at publicized walk-in service centers.

The Task Force expressed concerns that the *Standards Relating to Noncriminal Misbehavior* downplay the tragic, painful and dangerous clinical situations which are described as merely evidences of conflict within the family, school or community. There appears to be a casual reliance on insufficient and ineffective community-based services despite the expectations of the authors of the *Standards* that eliminating jurisdiction will force growth of existent community agencies and establish new ones. Where court services are adequate, compliance with the *Standards* would require termination of those services. The Task Force reads the anticommingling standard as preventing the treatment of noncriminal youths in residential facilities which serve delinquents, even where such a facility can appropriately treat the psychosocial problems of either youngster (90).

PRESENT STATUS OF THE JUVENILE JUSTICE STANDARDS PROJECT

In February, 1979, 17 volumes of the *Standards* were ratified by the American Bar Association House of Delegates. Six of the most controversial volumes were withdrawn by Judge Kaufman since the debate was "raucous" (91). They included the volumes on *Noncriminal Misbehavior, Court Organization And Administration, Probation* and *Juvenile Delinquency And Sanctions.* The *Abuse And Neglect* and *Schools And Education* volumes were not submitted.

In the February, 1980 American Bar Association House of Delegates midwinter meeting the battle continued between the Juvenile Justice Standards Commission and the opposition, led by the National Council of Juvenile and Family Court Judges. By voice vote, the House of Delegates voted against a resolution which would have had the effect of rescinding last year's vote adopting the first 17 volumes of *Standards.*

Judge Irving Kaufman, Commission Chairman, stated that the adoption of the *Noncriminal Misbehavior* volume was the most important result of the Commission's work. But the House of Delegates refused to support the volume, voting 145 to 142 to defer action indefinitely. While rejecting the volume on *Noncriminal Misbehavior,* the delegates adopted three other volumes of *Standards* resubmitted by the Commission—*Court Organization And Administration, Probation* and *Juvenile Delinquency And Sanctions.* After revision, the *Abuse And Neglect* volume will be submitted to the House of Delegates in the course of the August, 1980 meeting (91a).

A PERSPECTIVE ON STATUS OFFENDERS

Throughout this chapter we have endeavored to present the countervailing arguments in the retention-elimination controversy surrounding juvenile court jurisdiction over status offenses. Where the arguments of either side have been moralistic, specious, poorly supported by existent data or harshly polemical, we have not been reluctant to identify their frailties. Up to this point we have sought to inform and not persuade our collegial audience of the complexity and subtlety of the issue, emphasizing the social, legal and political vectors impinging on its resolution. In the real world, the views of child care professionals about the controversy have been muted for some of the reasons noted in an introductory section. This phenomenon has been reflected in this chapter thus far and in the voluminous status offender literature predominantly written by legal professionals and sociologists, most of whom have never experienced long-term clinical responsibility.

We reaffirm that it is necessary to have different laws, courts, definitions and procedures for children from those for adults. Children are not homunculi and are subject to the vicissitudes of growth and development in every dimension—in their emotional, physical and social components. Thus, there is no question about the continuing need for a juvenile justice system, one that is firmly rooted in the treatment or rehabilitation model. And within that model there is an important place for the child psychiatrist and allied professionals, provided we are willing to assume our professional and citizen responsibilities.

The history of the rehabilitation model in the juvenile court has been alluded to early in the chapter. In the 19th century, Isaac Ray wrote about the relationship between criminal responsibility and psychiatry (92). Freud, in his famous essay on "Those Wrecked By Success," shed fresh light on the psychology of crime (93). Physicians and lawyers were convinced that offenders could be reformed, remolded and resocialized. So the law was changed from the punishment model, which was best defined in the 18th-century writings of Cesare Beccaria, who saw that the certainty of punishment deterred the wrongdoer. The rationale of the treatment model in adult and juvenile systems held sway until the 1960s, when intervention models from individual to group therapy and reduced caseloads for probation officers did not reduce recidivism (94). The Kent v. U.S. decision in 1966 emphasized that the child was not receiving "solicitous care and regenerative treatment" (12). Gault, in 1967, identified the failure of the rehabilitation model (13). Thoughtful reports by distinguished authors impugned the treatment effects on recidivism, called for uniformity in sentencing and a decrease in judicial discretion (95, 96).

In the light of attention called to violent crime, it was discovered that six percent of a cohort of 10,000 boys born in 1945 and followed from the age of 10 to 18 were responsible for the street crimes which terrify the public (97). This study contributed to a hue and cry in the media to revise the juvenile justice system. Currently, the benevolence of the treatment model, which for some changed 17th-century sin to illness, is in the decline. The depredations of the IJA/ABA Project notwithstanding, there still reside strong therapeutic influences within the confines of the resurgent classical retribution model, a model which has begun to infect the juvenile justice system. We still buy into the idea of rehabilitation but the principle of noncoercive intervention with children and adolescents is beginning to make inroads.

The trend of the juvenile court system is to send violent offenders up to the adult court, to not only deinstitutionalize but to move gingerly in the direction of eliminating the status offender jurisdiction, and then to subject the residual group of delinquents to uniform sentencing relatively devoid of individualized treatment.

Our view of the management of status offenders largely concurs with the product of Task Force on the IJA/ABA *Standards* of the APA (89) .* Status offenders should not be subject to the delinquency jurisdiction of the juvenile court, ought not to be labeled delinquents, and should not have sanctions applied to them as if they were delinquent. Status offenders are not a homogeneous group. The arguments for elimination too frequently portray them as healthy adolescents experimenting with adaptations unacceptable to a society vigilant about the dangers of street crime. Surely those who truant once, who are short runaways in response to familial adversity, for example, ought not to be subject to the court's jurisdiction. We emphasize that the label of this heterogeneous group is a function of how the youngster comes to the attention of the clinic, agency, service, police or court. There are few adults who cannot recall committing a status offense in their youth and most of them have not been identified by schools, parents, police and courts. A critical point is that by the time most status offenders are referred to court they display entrenched social, educational and emotional troubles which are difficult to approach with our present training and clinical skills. The literature redounds with citations from experienced judges on both sides of the controversy that dealing with a delinquent is far more preferable than treating the stubborn and complicated issues revealed in status offenders. Their management problems often are outsize and sometimes defy the resources of structured shelters and other court remedies. We must underscore the fact that while many status offenders do not develop more serious problems, seriously delinquent youth, in most instances, have a prior history of status offenses. Diversionary programs for status offenders require specific treatment planning tailored to the needs of these youngsters and such programs, unfortunately, are in short supply since they are costly and difficult to mount with qualified staff.

---

* See page .... of this chapter for Task Force Recommendations.

We return once more to the anguish and tragedy attached to the status offenders who exceed the capabilities of community-based services and arrives in court. They are not mere examples of expectable adolescent turmoil, strivings for autonomy and independence and rebellion against authority who have found expression in their conflict with school, family and community. They are wretched, in pain worsened by family disorganization. Do these children and families not merit treatment by the state instrument of last resort in our society? With the past histories of failed interventions, can we assume that parents can redeploy their own depleted energies and strained resources to effectively address the conflict? If we stand under the banner of family autonomy, can we still assert that the state has no right to intervene to protect children and adolescents from genuine endangerment?

We recognize that coercive intervention by the courts in the service of the child's ego may involve costs as well as gains in that such moves may intrude into delicate family ties and erode the rights and responsibilities of parents in caring for their children. We have a strong presumption for family autonomy and view court action as an *exceptional* case. So we see retention of the status offender jurisdiction, somewhat modified, reflected in the Task Force's summary statement in an earlier section, as preservative of the family's interests and strengthening of the parent-child bonds. Where there is a choice of coming down on the side of the child or his or her parents, our choice is for the developing child who may need the protection of the state.

As noted many times in this chapter, the juvenile court is the last resort for children and families who have refused or not benefited from community-based voluntary services. Where these services have failed or have proven insufficient, withholding the court's powers is to ignore the court's historic preventive and rehabilitative functions which have been unfairly sullied in the polemics. We can document over and over again that where there has been a commitment to comprehensive systematic services, there are remarkable records of success with young people who were referred to the courts (98). The public has unknowingly and wrongly ascribed the paucity and ineffectiveness of these services to the juvenile court. Such comprehensive services are usually beyond the command of the court and rest within other state departments. Thus the court's treatment function is closely tied to services outside of its control. Even advanced states lack the array of programs essential to satisfy the critical needs of these youngsters and the court is often hard-pressed to make a constructive disposition. It is beyond belief that eliminating the status offender jurisdiction will compel the states to develop resources to address these youngsters.*

The argument set forth by some that the very existence of the court and its allied facilities has stunted the growth of community resources is specious. Judges have been outspoken leaders in pleading with legislatures for funds and community programs based upon their documented experience. They have failed in their quest because the poor and the young have no political power and faith in rehabilitation has declined. To eliminate the court's jurisdiction over those youngsters in need is to ensure that they will be society's victims, unprepared to survive. With elimination of the jurisdiction, will the state invest in enough residential and outpatient psychiatric care, independent living arrangements, vocational training, day treatment programs, which include education, recreation, drug and alcohol counseling? Will the state awaken interests, nurture talent and provide occupational opportunity? Will the state and the community voluntary agencies orchestrate competitive planning and programs and increase needed comprehensive services for these youngsters? Presently, we think not.

REFERENCES

1. *Hawaii* v. *Standard Oil Co.*, 405 U.S. 251, 257, 1971.
2. *Mormon Church* v. *United States*, 136 U.S. 1, 57-58, 1899.
3. Fox, S. J. (1970). Juvenile Justice Reform: An Historical Perspective. *Stanford Law Rev.*, Vol. 22, No. 6, June.
4. TEITELBAUM, L. & HARRIS, L. (1977). Some Historical Perspectives on Governmental Regulation of Children and Parents. In *Beyond Control: Status Offenders in the Juvenile Court*, L. Teitelbaum and A. Gough (Eds.). Cambridge: Ballinger Publishing Co., pp. 1-35.
5. PLATT, A. M. (1969). *The Child Savers*. Chicago: University of Chicago Press.
6. ORLANDO, F. A. (1977). The Juvenile Court and the Status Offender: A Dilemma. Paper Presented at Panel *Child Psychiatry Views the Status Offender*, American Academy of Child Psychiatry, St. Louis, Missouri, October 23.

* An inexact but instructive parallel is seen in the deinstitutionalization of adult psychiatric patients. The dumping of patients into communities was justified on the grounds of cost-effectiveness, restoration of legal rights and an opportunity for increased patient autonomy and independence. The rehabilitation failures in the psychiatric hospitals were geometrically increased by the states promising but utterly failing to provide resources in the communities. Freed from institutionalization, the patients have been led into new prisons of exploitation and despair. State auditors report savings to the legislatures; the departments of mental health report the disappearance of "cases" in the community. The same balletic sequence has been seen in status offender deinstitutionalization in Florida with the apparent disappearance of 18,000 cases from the court. But deinstitutionalized children and adolescents are surfacing in neglect and abuse cases and the child welfare system rolls.

7. STILLER, S. & ELDER, C. (1974). PINS: A Concept in Need of Supervision. *Am. Crim. Law Rev.*, Vol. 12, No. 1, p. 33, Summer.

8. *Report on Deinstitutionalization of Status Offenders Project,* State of Connecticut, Department of Children and Youth Services, October 11, 1978.

9. MACK, J. (1909). The Juvenile Court. *Havard Law Rev.*, Vol. 23, No. 2, pp. 104, 107, 119-120, December.

10. *Commonwealth* v. *Fisher,* 213 Pa. 48,62 A.H. 198,200, 1905.

11. RECTOR, M. (1970). Statement Before U.S. Senate Sub-Committee to Investigate Juvenile Delinquency. *Crime and Delinquency,* Vol. 16, pp. 93, 96.

12. *Kent* v. *United States,* 383 U.S. 541, 556, 1966.

13. *In re Gault,* 387 U.S. 1, 1967.

14. HUFFORD, H. & BIRDSALL, W. (1974). Juvenile Justice in Arizona. *Arizona Law Rev.*, Vol 16, No. 2, pp. 247-263.

15. ORLANDO, F. & BLACK, J. (1974). Classification in Juvenile Court: The Delinquent Child and the "Child in Need of Supervision." *Juvenile Justice,* p. 15, May.

16. GOLDSTEIN, J., FREUD, A., & SOLNIT, A. (1973). *Beyond the Best Interests of the Child.* New York: The Free Press, p. 8.

17. WHEELER, S. & COTTRELL, L. (1966). *Juvenile Delinquency, Its Prevention and Control.* New York: Russell Sage Foundation, pp. 22-27.

18. CULBERTSON, R. (1975). The Effect of Institutionalization on the Delinquent Inmate's Self-Concept. *J. Crim. L. and C.,* Vol. 66, p. 88.

19. MAHONEY, A. (1974). The Effect of Labelling on Youths in the Juvenile Justice System: A Review of the Evidence. *Law and Soc. Rev.,* Vol. 8, No. 4, p. 583, Summer.

20. THOMAS, C. (1977). *The Effect of Legal Sanctions on Juvenile Delinquency.* A Comparison of the Labelling and Deterrence Perspectives. Bowling Green: Bowling Green State University, October, p. 136.

21. KLEIN, M. (1976). Labelling, Deterrence and Recidivism: A Study of Police Dispositions of Status Offenders. *Social Problems,* Vol. 24, No. 2, p. 301.

22. FOSTER, J., DIMITZ, S., & RECKLESS, W. (1972). Perceptions of Stigma Following Public Intervention for Delinquent Behavior. *Social Problems,* Vol. 20, No. 2, p. 205.

23. Uniform Juvenile Court Act 2 (4) (1968).

24. BURKHART, K. (1975). *The Child and the Law—Helping the Status Offender.* Public Affairs Committee, Pamphlet No. 530.

25. GOUGH, A. (1977). Beyond-Control Youth in the Juvenile Court—The Climate for Change. In *Beyond Control: Status Offenders in the Juvenile Court,* L. Teitelbaum and A. Gough (Eds.). Cambridge: Ballinger Publishing Co., pp. 275-276.

26. *Gesicki* v. *Oswald,* 336 F. Supp. 371 (S.D.N.Y. 1971, off'd *Oswald* v. *Gesicki,* 406 U.S. 913) (1972).

27. 416 U.S. 918, 1974.

28. Institute of Judicial Administration/American Bar Association Juvenile Justice Standards Project. *Standards Relating to Noncriminal Misbehavior.* Introduction, p. 11, (hereinafter cited as IJA/ABA Standards).

29. *Robinson* v. *California,* 370 U.S. 660, 1972.

30. ARTHUR, L. (1977). Status Offenders Need a Court of Last Resort. *Boston University Law Rev.,* Vol. 57, No. 4, pp. 641-643, July.

31. GOLDSTEIN, J. (1976). On Being an Adult in Secular Law. In *American Civilization: New Perspectives, Daedalus, Journal of the American Academy of Arts and Sciences,* Fall, p. 73.

32. LEMERT, E. (1967). The Juvenile Court—Quest and Realities. In President's Commission on Law Enforcement and Administration of Justice, *Report of the*

Task Force on Juvenile Delinquency: Delinquency and Youth Crime, pp. 91, 93.

33. NATIONAL COUNCIL ON CRIME AND DELINQUENCY. (1975). Jurisdiction Over Status Offenses Should Be Removed from the Juvenile Court. *Crime and Delin.*, Vol. 21, p. 97.

34. ERIKSON, E. (1968). *Identity: Youth and Crisis.* New York: W. W. Norton Co., p. 132.

35. BAZELON, D. (1970). Beyond Control of the Juvenile Court. *Juv. Ct. Judges.*, Vol. 21, p. 44, Summer.

36. KETCHAM, O. (1977). Why Jurisdiction Over Status Offenders Should Be Eliminated from Juvenile Courts. *Boston University Law Rev.*, Vol. 57, No. 4, p. 653 (footnote 27), June. *Compare with IJA/ABA Standards.* Introduction, p. 18.

37. ARTHUR, L. (1977). Should Status Offenders Go To Court? In *Beyond Control: Status Offenders in the Juvenile Court*, L. Teitelbaum and A. Gough (Eds.). Cambridge: Ballinger Publishing Co., pp. 238-239.

38. *Report of the California Assembly Interim Committee on Criminal Procedure.* (1971). Juvenile Court Processes.

39. *Report of the California Assembly Select Committee on Juvenile Violence.* (1974). Juvenile Violence, pp. 56-57.

40. National Council of Juvenile Court Judges. *Juvenile Court Newsletter*, p. 2, July, 1975.

41. POLIER, J. W. (1975). Future of the Juvenile Court. *Juvenile Justice*, Vol. 26, No. 2, pp. 7, 8, May 1.

42. PAULSEN, M. (1966). Juvenile Courts, Family Courts and the Poor Man. *Calif. L. Rev.*, Vol. 54, No. 2, pp. 694-696, May.

43. Connecticut Department of Children and Youth Services. *Deinstitutionalization of Status Offenders Program*, April, 1977.

44. BLACK, D. & REISS, A., JR. (1970). Police Control of Juveniles. *Am. Sociol. Rev.*, Vol. 35, No. 1, pp. 63-77, February.

45. COLLINS, J. P. (1977). *Hearing of the Connecticut Juvenile Justice Commission*, November 22.

46. CHESNEY-LIND, M. (1977). Judicial Paternalism and the Female Status Offender. *Crime and Delin.*, Vol. 23, No. 2, April.

47. BAYH, B. (1977). New Directions for Juvenile Justice. *Trial*, Vol. 13, pp. 20-22, February.

48. *Status Offender Forum*, DSO Project, Connecticut Department of Children and Youth Services, Vol. 1, No. 3, p. 3, 1978.

49. ANDREWS, R. H., JR. & COHN, A. (1974). Ungovernability: The Unjustifiable Jurisdiction. *Yale L.J.*, Vol. 83, No. 7, pp. 1383-1407, June.

50. SACK, H. S. (1977). III. The Status Offender, Task Force on the Juvenile Justice System. *Summary Report of Studies Undertaken 1975-1977.* Connecticut Council of Child Psychiatrists, pp. 16-19.

51. BREEN, III, T. & SERGI, T. (1979). Classification and Incidence of Connecticut Youth Out of School. *Memorandum to the Connecticut Juvenile Justice Commission from the Department of Education*, February 26.

52. YUDIN, L. W., RING, S. I., NOWAKIWSKY, M., & HEINEMANN, S. (1973). School Dropout or College Bound: Study in Contrast. *J. of Ed. Research*, Vol. 67, pp. 87-93.

53. SYKES, G. M. & MATZA, D. (1957). Techniques of Neutralization: A Theory of Delinquency. *American Soc. Rev.*, 22: Vol. 22, No. 6, pp. 664-670, December.

54. LOGAN, C. (1978). *An Evaluation of Connecticut's Deinstitutionalization of Status Offender Project*, University of Connecticut, p. 92, June.

55. SHEDD, M. (1977). Commissioner of Department Education, State of Connecticut, *Hearing of the Connecticut Juvenile Justice Commission*, October 5.

56. National Education Association (1967). *Research Summary 1967-1971*. School Drop-outs. National Education Association, Washington, D.C.

57. DHEW (1974). *Behavioral Patterns in School of Youths 12-17 Years Old*. DHEW publication No. (HRA) 74-1621.

58. JUSTICE, B., JUSTICE, R., & KRAFT, I. A. (1974). Early Warning Signs of Violence. *Am. J. Psychiatry*, Vol. 131, No. 4, pp. 457-459, April.

59. ROBINS, L. N. (1966). *Deviant Children Grown Up*. Baltimore: Williams & Wilkins, 1966.

60. NIELSON, A. & GERBER, D. Psychosocial Aspects of Truancy in Early Adolescence, accepted for publication by *Adolescence*.

61. *Compact Edition of the Oxford English Dictionary*, Vol. II, Oxford University Press, United States: p. 3418, 1971.

62. *Memorandum to the Connecticut Juvenile Justice Commission*, the Department of Education, February 26, 1979.

63. *Newsweek*, p. 67, October 11, 1976.

64. SACKS, H. S. (1976). Suspension and Expulsion of Students. *Report of the Connecticut Juvenile Justice Commission*, December 1.

65. *New Haven Advocate*, Vol. IV, No. 37, p. 8, May 2, 1979.

66. Connecticut General Assembly, Office of Legislative Research, In-School Suspension. *Memorandum to the Connecticut Juvenile Justice Commission*, February 13, 1979.

67. SB 1447, *An Act Concerning In-School Suspensions*, Connecticut General Assembly, March, 1979.

68. AMBROSINO, L. (1971). *Runaways*. Boston: Beacon Press, Dedication page.

69. *Federal Register*, Youth Development Bureau, DHEW, February 23, 1978.

70. *Runaway Youth Act*, 42 USC, 5701-5751, 1974.

71. FEDERAL BUREAU OF INVESTIGATION. *Uniform Crime Reports*, 1976.

72. *Deinstitutionalization of Status Offenders Program Report*, DSO Project, Connecticut Department of Children and Youth Services, p. 11, 1978.

73. MILLER, D. (1976). *Typologies of Runaway Youth Services*. Social and Rehabilitation Service, DHEW.

74. BRENNAN, T., BLANCHARD, F., HOZINGA, D., & DELBERT, E. (1975). *The Incidence and Nature of Runaway Behavior*. Office of the Assistant Secretary for Planning and Evaluation, DHEW May 30.

75. *Information and Data Gathering*. Project on Behalf of Runaway Youth and Their Families, Office of Education, DHEW, 1976.

76. *First Year Report of the National Runaway Switchboard, 1974-1975*. Metrohelp, Chicago, Illinois, December, 1975.

77. BEASER, H. (1975). *The Legal Status of Runaway Youth*. Educational Systems Corporation for the Office of Youth Development, DHEW, April.

78. PALMER, J. A Profile of Runaway Youth. *DHEW Youth Reporter*, pp. 5, 6, March, 1975.

79. Office of Youth and Development, DHEW, *Model Acts for Family Courts and State-Local Children's Programs*, 14-15, 1974.

80. *Juvenile Justice and Delinquency Prevention Act of 1974*, 42 USC 5633(a) (12), Supp. IV, 1974.

81. HALLER, A. (1975). California Runaways. *Hastings, L.J.*, Vol. 26, No. 4, pp. 1013, 1043, February.

82. National Institute for Juvenile Justice and Delinquency Prevention: *Status Report*, August 15, 1975, LEAA, U.S. Department of Justice.

83. 42 USCA 5633A, Cumulative Supp., 1979.

84. TATE, M., BURKE, P., HELM, J., & WHITE, J. *Cost and Service Impacts of Deinsti-tutionalization of Status Offenders in Ten States: Responses to Angry Youth.* Arthur D. Little, Inc., Washington, D.C., October, 1977.

85. *A Policy Paper on the Proposed Revision of Status Offense Legislation.* Con-necticut Justice Commission and the Department of Children and Youth Services (DCYS), December 12, 1978.

86. S.B. 1619, *An Act Concerning Families With Service Needs.* Connecticut General Assembly, January, 1979. With the passage of the bill by the General Assembly, the law is now identified as 79-567.

87. TATE, M. *Connecticut: A Case Study of Deinstitutionalization of Status Offenders.* Arthur D. Little, Inc., Washington, D.C., August, 1977.

88. *Juvenile Court Annual Report,* State of Connecticut, Judicial Department, 1976.

89. *American Psychiatric Association Response to Juvenile Justice Standards Project of the Institute of Judicial Administration/American Bar Association,* Ad Hoc Task Force of the American Psychiatric Association Council on Children, Adolescents and Their Families, pp. 41-44, April 1, 1978.

90. DERDEYN, A. (1979). *The Juvenile Justice Standards Project: Issues and a Critique, Brief Summary,* Ad Hoc Task Force of the American Psychiatric Association Council on Children, Adolescents and Their Families, pp. 5-6, (unpublished).

91. GREENHOUSE, L. "Pragmatism" Brings Changes in the Juvenile Justice System. *New York Times,* News of the Week in Review, p. 4, February 18.

91a. GREENHOUSE, L. Bar Group Opposes Plan to End Court Role for Problem Chil-dren. *New York Times,* February 5, 1980, p. A18.

92. RAY, I. (1838). *A Treatise on the Medical Jurisprudence of Insanity.* Boston: Little Brown.

93. FREUD, S. (1916). *Some Character Types Met With in Psychoanalytic Work, II. Those Wrecked By Success,* Standard Edition XIV. London: Hogarth, 1957, pp. 316-332.

94. HOOD, R. G. (1967). Research on the Effectiveness of Punishments and Treatments. In *Collected Studies in Criminologic Research,* Vol. 1. Strasbourg: Council of Europe, pp. 74-102.

95. LIPTON, D., MARTINSON, R., & WILKS, J. (1975). *The Effectiveness of the Correctional Treatment: A Survey of Treatment Evaluation Studies.* New York: Praeger, 1975.

96. *A Working Party of the American Friends Service Committee Struggle for Justice.* American Friends Service Committee. New York: Hill & Wang, 1971.

97. WOLFGANG, M., FIGLIO, R., & SELLIN, T. (1972). *Delinquency in a Birth Cohort.* Chicago: University of Chicago Press.

98. WOLFF, E. & FISHER, B. Letter: On Juvenile Justice. Still Hoping for Rehabilita-tion. *New York Times,* p. A-18, March 12, 1979.

13

THE JUVENILE MURDERER

THEODORE A. PETTI, M.D.

Few childhood disorders are as disturbing to the general public or to mental health workers as the truly homicidal school-age child. The incidence of attempted and completed homicide by children and young adolescents is difficult to determine because many homicidal incidents go unreported or are treated as accidents (18).

THEORIES AND TYPOLOGIES

Various reviews (2, 29) and case reports (5, 10, 12) have cited a variety of etiological factors that result in the homicidal act committed by children; most describe the social and psychic lives of such children, but few agree upon any set of predictive criteria (23). The majority of reports and case histories in the literature refer to the violent adolescent (9, 17, 19, 27, 28, 29).

The few works that deal with the homicidal five- to 12-year-olds attribute causality to a wide spectrum of socioeconomic, psychosocial, and cognitive disturbances which include: normal children who unintentionally kill another child in the course of play or mischief; the normal child who only means to hurt or punish the murder victim; the child who feels no other recourse but to kill a frustrating person and is acting from a sense of hopelessness and helplessness; the child who has experienced violence from early childhood and is only acting on what he/she has seen or been taught; the child who projects his/her aggressive feelings onto another person to protect his/her own fragile ego and then acts out of fear; the child who feels the need to kill in order to gratify the needs and impulses of others, as an agent to provide vicarious pleasure or relief from a distressing situation for an adult; and the child with severe developmental deviations and organic, borderline or psychotic disorders (23).

194

Bender and Curran report that death caused by the first eight homicidal children they studied was always accidental and unexpected by the child (5). In studying an additional 26 cases, Bender noted the following necessary configuration to be present for a homicidal action: 1) a disturbed, poorly controlled, impulsive child; 2) a victim who serves as an irritant; 3) absence of a supervisory person who could have stopped the action; and 4) availability of a lethal weapon (4). Bromberg describes seven child and adolescent killers and reemphasizes Bender's point, that the murder is never premeditated and usually follows an event marked by envy, frustration, or humiliation (6). Bromberg relates the act to the "play experience" nature of the urge and attempts to draw an association to motoric expression of anxiety by both hyperkinetic children and adolescent delinquents.

Paluszny and McNabb relate the therapeutic progress of a six-year-old girl who killed her younger sib by severely banging her head against the floor (21). Prior aggressive behavior toward the sib had occurred, but the mother left the two unattended for a prolonged period. Psychological testing demonstrated ego disruption and regression into themes of violence, rejection, and brutalization. The four necessitites for successful homicide hypothesized by Bender were present.

Bender lists six dangerous psychiatric symptoms which should alert the clinician, particularly if they occur in combination: 1) organic brain damage with an impulse disorder, or abnormal EEG and seizures, 2) childhood psychosis with preoccupation with death and killing in mid latency or with antisocial paranoid preoccupations in later childhood, 3) compulsive fire setting, 4) reading disability, 5) severely deviant home and life experiences, 6) a personal experience with violent death (3). The latter two factors are frequently referred to as major contributing conditions (18, 28). Easson and Steinhilber note that the approval of violence may have been just as critical for the eight murderous latency and adolescent boys they describe, as the actual exposure to physical violence (10). In two studies, violence, child abuse, and neglect perpetrated by care givers were prominent in the history of potential and real child killers (21, 30).

Murder attempted or committed in an effort to gratify the wishes of others is frequently attributed as an etiologic agent in violent aggression (10, 15). Esquirol in the early 19th century described the active attempts of a seven-year-old girl at murdering her mother; her grandparents were the instigators (10). Tooley describes two "small assassins," a boy and a girl, six years of age who acted out their mother's unconscious murderous wishes and needs. Both the children and their mothers perceived the younger sibs as a disruptive psychic burden to the emotional well-being of the homes. Getting rid of the unwanted sib meant reunion or a more favorable position with the favored family member (30). A similar dynamic operated in the case of the 14-year-old boy who killed his mother in order to get closer to his father (27).

Sargent (26) utilizes the concept of superego lacunae developed by Johnson (16) to explain the homicidal acts committed by nine children referred for court action in a period of one year. He elaborates on a hypothesis that the murderous child acts as the lethal arm of an adult (usually a parent) who unconsciously urges the child on to murder in order to vicariously derive pleasure from the occurrence. He suggests that the adult fosters the latent hostility the child feels toward the victim, and that the success of this prodding is dependent on the immaturity of the child's ego and the child's special psychic tie to the unconsciously vengeful adult. A recent case of attempted murder of his father by a 10-year-old boy nicely illustrates this hypothesis (31).

Fear of the intended victim is another precipitant to homicidal behavior. Frequently this fear turns to terror and a sense of hopelessness ensues as nonviolent efforts fail (9). King relates the constant reference of nine homicidal youths, average age 14 years, to feeling that their social environment was both hostile and unpredictable (17). Expecting to be harmed in any social contact, they anticipated the hostile behavior of others and then acted precipitantly.

An excerpt from the psychological test results of a 15-year-old murderer helps illustrate this factor: "His general feeling of hopelessness out of which stems his attitude of not caring what happens to him results in his conviction that it is impossible to receive or to obtain from his environment enough support to sustain him in life" (29, p. 313). The murderous act is hypothesized as an ego failure, which, though superficially incongruous with the rest of his life, is really a defense against psychic disintegration. Heacock asserts that the primary drive expressing aggression and vengeance in deprived children is an effort toward mastery which is born from the frustration, helplessness, and humiliation of that deprivation (14). Rothenberg notes that arguments have been made that when a culturally prescribed goal or need is incompatible with the ability to achieve it, a condition of normlessness ensues, with a feeling that socially unapproved behaviors are the necessary tools to effect those needs, and that socially isolated people, when convinced of their isolation, become "apathetic, ignorant, and/or volatile" (25).

Major emphasis on the violent individual's sense of hopelessness and helplessness has been depicted for adolescents (19, 27) and adults (1). The concept of the helplessness, fear and a lack of control over his destiny has been related to the perception of an external locus of control by Petti and Davidman as differentiating homicidal from other behaviorally deviant children (23).

The case cited by Petti and Davidman of one child of nine who not only actively contemplated, planned and attempted to kill another individual but actually succeeded in this endeavor demonstrates this concept of "nothing left, but . . . murder." Each of the nine children were matched to similarly deviant children for sex, age (72-138) months and IQ (73-109) and differed significantly only in their cognitive style. As a group, they perceived themselves as significantly less in control of their destiny than the matched controls. There was no significant difference in race, national background, birth order, type home, history of child abuse, pre- and perinatal or psychiatric problems, or family history of psychiatric disorder. The failure of the other eight children to be successful killers was due to the weapon being insufficiently lethal, the child lacking adequate strength, or a supervisory person appearing to terminate or interrupt the attempt. One of the eight children became frightened of what he was doing and aborted the homicidal act himself (23).

Zients and Zenoff relate the behavior of older children and adolescents under 16 who have killed to the degree of intrapsychic structuralization (32). On one end of this continuum exist youngsters who have an undifferentiated intrapsychic structure, are narcissistic, nonempathic, impulsive and deficient in synthetic and integrative functions. Conflict is experienced in response to environmental frustration. On the other end of the continuum, Zients and Zenoff found youngsters who were psychologically more sophisticated with a differentiated intrapsychic structure but with major sexual identity conflicts. The latter group often showed subtle effeminate characteristics, were often taunted, and hence, felt the need to react aggressively to counteract their propensity to passivity in order to maintain their sense of masculinity. They needed to use a weapon to diminish their intense anxiety. These children were favorites of teachers and adults but not accepted by their peers. This fact, plus the disturbing changes engendered by adolescence, is hypothesized in conjunction with conscious homosexual thoughts to push the youngster to a panic state which, in a moment of passion, culminates in the murder. This group comprised six of the 19 children studied.

The seven undifferentiated, nonempathic youthful murderers all had prior histories of assaultive behavior, low-normal to borderline intelligence and lacked the skills to deal with stress. Those murders that did not occur during a robbery were without obvious provocation.

The remaining seven children were designated as "innocent murderers" for whom the act was either the result of an accident or the attempt at self-defense. No significant psychopathology was found in five of these children, one was considered neurotic, and one fit the nonempathic class of intrapsychic development.

ASSESSMENT

The assessment must be comprehensive in evaluating the homicidal child and must recognize that differences exist between children who kill accidentally in play or in self-defense and children who kill as a response to an overwhelming sense of frustration, or who kill as a response to overt and covert messages from meaningful adults. Distinguishing the child with severe characterological or other developmental deviation who kills from other violent children is also important. The evaluation must also recognize that the child who plans and carries out a homicidal attempt differs from those who are unsuccessful only as related to the presence of a supervisory person and insufficient lethality of his/her methods.

Assessment of the degree of depression, anxiety, and alienation and also the evolving character structure is critical for determining therapeutic interventions and for making recommendations to the court (11). The family must also be evaluated regarding their contribution to the total picture (13). Areas that demand exploration include parenting skills, family interaction relationships and community support systems. These areas are often pivotal and require diligent investigation.

A detailed developmental, social, medical and educational history from both the child and his/her parents is critical in highlighting areas of past and present dysfunction. A complete physical and neurological examination in conjunction with this history is helpful in differentiating the child with an organic problem, including episodic dyscontrol and a clear seizure disorder, from the psychotic child or the child with developing characterologic problems. A thorough psycho-educational battery is essential for determining cognitive capacities, delineating areas of inadequate functioning and, through projective testing, for illuminating dynamic factors. This is unfortunately an area which is often overlooked, and superficial appearances of competence and a tough veneer hinder adequate evaluation and treatment.

Defining the type of intrapsychic structure and determining the degree of empathy are also crucial for assessing the potential for rehabilitating the youthful murderer and predicting future dangerousness (32).

The child who "accidently" kills must be evaluated as comprehensively as those whose murderous act falls under another etiologic category to determine the effect of the death and subsequent court, family and community responses (22, 24, 32). Except for victims of the nonempathic murderer described by Zients and Zenoff, the deceased is often a close associate or relative, and the ensuing guilt, depression, and family/community responses must be assessed as they will be important in future efforts at intervention and prevention of unnecessary, destructive sequellae.

INTERVENTION

The specific therapeutic strategies for the homicidal child depend mainly on whether the homicide has been completed and on the dynamics of the individual case.

Jail is never the answer! Since incarceration only provides a time-limited external set of restraints, once those restraints are lifted, earlier dynamics come to the fore and a potential agent for further violence is released (17). Short-term hospitalization is generally helpful in sorting out the pieces and instituting appropriate interventions.

It is important that court involvement, whether required or desirable, be expedited as quickly as feasible. The anxiety of a court hearing and the uncertainty of outcome can contribute much to deviant behavior and hamper the expeditious inception of therapy and dispostional planning. The child should be prepared for the process by using language that is comprehensible, should have his apprehensions explored, and should be encouraged to role play if this proves necessary (24, 32).

Extensive work with the family or care givers who will ultimately be responsible for the child must be started immediately and be continued through the time after the child is returned to a home setting. This includes supportive work around the issues of having a homicidal child, assisting the parents in understanding the forces leading the child to a homicidal posture and training them, when necessary, in appropriate parenting skills. For the child who has accidentally killed, support to the family in dealing with community reactions, helping them through their own reactions to the death, and assisting them to make the necessary changes for their child to deal with the death and the continuation of life need to be provided (8, 11, 24).

Harbin describes a successful family therapy approach for the adolescent with episodic dyscontrol (13). He illustrates two typical family patterns, emphasizing the importance of family as well as individual dynamics, and details the utility of such an approach, particularly when the violence is directed toward a family member. An active and directive approach is advocated by Harbin to change the violent behavior through a shift in the family structure. By systematizing the family's response to violent behavior, including calling the police for instance, he hopes to decrease the family's fear, open communication between the family and the youngster, clarify generational boundaries, and lessen the adolescent's fear of losing control. Once this is accomplished, communication problems and other family dynamics can be addressed in therapy. A major goal with this approach is again making the violent youngsters responsible for their actions. This is especially true for the individual with seizures or organic abnormalities.

For the children who have an organic basis for their homicidal behavior, appropriate medical and possible behavioral treatment should be instituted promptly (13). For those who are psychotic, appropriate psychotherapy and medication should be individualized for the child's needs. Antidepressant medication is often very useful in providing the child, in a state of clinical depression, the means to benefit more fully from other therapeutic modalities (22, 23, 24).

For both the juvenile and the adult killer, the development of a sense of control over, and responsibility for, his/her destiny may be of pivotal importance. King relates the need for a two-pronged approach of academic education and training in the "legitimate operations of feelings" as one way of completing this task. The training of psycho-educational skills provides mastery over elementary symbols and decreases the glaring educational deficits most of the children demonstrate (17). Cognitive training provides the tools for sequencing thought rather than action after an emotional feeling, thus providing the child with a sense of mastery over what had formerly been a frustrating, unpredictable and frightening world. Specific methods of effecting these changes are more fully described elsewhere (22, 24) as is a rationale for justifying this type of extensive intervention (23).

Finally, for many homicidal children, the home environment is so destructive in a multitude of ways that placement away from home is desirable or necessary (8, 18, 23, 26). The placement should be structured but not simply for purposes of containment. It should have the facilities to provide a therapeutically socially and educationally enriching environment to allow the child to develop a greater sense of mastery over his environment and of responsibility for his life. The child who is prone to homicidal or violent actions must learn to perceive outcomes as personally determined to a significant degree and to develop the skills to function effectively in stressful situations. The dynamics described for the juvenile murderer have recently been described in an analogous way for young—ages 15-23—male murderers (7). To counteract a youth killing again, we must provide a warm, accepting environment which will nurture the youth's sense of responsibility for himself and his future. We must, however, recognize the differences between the various types of killers and gauge the degree of structure and intensity of treatment to the needs of the child.

It is clear that the nonempathic killer described by Zients and Zenoff (32), and the hardened adolescent require a more secured setting than does the child who kills for other reasons (17). Since many homicidal children are placed away from home for months and sometimes years, the family also needs assistance in reassimilation of their child back into the home.

COURT TESTIMONY

In the author's experience with the juvenile murderer under 13 years of age, the court is more interested in what can be done for the child and his/her family than in punishing the act. However, this is not a universal experience (32). Testimony should be clear and precise. A diagnosis with qualifiers is necessary to put the problem within a contextual framework. Often, explicating material is requested to describe what may have led to the homicidal action and to depict how such a situation might be prevented in the future. Zients and Zenoff stress the point that the court needs to be provided the data which can assist them to place the child within a context that elucidates the complexities of growth and development as they relate to the child's situation (32). This is particularly true for the adolescent who uses suppression and denial as a means to deal with his role in the death. Requests for dispositional recommendations are a high priority and the psychiatrist must be prepared to present a list of alternatives ranging from the ideal to the barely acceptable. For families with marginal histories of compliance with professional recommendations, extended involvement of the court as an overseer can prove to be a great asset in assuring compliance in an ongoing therapeutic program (24).

Markus and Cormier advocate maintaining adolescent murderers within the social welfare court in Canada to allow the youth sufficient support to be released to society by 21 years of age (20). They also opine that adjudicating the older adolescent as an adult with a long prison sentence deprives him of the normal experiences of youth, causing a loss of both adolescence and early manhood, and creates an overwhelming and stressful situation for him when he is released.

In summary, the child needs an advocate in court who can assist in constructive planning for his/her future. The child psychiatrist must impress the court with the psychic and social life of the youthful offender as a process rather than allow it to be frozen at the time of the lethal event.

REFERENCES

1. ABRAHAMSEN, D. (1973). *The Murdering Mind*. New York: Harper & Row.
2. ADAMS, K. A. (1974). The Child Who Murders. *Criminal Justice & Behav.*, 1:51-61.
3. BENDER, L. (1959). Children and Adolescents Who Have Killed. *Am. J. Psych.*, 116:510-513.
4. BENDER, L. (1974). Aggression in Children. *Research Publication Association For Research in Nervous & Mental Disorders*, 52:201-208.
5. BENDER, L. & CURRAN, F. J. (1940). Children and Adolescents Who Kill. *J. Crim. Psychopathol.*, 1:296-322.
6. BROMBERG, W. (1961). *The Mold of Murder*. New York: Grune & Stratton.
7. BROWN, S. (1978). The Violent Patient: Assessment and Management. Paper presented at The Annual Meeting of the California Medical Association, in *Audio Digest* 7, No. 8.
8. CAREK, D. J. & WATSON, A. S. (1964). Treatment of a Family Involved in Fratricide. *Arch. Gen. Psych.*, 11:533-542.
9. DUNCAN, J. W. & DUNCAN, G. M. (1971). Murder in the Family. *Amer. J. Psych.*, 127:1498-1502.
10. EASSON, W. M. & STEINHILBER, R. M. (1961). Murderous Aggression by Children and Adolescents. *Arch. Gen. Psych.*, 4:1-9.
11. FOODMAN, A. & ESTRADA, C. (1977). Adolescents Who Commit Accidental Homicide: The Emotional Consequences to the Individual, Family and Community. *J. Amer. Acad. Child Psych.*, 16:314-326.
12. GARDINER, M. (1976). *The Deadly Innocents*. New York: Basic Books, Inc.
13. HARBIN, H. (1977). Episodic Dyscontrol and Family Dynamics. *Am. J. Psych.*, 134:113-116.
14. HEACOCK, D. R. (1976). The Black Slum Child and the Problem of Aggression. *Am. J. Psychoanal.*, 36:219-226.
15. HELLSTEN, P. & KATILA, O. (1965). Murder and Other Homicide by Children Under 15 in Finland. *Psych. Quart. Supp.*, 39:54-74.
16. JOHNSON, A. (1949). Sanctions for Superego Lacunae of Adolescents. In: *Searchlights*

on *Delinquency*, K. R. Eissler (Ed.). New York: International Universities Press, 225-234.

17. KING, C. H. (1975). The Ego and the Integration of Violence in Homicidal Youth. *Am. J .Orthopsych.*, 45:134-145.
18. MACDONALD, J. M. (1961). *The Murderer and His Victim.* Springfield: Charles C Thomas.
19. MALMQUIST, C. P. (1971). Premonitory Signs of Homicidal Aggression in Juveniles. *Am. J. Psych.*, 128:461-465.
20. MARKUS, B. & CORMIER, B. M. (1977). A Preliminary Study of Adolescent Murderers. Paper presented at the 27th Annual Meeting of the Canadian Psychiatric Association, Saskatoon.
21. PALUSZNY, M. & MCNABB, M. (1975). Therapy of a 6-Year-Old Who Commits Fratricide. *J. Am. Acad. Child Psych.*, 14:319-336.
22. PETTI, T. A. (1979). Three Types of Children Who Kill. In Preparation.
23. PETTI, T. A. & DAVIDMAN, L. (1977). Homicidal School-Age Children. Paper presented at the American Academy of Child Psychiatry 29th Annual Meeting, Houston, Texas.
24. PETTI, T. A. & WELLS, K. (1978). Crisis Treatment of a Preadolescent Who Accidentally Killed His Twin. Paper presented at the American Academy of Child Psychiatry 30th Annual Meeting, San Diego, California.
25. ROTHENBERG, P. (1968). *Locus of Control, Social Class, and Risk Taking in Negro Boys.* Ann Arbor: University Microfilms, Inc.
26. SARGENT, D. (1962). Children Who Kill. *Social Work,* 7:35-42.
27. SCHERL, D. J. & MACK, J. E. (1966). A Study of Adolescent Matricide. *J. Am. Acad. Child Psychiat.*, 5:559-593.
28. SENDI, I. B. & BLOMGREN, P. G. (1975). A Comparative Study of Predictive Criteria in the Predisposition of Homicidal Adolescents. *Am. J. Psych.*, 132:423-427.
29. SMITH, S. (1965). The Adolescent Murderer. *Arch. Gen. Psych.*, 13:310-319.
30. TOOLEY, K. (1975). The Small Assassins. *J. Am. Acad. Child Psych.*, 14:306-318.
31. TUCKER, L. S. & CORNWALL, T. P. (1977). Mother-Son Folie à Deux. *Am. J. Psych.*, 134:1146-1147.
32. ZIENTS, A. B. & ZENOFF, E. H. (1977). The Juvenile Murder. Paper presented at the American Academy of Child Psychiatry 29th Annual Meeting, Houston, Texas.

Part IV
SPECIAL ISSUES

14

THE CHILD AS A WITNESS

LENORE C. TERR, M.D.

An interesting and up to now neglected function of the child psychiatrist is to help the court or the police to qualify a child as a witness to a crime or to an act of negligence or fault. To date, no reports appear in the psychiatric literature on this subject. There are a few striking literary examples of children who purposely or inadvertently bear false witness with tragic results—Lillian Hellman's "The Children's Hour" (4), Henry James's *The Turn of the Screw* (5), and Arthur Miller's "The Crucible" (8). The girls of "The Children's Hour" and "The Crucible" are motivated to "witness" against others because of vengeance for prior punishments and in order to divert attention from their own misdeeds. Miles's motives for "telling stories" are purposely left vague by Henry James.

This chapter will discuss and provide clinical examples of children who serve as witnesses to crimes against themselves or others and those who witness injury to themselves or others. Two closely related issues will be discussed: competency of children to be witnesses, and the weight given to a child witness' testimony. The legal requirements establishing competency of a child witness will be reviewed. The special functions of the expert child psychiatric witness which enable the court to bypass the child witness's direct testimony will be covered. Particularly regarding the weight given to testimony, those psychic factors which enhance and those which interfere with the child's ability to testify will be reviewed.

The legal requirements for competency of a child to testify and the psychiatric requirements for verification of a child's story are quite different (see Table 1). The law concerns itself with intelligence and an understanding of the moral importance of telling the truth. Psychiatry considers cognitive functioning, defense mechanisms, behavioral reenactments, play, dreams, and consistency as verifications of whether the child saw or experienced what he/she says happened.

TABLE 1

Similarities and Differences at the Interface of Law and Psychiatry Regarding Child Witnesses

Characteristic of Child	Law	Child Psychiatry
1. "Intelligence"	Child must be able to verbalize	Nonverbal child may "show" behaviorally what occurred. "Verbal" child may have no vocabulary for the event which occurred especially if sexual or involving emotions for which the child has no words.
	"Retarded child" can be disqualified	"Retarded child" may verbally or motorically indicate accurately what occurred.
2. Chronological age at time of trial	Age 3 minimum	Infant under 12 months may *behave* in a fashion indicating what occurred.
	Children age 10 or 14 accepted by most states as witnesses without extensive judicial examination	Children *any* age can be witnesses if observations are verbalized, or if "reenactment" interpreted by expert psychiatric witness occurs.
3. Chronological age at time of crime or negligent act	Age at which incident(s) occurred *not* a factor	Age at which incident occurred determines whether memory is "verbalized" or is sensory-motoric.
4. Ability to tell the truth	If a child understands punishments for lying, he will tell the truth	Child will lie regardless of punishments, if there are strong emotional "reasons" for lying, i.e. loyalty conflicts, shame, vengeance, and fear of being blamed or hurt.
5. Accuracy of perception	May be a legal concern in weighing evidence	Child-victim may experience distorted perception during traumatic event leading to inaccuracy as a witness.
6. Verbal consistency and naivete	May be a legal concern in weighing evidence	Over time, a child should tell a story in naive language which varies each time the *same* story is told.
7. Defense of "denial"	Not a legal concern	Traumatized children do not "deny" reality as adults do, and therefore may remember more details of a traumatic event than adults would.

TABLE 1 *(continued)*

Characteristic of Child	Law	Child Psychiatry
8. Loyalty conflicts	Court may consider child a "biased" witness and give less credence to his/her testimony	Food, shelter, and parenting more important to child than violence, therefore child may opt for survival and lie about a violent or sexually abusive parent/guardian. Children may identify with aggressors and attempt to protect a criminal on this basis.

THE LEGAL REQUIREMENTS FOR COMPETENCY OF CHILD WITNESSES

The state laws regarding competency of child witnesses generally deal with the child's ability to understand the facts about which he/she will testify and the child's ability to understand the concept of telling the truth (1). It is the "intelligence," not the age, of the child which is the usual test of competency as a witness. This holds true in both civil and criminal cases. There are exceptions and "fine points" established in certain states. For example, if a child were 12-years-old at the time of trial, but 4-years-old at the time of injury, the question of the child's competency to testify is decided at the time the child is offered as a witness, not at the time when the injury occurred (6). A case with similar court findings in which an 8-year-old girl was declared competent to testify about an injury she sustained at 3 years 3 months is Malchanoff v. Truehart (7).

There is considerable attention in the courts as to whether a child understands what it is to "tell the truth" and what punishments will ensue if he/she does not. It is not necessary for a child to understand the word "oath" (10), nor is it necessary for a child to understand "perjury" (3). There is disagreement in the courts as to whether a child must fear some sort of divine punishment to be qualified as a witness. In State v. Belton (12), a child who had not heard of God was found to be incompetent to serve as a witness, whereas in People v. Zeezich (9) a child witness who had never heard of God was allowed to testify.

The common law presumes that a child over 14 is competent to be a witness and it conversely assumes that under 14 there must be judicial inquiry as to the mental capacity of the child (1). Although no minimum age of competency has been firmly established, in Wheeler v. United States (15) it was noted that "no one would think of calling as a witness an infant only two or three years old." On the other hand, many states have statutes which assert that children under 10 who appear incapable of receiving "just impressions" of the facts about which they are examined, or of relating them "truly," are incompetent to testify (1). California had such a statute until 1967 (2).

The competency of a child to serve as a witness is determined by the trial judge who examines the child without interference from the attorneys. If the judge is satisfied that the child is competent, he/she cannot be forced to submit the child to a commission of medical experts to confirm or reject his decision (13). On the other hand, the opinion of a medical expert may be voluntarily sought by the judge in order to help him/her determine the child's competency. The examination and the discretion whether to ask for medical consultation are solely up to the judge. With or without medical consultation, the judge is required to examine the child in court, not privately, prior to determining the child's competency to testify (16).

In order to satisfy the requirements of the law, the following type of judicial examination of a child might occur. This excerpt is a "typical judicial examination" which was hypothesized in a book aimed at preparing witnesses for trial (11).

Q. [Judge]: How old are you, Matthew?
A. Seven.
Q. Pretty big boy for seven! Do you go to Sunday School?
A. Yes, sir.
Q. What do they teach there?
A. Everything.
Q. Do you know what a lie is?
A. Yes, sir.
Q. What is a lie?
A. If you don't tell the truth.
Q. Good boy! And what happens to little boys who tell lies?
A. You get a sin.
Q. Anything else?
A. And you get punished and you don't go to Heaven.

Rose concludes that "Matthew" successfully qualified as a competent witness by his answers to this judicial examination.

CHILD PSYCHIATRIC EXPERT TESTIMONY WHICH BYPASSES THE CHILD WITNESS'S DIRECT TESTIMONY

On many occasions, the child tells his/her story to the psychiatrist or mental health worker, and in this fashion the child's direct testimony is bypassed. The expert witness tells it "for the child." This is a particularly common practice in custody hearings and child abuse or neglect trials. Because the expert witness is asked to report upon his/her examination as the basis for his/her opinion, the expert may recite the "history" the child told him/her which relates to the psychiatric opinion.

David, age seven, was evaluated in a custody-visitation suit in which his mother claimed that visits with the father caused David to be hyperactive, upset, tearful, and disorganized. In his psychiatric interview, David told me that on visits at his father's home, people came to the house, paid money to his father for "pink powder" and along with his father put the powder into their noses. They used their fingers to sniff the powder. When asked to show the color "pink," David pointed to the white office walls and to a white picture mat. David wished to have more, not fewer, visits with his father. The powder-sniffing was mentioned in passing, as an activity that frequently took place at his father's home. David had no conscious reason to sabotage his paternal visitation. As a matter of fact, he protested that he wished to continue the visits. In David's case the "pink powder" description appeared to me to be valid observation. The naive mistake "pink" ruled out coaching from the mother. Furthermore, when asked, the mother was outraged and shocked about any possible cocaine usage by the father in the presence of the child. The child's description was provided both in my psychiatric courtroom testimony and the psychiatric report. The father was reprimanded by the judge who believed the child's story as reported by the expert psychiatric witness.

Child psychiatrists understand that children may show nonverbally what has caused them anxiety. Even well below the minimum age for legal competency to testify noted in Wheeler v. United States, an infant may illustrate through its actions what it had experienced traumatically. It is the child psychiatrist's function as an expert witness to explain this type of "reenactment" or "traumatic play" (14) behavior to the court.

In one such instance, two infants who obviously were too young to serve as witnesses exhibited signs upon psychiatric evaluation that they had been victims of a satanic ritual. A 15-month-old girl began losing weight and her seven-month-old boy cousin was discovered with a straight, deep clean cut under his foreskin. Both babies acted "fussy" and stopped sleeping. Within a week or two, the 15-month-old girl developed a habit of "sitting" on the seven-month-old's head. Both mothers had used a babysitter, who admitted to them in a letter that he had become involved in satanism. Furthermore, the mothers themselves had been raised by parents who practiced satanic rituals upon them. Sitting on the victim's head, a practice in some satanic rites, had been repeated in action (reenactment) by one of the current victims, a 15-month-old baby. In this case, the very unusual behavior of the toddler could be interpreted to the police by the child psychiatrist. The identity of the perpetrator(s) could not be established by the baby witnesses, but the fact that the infants had indeed been victims had been demonstrated by the infants themselves.

Despite the fact that the child psychiatrist can tell the child's story as part of his or her expert testimony, there are instances in which the child must tell the story for himself or herself, particularly if the child accuses another individual of a crime (murder, rape, kidnapping, assault) or of negligence (when another child or the witness child himself is injured through another's fault). In these instances, a child psychiatrist may be asked to evaluate the child witness for veracity (truthfulness), accuracy of memory, and correctness of the original perception or cognition, but the child himself/herself will be required to "take the stand" and to testify.

FACTORS ENHANCING A CHILD'S COMPETENCY OR BELIEVABILITY AS A WITNESS

When a crime is committed against a child, assuming that the crime is major, such as attempted murder, rape, kidnapping, assault with bodily harm, the psychic mechanisms of immediate response to trauma take place. My study of 23 Chowchilla kidnap victims (14) reveals that the important initial responses of children to psychic trauma were immediate fears of death, separation, and further trauma, retrospective search for omens and portents, misidentification of perpetrators, and/or hallucinations. Later thinking errors exhibited in this group of children were time distortions and additional misidentifications and overgeneralizations. "Reenactment" and "traumatic play" motorically illustrated the type of trauma to which they had been victims. These symptoms can both aid and interfere with the veracity of traumatized children as witnesses.

Reenactments and Play

Children's reenactments and traumatic play are very close to the actual traumatic circumstances to which they were subjected. Their repeated dreams describe the same story which they reiterate to the police and investigators during the day. Verifications for their official statements are found in the nature of their play, reenactments, and repeated dreams. These items are important clues to what actually happened to the child.

In order to illustrate the verification a psychiatrist can glean from reenactment behavior, a nonlegal example follows. Andrew, a 6-year-old part Chicano boy from an economically deprived family, was observed repeatedly placing his toddler brother in a toy chest and shutting the top. Andrew's mother, fearful that he might smother his brother, phoned me. In his psychiatric interview, Andrew was asked, "Did anyone ever put you in a box and frighten you?" "Not a box, a clothes dryer," Andrew replied. "Jeremy [older brother] and his friends bet me five bucks that I could get into a dryer. When I got in, they banged the door shut and left. I thought I would die in there. I punched and punched the door. Almost broke my hand. I screamed. Nobody came. Finally I got out. They never paid me the five bucks!" Andrew had been traumatically frightened by being locked and abandoned in the clothes dryer. His reenactment behavior was the first indication that this had happened. Andrew had never verbalized the incident until asked about it by the psychiatrist.

Absence of "Denial"

The fact that children barely, if at all, employ the defense of "denial" during a trauma, as illustrated by the 23 Chowchilla victims, enables the child to give a complete and detailed picture of what happened to him/her. Even though the child may misperceive *who* did it, and in what order it occurred, all the incidents are remembered. There is no amnesia. In this respect, children make better witnesses than adults who often employ massive denial when traumatized.

Doris was 4 years old when she saw her little brother bouncing up and down on his bed. His bed had been next to the window, and when he stopped bouncing, he stood up to the window, put both hands on it, and looked out. The slum apartment window gave way, fell outwards, and the small boy tumbled out. There was a lawsuit following evidence of the brother's permanent brain damage. Since Doris was the only witness to the fall, her testimony would be a key factor in the upcoming trial. I saw Doris three times prior to the trial, at age eight, age 10, and age 11. On each occasion she provided the same account, although her words (written down each time) varied. She had not memorized something she had been coached to say because: 1) her statements were in child's wording; 2) the wording was different, but the story was the same in three widely spaced interviews; 3) there was verification for her story in her dreams. Doris had *repeated* dreams of a baby falling out of a window, most likely caused by the actual experience, not simply hearing a story. I wrote a letter vouching for Doris' accuracy as a witness, and a large settlement on her brother's behalf ensued shortly thereafter.

Carolyn, who was attacked by a German Shepherd dog, remembers every detail of the traumatic event which occurred when she was seven. Her mother, who pulled the dog off her child's slashed throat, cannot remember how she got the dog off and what she did next. Carolyn remembers exactly what her mother did, and testified about this more accurately in the trial (verified by witnesses) than her mother was able to do. In this instance, as in the Chowchilla kidnapping, the child did not employ the psychological defense of "denial," which accounts for partial "blanking out" or "amnesia" in many traumatized adults.

FACTORS DIMINISHING THE CHILD'S COMPETENCY
OR BELIEVABILITY AS A WITNESS

Perceptual and Cognition Distortion

Distortions in cognitive functioning, i.e., poor time sense, misidentification, hallucination, and overgeneralization, diminish children's accuracy as witnesses. Of 23 child victims interviewed after the kidnapping in Chowchilla, five initially misidentified a kidnapper, three hallucinated an entire scene, and six others eventually formulated theories of a fourth kidnapper at large or believed that they had recently seen one of the kidnappers in a TV show or a movie. These cognitive and perceptual distortions are, in my opinion, one of the primary observable signs of an ego which has been traumatically disrupted. (It is likely that traumatized adults also suffer disordered perceptions when experiencing exceptional fear.)

Benji, 6 years old at the time he was kidnapped in Chowchilla, believed he had seen a "black man" among the individuals who hijacked his school bus. Although months later he lost his conviction that the kidnapper was black, he believed 13 months after the kidnapping that a fourth kidnapper remained at large. In his last interview he asked the author, "Have you noticed a man with a long nose?" Benji knows exactly what was done to him. He remembers the events of the kidnapping and what other children did and said. He elaborates upon what he himself did and said, hoping that he was more heroic than he actually was. He loses his accuracy in the field of perception, the ability to recognize the perpetrators, and in the field of cognition, understanding his own role in the traumatic event. Benji does not lie, or purposely change facts. He distorts the perception of the men themselves because he was so suddenly and intensely frightened when he saw them. He distorts his own role because his true helplessness is unacceptable to him and too remote from his ideals of strength and control to be tolerated.

Loyalty Conflicts

Another factor which may interfere with a child's ability to testify accurately against someone who has harmed him/her is the occasional presence of the defense mechanism "identification with the aggressor." Because the child is severely stressed, any number of defense mechanisms may be elicited, but this particular defense places a child in a loyalty conflict when he/she testifies. Particularly in kidnapping, when the kidnapper has spent time with the child, this mechanism may be observed. Three young boys were taken hostage in their own home and held by an escaped convict for 12 hours until the boys escaped. In interviewing two of the boy victims, the author learned that the kidnapper had confided to his victims a story of lifelong ill treatment and failure. The boys, very open to what they saw and heard because of their extreme anxiety, developed a liking for the criminal. They identified with his years of bad luck and ill treatment, probably through memories of their own unearned punishments and bad luck. (Actually they came from a well adjusted family, but every child feels victimized at times.) Even though they had been held for hours at gunpoint and one of them had been sexually fondled, both boys felt reluctant to face the kidnapper in court and to report what he had done. They referred to the kidnapper by first name and they reported that he is a friend.

Loyalty conflicts are the most intense in children when they have witnessed a crime perpetrated by someone upon whom they are truly dependent for nurturance (life).

An extreme example of such a loyalty conflict is Sarah, who witnessed a scene in which she believed she saw her father murder her mother. She testified against her father, who was subsequently acquitted. After the trial, the child was returned to her father, a situation of helpless dependence upon the very person against whom she had served as a witness.

Family homicides and other family assaults often place a child in the extreme loyalty conflict illustrated above. Life-nurturance vs. accurately testifying against a parent can be a virtually suicidal dilemma. One wonders whether children can testify honestly under such circumstances. Should they be protected against such conflicts by rules such as those adopted in many states providing that a wife cannot be forced to testify against her husband? Medical testimony or other testimony regarding vaginal or rectal tears or the presence of semen may be used to validate incest charges instead of the testimony of the child herself/himself. The type of weapon, time of death, etc. might be employed by police to convict a parent-murderer rather than the "key testimony" of a child witness. Whenever possible such supporting evidence should be used, as opposed to the testimony of the child himself/herself against his/her parent. If the child's story is essential at trial, one wonders if the expert psychiatric testimony which bypasses direct testimony described earlier in this chapter might be preferable to the child's own testimony. This may both protect the child from a potential attack by the parent and/or it may protect the court from a child forced to lie because of fear of parental retribution.

THE CHILD WHO LIES

Lying is not easily detectable by a psychiatrist. Even those psychiatrists who employ hypnosis or sodium amytal interviews believe that an individual who strongly wishes to lie may do so under hypnosis or under the influence of "truth serum."*

How then can a child's story be believed? Even though there is no sure way, some of the following techniques may be helpful: 1) Verification over time. Have the child tell the story in several different interviews. Tape or take written word-for-word notes. The wording should vary, but the child's facts should remain the same. 2) Verification through dreams, reenactment, or traumatic play. These items should repeatedly coincide with the facts the child tells. If a child were a victim or a close observer to a serious crime or act of negligence, the child would be severely stressed and should show one or all of these "traumatic signs." 3) Verification through outside "clues" or facts. Does the individual the child accuses have a record of other such crimes? Did the criminal leave a verifying clue? Not only should there be internal verification within the child, but external verification through police investigation. 4) A history of reliability in the child witness. School records, family history,

---

* Private communication, L. Jolyon West, Professor of Psychiatry, U.C.L.A.

the child's history should be checked for past incidents of lying or cheating.

Two examples will illustrate the problem of lying. Andrea, age 14, was accused by her best friend, Arlene, also age 14, of murdering four of Arlene's relatives in a mass murder. Arlene also accused her male cousin, Harvey, age 19, and her cousin's girlfriend, Susie, age 14, of joining in the murder. Arlene had "kept quiet" about the entire crime for four months until a series of dreams caused her to go to the police, who up to then had few, if any, clues. Arlene's story under hypnosis was consistent with her dreams. It was consistent with Harvey's history (both of Harvey's parents had died mysteriously, very possibly murders), and with Susie's history (Susie had been extremely rebellious, a runaway, school truant, aggressive, and promiscuous). Arlene's story, however, was not at all consistent with Andrea's history. Andrea had been a good student, reliable member of her school, good daughter to her mother, and an unusually easy to handle and flexible member of the juvenile detention home facility, once she was confined there. Andrea had had no contact with Harvey and Susie except in Arlene's company. The police found a few clues linking Andrea to the dead family. (A pillow case in Andrea's home belonged to a murder victim, but Andrea insisted it had been given to her. Andrea's ring was found in the bedroom of the dead family, but she had visited there many times.) On the basis of Arlene's very strong testimony, Harvey and Susie were convicted of murder and Andrea was found to be an accessory to murder.

In this instance there was no psychiatric evidence that Andrea could have been involved in this incident. She had no rage, no anger at her own family or at school or society at large. There was no thinking defect. She had no memory of any such event. Although a psychiatrist is not in a position to prove innocence, Andrea lacked any of the qualities a professional would have expected in a mass murderer. On the other hand, Arlene's key witnessing seemed suspect. She had caused several teenage workers to be fired the previous summer by "telling a tale" about some teenage infighting to the work supervisors. It was Arlene, not Andrea, who had had a strong relationship with Harvey and Susie. It was Arlene who had withheld the story for four months until her dreams sent her to the police.

Because the supporting evidence was far stronger in Arlene's accusations of Harvey and Susie, they were both convicted of murder. The juvenile court judge who heard Andrea's case convicted her of being an accessory and set a light sentence. Most likely his response was similar to the author's, because Arlene's veracity as a witness against her "best friend" could not be fully established.

The second example of questionable child witnessing is the case of 11-year-old Serena whose cousin Adele, also 11, was strangled. Serena and Adele had left a Little League game and they were attempting to find a stray cat Serena had previously spotted in the underbrush near the baseball field. When they found the cat, Adele asked Serena to buy cat food while she watched the kitten. Serena was delayed getting money and when she returned, Adele was gone. Adele's body was later discovered in the same spot the girls had originally found the cat. Serena testified to the police that she had seen a neighbor teenage boy, Jim, pass by about three times before and after she left Adele to get the cat food. The police, who had no other clues, began questioning the boy intensively. Jim had been known as an outstanding student, reliable worker, and a morally upright individual.

Serena was seen for three psychiatric interviews within one week. In each succeeding interview, the story of seeing Jim became more and more vague. In asking Serena to go over the story again she could not be sure from which direction Jim had come, whether by foot, car, or bicycle, or whether he had been there at all. At first, Serena recalled he had said "hi" and on another occasion he had said "Don't tell anyone I was here." Later she could not recall what he had said. Finally she admitted that she could not be sure she had seen or spoken to Jim at all.

Serena had a history of lying in the past. She experienced a series of dreams during the first week post murder relating to being strangled herself. There was no identifiable strangler in the dreams. Jim was not present in any of her dreams. Serena had been psychically traumatized by her cousin's murder. She identified with the murder victim, as evident in her dreams. She was most anxious, too anxious to be helpful, to find the perpetrator. She hoped that she could aid her aunt and uncle's family by being the "key witness." Furthermore, she felt guilty for leaving Adele alone, and she had lied on previous occasions when she felt guilty or accused. In Serena's case, her account of Jim's involvement was not internally consistent, nor did it correspond with external "clues." The investigation of Jim was terminated and the case remains unsolved.

THE CHILD WITNESS WHO CANNOT OR WILL NOT SPEAK

Nonverbal infant witnesses may illustrate what happened to them through their behavior. The example of the two babies who underwent satanic rituals illustrates how a child psychiatrist can interpret infant behavior to police investigators. In this way, the child psychiatrist may be able to put words into infants' nonverbal experiences.

There are instances in which a verbal child does not have the words to describe an experience or crime. This often applies to a crime or incident involving sex practices or sexual anatomy for which the child knows no words. Many children do not know the words for their sexual anatomy, and are embarrassed and/or inaccurate in their use of "street language." Most street language is learned through common child usage, and often conveys inaccurate information about explicit sexual practices.

Jennifer was nine when she stepped over an out-of-control high pressure hose at her apartment house in an attempt to stop the water. Her uterus, vagina, and abdomen were severely injured. She was unable to tell her attorney any part of what had happened. The attorney consulted the author because Jennifer had been unable thus far to assist in her own lawsuit. She had failed to cooperate with pelvic examination following her emergency surgery, and it had been impossible to assess any remaining damage.

Jennifer was much the way her attorney described when first seen psychiatrically—pale, apprehensive, and unable to tell her story. The author first worked with Jennifer discussing normal female anatomy and the words for internal organs which the child had never learned. Gradually, after going over a diagram, Jennifer was able to recount what had happened to her. She described her horror at seeing the blood coming from inside "a part" she had not fully realized existed. She experienced relief in discussing with the child psychiatrist her heretofore undiscussable terror. After three interviews, she was able to allow both a vaginal examination and an examination under anesthesia which revealed that all physical damage had been surgically corrected. Jennifer's relief was even more marked following the good news about her gynecological future.

In Jennifer's case, there is a situation in which the attorney might have been able to claim greater damages on behalf of the child if he had ignored her silence and made his claims on the basis of the findings in emergency surgery. His action in making sure the child understood what was happening surely limited the huge damages Jennifer might have collected. On the other hand, the psychic trauma was minimized because of the prompt psychiatric intervention. The attorney's referral is, in my opinion, an example of the true professionalism of a lawyer acting in the best interests of his/her client.

The final example of the child witness who would not speak is the case of Christine, age 14, who was raped by a gang of boys in her school-yard. Christine had been "thrown out" of a school dance for smoking and was forced to leave the building by the principal, even though she protested that her parents were not available to drive her home. Christine, although hostile after the attack, was quite verbal to her parents, her attorney, and to the child psychiatrist until her deposition. During the deposition the attorneys representing the school implied that Christine had had prior sexual experiences. Even though there is a California law which protects rape victims from such questioning in criminal trials, this law could not be extended to cover Christine's rights while undergoing deposition in a civil suit. This line of questioning so infuriated and frightened Christine that she absolutely refused to take the stand at her trial. As a result, a very small settlement from the school was accepted on Christine's behalf, and the school was never publicly exposed, as the parents had wished, for failing to protect a student at one of its functions.

DISCUSSION AND SUMMARY

It has been illustrated and described in this chapter how the law's requirements and the psychiatrist's assessment of a child's capacity to serve as a witness widely differ. There may be cut and dried instances in which a child witnesses something which does not cause any stress. In such cases, the legal requirements of intelligence and moral belief in the truth may suffice. On the other hand, the law habitually deals with strongly emotional issues, which people on their own cannot settle. It is in this context that the child psychiatric view of "trauma" or severe stress becomes very important. If the child psychiatrist is asked to evaluate a stressed child witness, both internal consistency and external consistency must be evaluated. In assessing internal consistency, the psychiatrist considers behavioral manifestations (reenactment, play), dreams, and the child's verbal "story" over time. Child-language is evaluated to make sure that it is consistent in its naiveté and does not appear inflexible, repetitive, or "coached" by adults. In assessing external consistency, the psychiatrist considers the child witness' story in context with the child's history, medical record, school record, and the "clues" and data provided by the police, D.A.'s office, and/or attorneys. Loyalty conflicts are assessed, and care is taken not to place a child witness in a position which threatens his/her future sustenance.

REFERENCES

1. *American Jurisprudence* 2nd Edition, 81 (1976), Witnesses, § 88-93. San Francisco: Bancroft Whitney Co.
2. California Statute CCP § 1800.
3. *Harrold* v. *Schluep* (Fla. App) 264 So 2nd 431.
4. HELLMAN, L. (1934). *The Children's Hour.* New York: Knopf.
5. JAMES, H. (1898). *The Turn of the Screw.* Avon, Conn: The Heritage Press, 1949.
6. *Knab* v. *Alden's Irving Park, Inc.,* 49 Ill. App. 2d 371, 199 NE2d 815.
7. *Malchanoff* v. *Truehart,* 354 Mass. 118, 236 NE2d 89.
8. MILLER, A. (1953). *The Crucible.* New York: Viking Press.
9. *State* v. *Zeezich,* 61 Utah 61, 210 P 927.
10. *Provost* v. *State* (Tex. Crim. App) 514 SW2d 269.
11. ROSE, A. (1941). *So You Are Going to Be a Witness!* New York: Institute Press Publishers, pp. 33-34.
12. *State* v. *Belton,* 24 SC 185.
13. *State* v. *Driver,* 88 WVa 479, 107 SE 189, 15 ALR 917.
14. TERR, L. (1979). Children of Chowchilla: A Study of Psychic Trauma. *The Psychoanalytic Study of the Child,* 34:552-623.
15. *Wheeler* v. *United States,* 159 U.S. 523, 40 L Ed 244, 16 SCt 93.
16. *Whitehead* v. *Stith,* 268 Ky 703, 105 SW 2d 834.

15

COMPETENCY AND CRIMINAL RESPONSIBILITY

JOSEPH J. PALOMBI, M.D.

INTRODUCTION

It is only within the past five to 10 years that the necessity for the consideration of competency and responsibility of the juvenile in court has become relevant. The Supreme Court of the United States handed down the famed Gault decision in 1967, which stated that every constitutional protection afforded to a given adult at any stage in a hearing after arrest must be afforded the juvenile (2). Thus, from a practical point of view, any juvenile may now ask for the determination of competence and examination in regards to use of the insanity defense, more widely known as a determination of responsibility for the act. The Gault decision, although raising many questions for lawyers, courts and psychiatrists, as well as for juveniles, for all practical purposes, did not significantly change the procedural aspects of juvenile courts throughout the country. It did, however, open the door for subsequent cases, procedural changes, and the necessity for such determinations in states such as New York and possibly Connecticut, where transfer of jurisdiction from juvenile to adult criminal courts either already exists or is contemplated. Thus, the child psychiatrist, who had previously only been utilized in an irregular fashion for dispositional determinations in the juvenile courts, is now thrust into the limelight of procedural hearings, much as the adult psychiatrist has escalated in importance in court proceedings over the past 10 to 15 years. This chapter will discuss the definition of competency and responsibility as generally understood, and their possible applicability in the juvenile court or in the situation where the juvenile is transferred to the adult court. In addition, an outline of the difference between competency and responsibility is proposed. The child psychiatrist's role in these procedures is also discussed.

It should be noted that, at this time in the development of psychiatry and the relationship between psychiatry and law, the areas of competency and responsibility are probably two of *the* most controversial areas of interchange. A recent Group for the Advancement of Psychiatry Report has explored the many issues dealing with competency to stand trial (3). In addition, one need only to pick up a newspaper over the past three to four years to realize that the "insanity" defense, which is more appropriately called a responsibility issue, has been criticized loudly from both the legal and the psychiatric community. Thus, although there is increasing controversy around both of these issues, there will undoubtedly be more demand from the legal system to provide these types of evaluations and input, specifically around juvenile issues as juveniles are held more responsible for more serious crimes at increasingly earlier ages. Two most recent clarifications of procedures which would increasingly involve the child psychiatrist with the courts have taken place in New York State. The Juvenile Justice Reform Act of 1976 outlined a completely new set of procedures with which to handle the adjudication of 14- and 15-year-olds who had committed more serious offenses. In addition, the Juvenile Offender Bill of 1978 in New York State extended down procedural safeguards to adolescents 13 and above who were accused of committing serious crimes. Further, Chapter 55 of the State of Texas Family Code details a well worked-out set of codes including a separate section on competency to proceed and a mental condition as a defense for a child as young as the age of 15 (6). One need only look back a few years in the history of adult criminal procedures to realize that the future undoubtedly holds an increased utilization of both competency and responsibility within the juvenile courts.

COMPETENCY

Definition

Competence is fundamentally a legal concept dealing with the mental capacity or ability of a child to perform an act. Capacity or ability is more often than not reflected in the cognitive-affective-behavioral pattern of the person, depending on the specific legal situation that is involved. Most psychiatrists or other physicians, and often lawyers and laymen, use the word "competence" to describe a level of judgment that is sufficient to make decisions. Thus, having the capacity or ability to perform is based on a concept of the integration of a person which usually is made up of the psychiatric triad of cognition, feeling, and conation, and which may be affected in many ways by either mental disease or defect.

The part of the definition which includes performance has a whole variety of meanings depending upon the context in which it is used. Indeed, in this part of the definition, one comes up against the most important departure from the everyday use of the word "competence," in that the psychiatrist is only trying to determine how one child is able to perform a certain specific act or in a given situation rather than his/her overall capacity to perform in general.

One should remember that the issue of competence is ultimately a legal one; although the child psychiatrist's report is welcomed and utilized by the court, the judge has the final decision concerning the competency of the child in whatever situation is being tested. The mental health professional has a limited role as an advisor and the recommendations, observations, and diagnoses are subject to specific legal guidelines and review.

Although there are innumerable areas of competence which are more relevant to the adult than to the child or adolescent, several most crucial to the work of the child psychiatrist will be explored in some detail. However, the base line in all these issues involved in competence is: Is there a mental disease or defect which affects the judgment decision-making power or behavior of the child? And, if there is, is it to such a degree that it meets the criteria of the legal standard regarding that specific issue? The child psychiatrist's professional background and training often enable him/her to be a very useful advisor in answering the first of these questions. The individual, however, who makes the ultimate legal decision will incorporate that information and opinion in some attempt to determine an answer to the second question.

Theoretical Issues and Contradictions in the Determination of Competency in Children

It is only within the past ten years that the issue of competency of the child has become an issue for evaluation and debate. English common law in its truest form held that the young person who had not reached an age of judgment was generally neither competent to decide significant issues nor responsible for his/her behavior. With the lowering of the age of majority to 18, by a Constitutional amendment, and the increasing visibility of teenagers in our society, coupled with their demands for a more active role in both their own behavior and determination of what they should be allowed to do, psychological, legal, and societal norms have come into conflict. One need only to study the psychology of Jean Piaget, as best outlined by Flavell (1), and the developmental aspects of adolescence as outlined by Malmquist (4), to realize that the psychological and psychiatric impressions of the formation of judgment and the capacity to comprehensively understand are still in question and quite variable. Thus, although a legal interpretation of the minor's capacity to understand and comprehend a given situation may be clear—whether it be in court or in other situations—society's and the psychiatrist's understanding of the adolescent's capacities might be quite different.

In fact, this is exactly part of the rationale and argument that has been utilized over the past five years in certain areas to call for the more adult-like treatment in court of the younger adolescent. In essence, society is stating that it is no longer appropriate for the 13-, 14- and 15-year-old to be treated as a juvenile in the juvenile court system, with its inherent philosophy of treatment, leniency, and nonresponsibility as has been the case in the past.

In addition, the two other major areas of importance in determining the competence of an adolescent are those of the minor's role in consenting to any type of medical treatment including psychiatric treatment and, specifically, in consenting to commitment to a mental institution. We will not explore either one of these areas as the principles of determination of such competence are similar to that in the court situation. This specific area of conflict between parental rights and children's rights has already begun to be an area of increasing litigation, and academic discussion by both lawyers and psychiatrists. Schowalter, in a recent publication, outlines comprehensively this special area of competence with regard to outpatient and inpatient psychiatric (5) treatment. Most importantly, he states that the age of 14 might be reasonably selected as the appropriate cutoff point between consideration as a minor and as an adult. He indicates that the individual determination of competency is superior to an arbitrary age. This reinforces the necessity for special skill in assessing the competency of, in particular, the younger adolescent in whatever legal situation this determination might be utilized.

Competency in Court Procedures

The determination of competence is applicable at many stages of the court process. Initially and probably of most significance is the question of competency to stand trial, or to proceed in whatever type of judicial process is in question. As mentioned earlier, incompetency to proceed in a juvenile proceeding under the Texas codes is essentially the same as incompetency to stand trial under an adult criminal proceeding. In jurisdictions, such as New York, where laws governing juveniles have built-in greater procedural safeguards, this has generally been the case. It would certainly seem just as unfair to subject a child who is incompetent to proceed to juvenile proceedings as it would be to subject an adult who was determined incompetent to stand trial on any criminal charge. The base line determination of competency in a case involving a child or adolescent should involve three specific issues:

1) Does the adolescent understand the nature of the proceedings in which he/she is about to take part?
2) Does the adolescent understand the charges, or in many situations, petition?
3) Is the adolescent capable of taking part in his/her own defense and cooperating with his/her attorney?

One can see that in the determination of competency to proceed, the aspect of cooperation and capacity to aid in one's defense is added to the more fundamental aspects of understanding and comprehension of legal situation.

Waiver

The other major area in the juvenile proceeding in which the child psychiatrist may be called upon to offer an opinion is in the area of transference of jurisdiction from juvenile to criminal courts—trying the juvenile as an adult. The juvenile laws of a number of jurisdictions recognize that certain extreme conduct necessitates different handling and provide "vents" for the system by allowing transfer of juveniles to regular criminal courts.

In order to "transfer" or "waive" juvenile court jurisdiction, laws in different jurisdictions set different standards. Usually these are criteria such as age, nature of the crime, and prior record and treatability. In some jurisdictions, such as New York, recently enacted laws remand juveniles who have committed serious crimes to the adult court.

The child psychiatrist might also be called upon to aid the court when the very important distinction between being tried as a juvenile and being tried as an adult is being considered. In fact, examination for determination of competency by the child psychiatrist might serve the continuation of the social welfare philosophy of most juvenile court proceedings and, undoubtedly, aid the court in serving both its own needs and society's needs in providing the rationale for some type of treatment intervention if indicated for the juvenile who might be incompetent. It should be noted that although many juvenile jurisdictions throughout the country require psychiatric evaluation of adolescents and children prior to dispositional hearings, or as an aid in the degree to which a proceeding will continue, the specific provision for determination of competency at a much earlier point in the proceeding is in most situations both an asset for the court as well as for the individual adolescent.

Some may argue, however, that the juvenile court generally has not been able to fulfill its obligations to treatment of the majority of adolescents coming through its portals. Although one might agree with that fact, per se, it is certainly worthwhile from most points of view that an adolescent be given the opportunity for some type of intervention such as outpatient treatment before the extreme of incarceration in either a correctional institution or a mental institution is mandated. In the long run, this may be, indeed, the most fruitful function and most positive outcome of introduction of a competency evaluation in the juvenile court proceeding.

RESPONSIBILITY

Definition

The use of the term "insanity" in a judicial procedure is not a medical term but, instead, a legal concept meaning that a degree of mental disorder relieves an offender of criminal responsibility for his action. Thus, when one speaks of responsibility in the juvenile court setting, one is speaking of an inherent contradiction. That is, because the overriding philosophy of the juvenile court is of a benevolent nature to provide treatment and deter others from similar acts, no determination of responsibility should be necessary. With the change of this philosophy in some juvenile court jurisdictions, the possibility of a responsibility defense both in juvenile court proceedings and in those adolescents who are tried in adult courts exists.

There are essentially two specific reasons for excusing persons from responsibility for their conduct. First, criminal culpability requires the presence of an intent to commit a criminal act. Thus, individuals who lack the capacity or "free will" cannot form a criminal intent and, therefore, do not meet this requirement for culpability. Secondly, the purposes of the criminal system, such as punishment, are not served by punishing those who do not have the capacity to make a free rational choice.

In essence, "responsibility" or more clearly "criminal responsibility" is a special type of competence which is based on a specific capacity to be held blameworthy for acts committed which are otherwise classified as criminal. The juvenile ordinarily is not considered to possess a *mens rea*, i.e., guilty mind. To reiterate, the only areas in which this type of determination would be applicable would be in those jurisdictions, such as New York, where recent changes in the law have made certain juvenile procedures more like criminal court, and when the juvenile has been transferred to adult court and is being treated as an adult.

Criteria for Using Mental Condition as a Defense

There is probably no greater area of controversy in psychiatry and law than that of the "insanity defense." The controversy has continued to rage even more actively in the past five years in light of the increase in utilization of this defense in adult courts. With this in mind, it would be useful to review the four tests of criminal responsibility that are used by the state and federal courts in an attempt to evaluate offenders suffering from a mental condition. The utilization of one's mental condition as a defense against responsibilty for a criminal act is by no means agreed upon in any area of the country, and each of these tests has its advantages and shortcomings. These tests are the M'Naughten Rule; the M'Naughten Rule with the irresistible-impulse test; the Durham or "Product" test; and the criteria for insanity promulgated by the American Law Institutes Model Penal Code or the ALI test.

The M'Naughten test was first formulated in the 1840s and remains the sole test in fewer than one-third of the states. An additional 15 states rely on a combination of the M'Naughten Rule supplemented by the irresistible-impulse test. Fundamentally, the M'Naughten Rule states that one needs to demonstrate that an offender did not know the nature and quality of an act that he/she was doing was wrong, and also that these conditions were present because of a "disease of the mind." In essence, the most prevalent form of the test emphasizes that the defendant had the capacity of "knowing right from wrong" as this knowledge relates to the specific criminal act.

As a response to a disenchantment over the M'Naughten Rule, approximately 15 states have adopted a second criteria or requirement along with M'Naughten. The irresistible-impulse test excludes from consideration those who cannot "control their emotional responses." According to this rule, an offender may know the difference from right and wrong but find himself under the influence of an overpowering impulse which drives him/her to commit the criminal act. Thus, this rule recognizes that the power of free will may be impaired even though the offender intellectually recognizes the nature of his act and knows it is wrong.

The Durham test or "product rule" was first established in a case in New Hampshire in the 1870s. In essence, this rule stipulated that a defendant was not held responsible for his/her act if this act was the "product of mental disease." As a result, this test permits the introduction of the complete psychiatric picture of the offender for consideration by the court and jury and consequently broadens considerably the classes of mental illness sometimes responsible for specific behaviors. It should be noted that, at this time, the Durham test is used only in New Hampshire, Maine, and the Virgin Islands. It enjoyed a period of popularity during the 1960s but was dramatically altered in 1972 when it was felt to be too broad a criteria.

Finally, the test of the American Law Institute, otherwise known as the ALI test, states that a person is not responsible for criminal conduct if "at the time of such conduct, as a result of mental disease or defect, he lacks a substantial capacity to appreciate the wrongfulness of his conduct or to conform his conduct to the requirement of the law." From the psychiatric point of view, what is most useful about the ALI test is that it helps to outline specifically what role the psychiatrist can take during the evaluation of the defendant. There are three specific aspects of this test that are important: first, a statement concerning the offender's intellectual ability to decide between right and wrong; second, an assessment of his/her volition from the perspective of whether he/she desired to commit the crime; and third, consideration of his emotional capacity to control his/her own conduct. Thus, this is the most recent and most comprehensive of the tests, although still not completely acceptable. It is utilized in approximately 15 states at this time. The ALI test does, however, more completely outline the role of the psychiatrist in the insanity defense and help clarify his function as an aid to the court.

Evaluation of the Adolescent for Competence

As mentioned, the fundamental issue in the determination of competence in the adolescent should be the determination of mental disease or defect, within the legal framework and in terms of level of competence being determined. Thus, from the outset, one needs to be relatively well aware of the criteria established in a given location for a level of competence to be determined. Some jurisdictions are relatively strict and limited in their definition, while others range fairly broadly in the determination. The evaluator should be acquainted with the local statutes and previous decisions of the jurisdiction within which he/she is working. This knowledge will go a long way in terms of establishing the expertise of the evaluator in the eyes of the court and specific judges, as well as helping the child psychiatrist be of most value in his advisory and evaluative role to the court.

Returning again to the most typical situation of the determination of competence of an adolescent, which is that of the determination of the competence or fitness to proceed to trial, it should be noted that the examination is specifically done at a time and place in order that a current evaluation of the individual's competence be available. In most situations the gathering of much preliminary data including family history, previous behavior and other treatment or hospitalizations is usually not necessary, but may be of some value. Although it can be of use to the child psychiatrist to have preliminary data—much of which is often not available—the court is specifically looking for a reasonable evaluation of the adolescent's present function and capacity to respond to the criteria already stated. Thus, the mental status and the short-term evaluation of the adolescent's present situation, under whatever stresses he might be suffering, and in whatever physical condition he/she might be, are essential to a true determination of his competence. It should be kept in mind that this determination again is specifically for the evaluation of competence and not for some other broader purpose.

It is important to test specifically those areas of the adolescent's mental status with which the child psychiatrist is experienced. Then he/she can be of a specific help through his/her knowledge, experience, and ways of formulating mental disease or defect in the adolescent. An understanding of specific developmental norms is also a very useful and practical part of the evaluation, since this is one area in which most general psychiatrists have little, if any, experience and is usually quite concretely and easily interpreted by the court in its final determination of competence. In fact, specific simple examples of the various direct statements from a mental status exam given by the evaluator can serve a very useful purpose by giving direct examples of the individual's current verbal, cognitive, and perceptual functioning. This, indeed, is the crux of the court's acceptance and utilization of the competency evaluation. Most judges look with some trepidation on reports and evaluations that are purely interpretive. They are very grateful and accepting of those evaluations which are easily understood, comprehensive, and offer current examples of the individual's behavior or verbalizations as evidence for the diagnosis and determination.

Important areas of the mental status examination of the adolescent include appearance, affect, orientation and perception, coping mechanisms and thought processes and verbalization. In addition, some inquiry as to the adolescent's awareness of his problem and some clinical intelligence quotient estimate should also be made. The areas of fantasy, superego, and concept of self are certainly more difficult to evaluate in the typical competency evaluation and are, indeed, less relevant for the function of this specific evaluation. It should again be emphasized that relevant statements in terms of both specific and anecdotal examples from the actual interview, and reasonably well known developmental comparisons should be part of the evaluation. These areas are usually less well known to even juvenile court judges, and are certainly less well known to most attorneys.

When evaluating an adolescent specifically for competence to proceed in court, consent to some specific medical treatment, or consent to psychiatric treatment or commitment, we should remember that the evaluation is done exclusively for determination at that point in time and under those circumstances. Although it is not usually the rule, the legal authority, whether it be a judge or an administrative officer, does have the right to ask for another determination by another individual, or another later evaluation by the same clinician. In fact, in most adult jurisdictions, the determination of competency to proceed to trial is usually automatically done by two psychiatrists who, if they do not agree, ask the opinion of a third colleague to break the tie. This is, however, not usually the case in a juvenile court setting where the court usually relies on a single evaluation. This does further demonstrate, however, the essence of the evaluation—that is, to provide the court with the type of information and evaluation that it can utilize in its eventual and final determination of competence from a legal point of view. Thus, the more specific, easily understood and relevant to the situation an evaluation is, the more acceptable and utilizable by the court it will be.

It is important to reemphasize that the rendering of an appropriate and relevant diagnosis is important. However, the demonstration by the child psychiatrist of the adolescent's understanding of the situation, whether it be charges against him/her or a potential of commitment to an institution, an understanding of the workings of the operation of the system, and the capacity to take part in those proceedings and to assist whatever counsel, and testify is essential. Thus, the clinician attempts to aid the court in making a quantitative determination of these several abilities, and tries to provide evidence and examples to demonstrate such.

Finally, it should be remembered that there is no absolute formula for the determination of competency. One must weigh the various aspects of the adolescent's mental status and present functioning in the light of previous clinical experience both within the court setting and with other adolescents. Additionally, one should not feel rejected if one's recomendations are not followed by the court. The evaluation may be at least a step in the direction of some consideration of the adolescent's mental status and capacities and how they may relate to his/her behavior.

Evaluating the Adolescent for Responsibility

It is not likely that even the average child psychiatrist who works in a court setting will have to carry out an evaluation for the responsibility defense more than three or four times in his/her career. Noting, however, that responsibility is, in essence, a very specific type of competence, one can keep the already outlined guideline in mind. In addition, the determination of responsibility does require a much more extensive documentation, demonstration, and probably a higher level of proof, in a legal sense, than does the routine determination of competence. It is inevitable that the child psychiatrist will be viewed by the court as being on one side or the other, thus losing to a major degree the more typical "friend of the court" or impartial evaluator status. It should be obvious that now the child psychiatrist is squarely in the adversary position, and will, in essence, be trying more diligently to convince either a judge or jury of the relevance and validity of his/her findings.

This conviction that the child should not be held responsible for his/her behavior should not only be sincere and believable, but needs to be supported with clinical data which are easily understood by all. This is imperative because there will, undoubtedly, be contradictory data and opinion on the other side of the issue. If the child psychiatrist is to be effective in his/her role for the defense, he/she must be more convincing and plausible in the opinions presented.

Initially, this may mean that such areas as fantasy, wishes, concept of self, including object relations and identifications, and superego integration will all become much more important areas of evaluation for the child psychiatrist. In addition to the other areas of the mental status, the child psychiatrist will be trying to demonstrate with a very high degree of certainty that not only is his/her diagnostic formulation correct but that, depending on the test utilized in a given jurisdiction, the individual adolescent cannot be held responsible for his/her behavior.

Additionally, one must attempt to determine and demonstrate the state of mind of the adolescent at the time of commission of the crime. It is only possible to do so with the cooperation of the defendant, and the more facile the clinician's interviewing skills, the better. However, it is not uncommon that the adolescent defendant is less than cooperative, even though he/she does understand that you are trying to help. Thus, skillful elicitation of the thought processes, fantasies, and delusions at the time of the crime and their incorporation into the already established diagnostic picture are crucial. Significant direct statements from the defendant, in addition to testimony from individuals who observed him/her both prior to and after the act, are helpful. Previous medical and police records, when admissible, may help to buttress the picture of an adolescent who has regularly become hostile, violent, disorganized or openly paranoid, perhaps during the period of drug or alcohol use and possibly for significant periods of time thereafter. In essence, a convincing picture of the state of mind at the time of the act which is compatible with previous psychopathology is often the most telling part of the testimony.

In many situations, even if the adolescent is not held responsible in one level of court within a given jurisdiction, he/she may then be remanded to a lower level such as to the juvenile or family court for disposition. This is similar to the adult situation where the individual is often remanded to a treatment situation or institution until such time as other than legal or corrections determination of his/her sanity allows release. Hopefully, with the adolescent, the appropriate type of treatment can be underscored and disposition to a specific treatment setting encouraged, thus providing a truly advocacy function for the adolescent in getting him/her the proper mental care.

Working with the defense attorney for the adolescent is a crucial aspect at any stage of a responsibility evaluation and defense. Since testimony in court is crucial, coordination of the defense for the better understanding and disposition of an adolescent is absolutely necessary. One might also hope that, in addition to the adversarial role that one is inevitably taking in this type of situation, some educational role for attorney, judges, and other court personnel might take place.

The utilization of psychological testing, especially sophisticated projective tests and specific tests for organicity, is strongly recommended in this situation. The Rorschach Test, the Thematic Apperception Test (TAT), and the Minnesota Multiphasic Personality Inventory (MMPI) are the most widely used. Interpreted by the trained clinical psychologist with experience in testing adolescents, they can be a great help in diagnostic evaluation. Questions regarding their reliability and validity will, undoubtedly, arise and it will depend on the court and the capacity of the examiner to eventually determine their acceptance and degree of acceptability during a trial. In the majority of situations it would, undoubtedly, bolster and support the clinical findings, and although sometimes not admissable, provides just the amount of confirmatory evidence that is necessary in some cases.

Finally, the child psychiatrist may, in addition, be called upon at a future time to reevaluate the given adolescent for proper disposition and treatment planning. Facilitating the appropriate treatment of the adolescent who has, unfortunately, had to interface with the justice system because of his/her behavior, might be a long range goal for the child psychiatrist who is initially asked only to evaluate competency and responsibility. Hopefully, this would further the goals of both society and the individual adolescent, and allow both the juvenile justice system and the mental health system to carry out their roles appropriately.

REFERENCES

1. FLAVELL, J. (1963). *The Developmental Psychology of Jean Piaget.* New York: Van Nostrand.
2. *Gault* v. *Ariz.,* 387, U.S. 6 May, 1967.
3. GROUP FOR THE ADVANCEMENT OF PSYCHIATRY REPORT (1974). *Misuse of Psychiatry in the Criminal Courts; Competency to Stand Trial.* New York: GAP, Vol. VIII, Report No. 89, February.
4. MALMQUIST, C. P. (1978). *Handbook of Adolescence.* New York: Jason Aronson.
5. SCHOWALTER, J. E. (1978). The Minor's Role in Consent for Mental Health Treatment. *J. Am. Acad. Child Psych.,* Vol. 17, 3, Summer.
6. Texas Family Code, Title III, Chapter 55, 1973, as amended in 1975.

16

COMMITMENT PROCEEDINGS FOR MENTALLY ILL AND MENTALLY RETARDED CHILDREN

JAMES ELLIS, J.D.

The manner in which the law allows children to enter institutions for the mentally ill and mentally retarded is a subject of much current debate. Courts (1), legislatures (2), legal scholars (3), and mental health professionals (4) have all weighed in with proposals on the subject in the last half dozen years. The intensity of this debate reflects not only our varying degree of trust in the institutions to which children are sent, but also our differing views on the nature of childhood and adolescence. The resolution of the debate may have an even greater impact on the law's overall view of children than it does on the mental health and retardation systems which are at issue.

THE REASONS FOR COMMITMENT HEARINGS

History of the Problem

Until the 1970s, it appears that very few children went through any kind of formal commitment proceeding before entering an institution. Most states, until recently, allowed parents to place their minor children in institutions as "voluntary" patients without any judicial action at all (5). The tenuous nature of the analogy between an adult admitting *himself* voluntarily and one party—here, the parent—consenting to the admission of *another* did not receive much attention, but the general system of parental consent was seen as consistent with the universally held view that parents made important decisions for their children. It was generally assumed that parents could and must consent to other forms of medical treatment for—and on behalf of—their children, and there is little suggestion in the literature that lawyers or doctors saw any reason to view mental health or mental retardation treatment any differently.

In the case of hospitalization for mental illness, the statutes which authorize parental "voluntary" admissions were largely enacted in the 1950s, following the suggested language of the National Institute of Mental Health's *Draft Act Governing Hospitalization of the Mentally Ill* (1951) (6). It is possible that in many states this legislation merely codified what had been informal practice previously. The statutes regarding mentally retarded children were, at least in some states, explicit about parents' rights decades earlier. In one state, parents were given the power to place their child in a retardation institution on their own initiative, but were required to obtain a court order to get their child *out*, once admitted (7). The more noticeable concern of legislatures in the institutionalization of mentally retarded children, as compared to mentally ill children, is probably a result of the pervasive fear, early in this century, of the social ills of crime, delinquency, disease, and immorality which were attributed to the "feebleminded." Strict segregation of the mentally retarded from the rest of society, along with eugenic sterilization, were the legislative remedies chosen (8). Even when this rather hysterical fear of retarded people subsided, legislation allowing parents to place their children was left intact.

Despite these apparent differences in the origin of laws authorizing parental admissions, the result was essentially the same: parents had the power to place both mentally ill and mentally retarded children in institutions without any form of judicial review.

The Constitutional Issue

Two major factors have brought about change in this legal arrangement. One is the increasing attention courts have paid to conditions in institutions. In a striking series of cases, federal courts have found conditions in institutions for the mentally ill (9), mentally retarded (10), and juvenile delinquents (11), to be below constitutionally minimal standards. This new scrutiny of institutions in which children live has led naturally to scrutiny of the procedures under which the children enter them.

The other major contributor to legal change has been a shift in the courts' view of the constitutional rights of children generally. Judge Wald's chapter in this volume clearly traces this constitutional development, and as she notes, the notion that children have rights independent of their parents is of recent origin. The clearest pronouncement in this area prior to 1979 was the Court's ruling that states could not give parents of a teenage woman a veto power over their daughter's decision to obtain an abortion (12). The rationale in that case was that the parents' interest in control of the upbringing of their child was outweighed by her privacy interest in making this important medical decision. This ruling was necessarily premised upon an assumption that in some instances the interests of parents and children may come into conflict. Lawyers for children challenging the "voluntary" commitment statutes contended that the same principle of conflict of interest between parent and child rendered parental admissions unconstitutional.

The specific request of the children's attorneys was that their clients be given a hearing to contest the necessity or appropriateness of the proposed commitment. Their argument was based on the fact that children possessed a liberty interest protected by the Due Process Clause of the fourteenth amendment of the U.S. Constitution (". . . nor shall any State deprive any person of life, liberty, or property, without due process of law . . ."). The Court had already held this to be true in its landmark case involving procedural rights in juvenile courts (13). Counsel argued that children were entitled to similar procedures before being placed in an institution by their parents. The lower courts agreed.

On June 20, 1979, the Supreme Court reversed the lower court rulings. In an opinion by Chief Justice Burger, the Court ruled that while states were free to provide formal hearings prior to admission, the Constitution did not require them to do so. The minimum requirement established by the Court provides that an "independent" examination of the child's need for institutionalization must be provided. "We conclude that the risk of error inherent in the parental decision to have a child institutionalized for mental health care is sufficiently great that some kind of inquiry should be made by a 'neutral factfinder' to determine whether the statutory requirements for admission are satisfied. That inquiry must carefully probe the child's background using all available sources, including, but not limited to, parents, schools and other social agencies. Of course, the review must also include an interview with the child. It is necessary that the decisionmaker have the authority to refuse to admit any child who does not satisfy the medical standards for admission. Finally, it is necessary that the child's continuing need for commitment be reviewed periodically by a similarly independent procedure" (14).

A concurring and dissenting opinion by Mr. Justice Brennan, joined by Justices Marshall and Stevens, argued that due process requires more elaborate and formal review of the child's need for confinement, and that this review should take place shortly after admission.

Several facts about the *Parham* opinion should be noted. First, the decision does not affect the laws of those states which have already chosen to provide hearings to children. Second, in California the state Supreme Court has already held that the *state* constitution requires formal hearings, and that interpretation is unaffected by *Parham*. Courts in other states may reach a similar conclusion. Finally, it should be noted that the *Parham* decision has been severely criticized by many lawyers and mental health and mental retardation professionals. The critics note that the majority places great weight upon the assumption that the admissions process makes few diagnostic and placement errors, and they argue that this assumption is not supported by scientific studies or by clinical experience. Even the position of the American Psychiatric Association would have provided formal hearings to a far larger number of children than did the majority opinion. Since the empirical basis for the ruling is arguably shaky, the critics believe that it may be overturned by a future Court, and that in the interim state legislatures should act to provide hearings for children who are at risk of erroneous institutionalization.

Policy Considerations

Independent of what the Constitution requires, there are strong policy arguments in favor of a state's providing commitment hearings to children who face residential treatment or habilitation in an institution. These policy considerations would argue for the provision of such hearings even if the Constitution does not require them, and should also serve as a guide to the states as they determine what kind of hearings to provide.

One major reason for due process hearings is to check for errors in the decision to institutionalize a particular child. This is not to suggest that those who currently serve in the admissions process of residential facilities are careless or uncaring. But no process in an area as uncertain as the diagnosis of mental illness or mental retardation in children is without a risk of error. And there may be particular difficulties for the admitting officer when a parent presents a child for institutionalization. In mental illness cases, there may be a question about the relationship between the pathology of the child and the pathology of the family which is proposing his admission (15). In mental retardation cases, the family often presents a description of serious family difficulties in coping with the child—difficulties which they can no longer physically or emotionally handle (16). In such situations, the admitting official may reasonably be moved by considerations other than the child's demonstrated problem and needs. And while studies are not available on the incidence of erroneous admission of children as either mentally retarded or mentally ill, anecdotal accounts of such errors are cause for concern (17).

In explaining when the Due Process Clause requires a hearing, the Supreme Court has said that the nature of the individual interest involved must be considered along with the risk of error without a hearing and the chance that a hearing will reduce the risk of error, and that these must be balanced against the state's interest in avoiding a hearing (18). Leaving aside constitutional questions, this same balancing test can serve as a useful guide in deciding as a matter of social policy whether hearings are warranted. In this case, the child's interest in avoiding *unnecessary* institutionalization is strong. There are numerous studies which demonstrate the risks of institutionalization to a child— developmental deprivation, stigmatization, etc. (19). When a child's condition requires residential treatment, these costs may be outweighed by the advantages to be gained from the treatment. But where the original determination of need was in error, there are no benefits to outweigh the harms of institutionalization. As for the risk factor in this balancing process, it is difficult to quantify the likelihood that, without hearings, a child will be incorrectly institutionalized. It is equally difficult to measure the likelihood that hearings would identify and correct such errors. But an analysis of the nature of the "voluntary" admissions process suggests that the admitting officer may not have all the relevant information to guide his or her judgment that the child requires placement, and indeed that such officers may also consider matters, such as the family's condition and needs, other than the medical or habilitation needs of the particular child. But it is in the nature of due process hearings that they are designed to sharpen the accuracy of the fact-finding process. The hearing is before (and the ultimate decision will be made by) an impartial tribunal. This fact-finder is assisted by the presentation of testimony, including expert testimony, on the condition and needs of the child. The utility of this testimony to the decision-making process is enhanced by subjecting that testimony to more careful analysis through questioning of an advocate of a different viewpoint. The child has a chance to be heard and to be assisted by a trained advocate. No fact-finding process can totally eliminate errors, but a due process hearing, tailored to the needs of mentally ill or mentally retarded children, can bring a more rigorous and consistent approach to individual cases, and therefore seems likely to reduce the risk of errors.

The state's interest in avoiding hearings is also difficult to evaluate. One element is surely the financial cost of the new procedures. But the evidence from states which currently provide hearings suggests that the cost would not be massive, and the additional dollars required would surely not be enough to outweigh the child's interest in avoiding unnecessary institutionalization. The more serious concern is whether there are other kinds of costs to a hearing system for children. One possible harm which is sometimes alleged by critics of due process hearings is that they would become countertherapeutic. This argument suggests that an open discussion of the reasons for the proposed placement would be disturbing to many children, and that the prospect of parents and children taking opposite sides on the question would damage family relationships. Neither of these possibilities should be casually dismissed.

The opening of family disputes and sensitive information about family relationships to outside scrutiny (even in hearings which could be kept closed to the public) represents a considerable intrusion into family privacy. To advocate a system which entails such an intrusion requires the showing of a strong countervailing interest. Such an interest does appear to be present in avoiding an erroneous parental decision to institutionalize a child. Parents who decide that their child requires institutional care may be operating from entirely understandable and even commendable motives, but those motives are not limited to the needs and best interest of the child (20). Parents may also have concerns about the effect of the child's presence in the home on other children in the family or on the parents' marriage. And even when they are correct in their conclusion (as they often will be) that they can no longer live with the child in the family under current conditions, they may be wrong in their conclusion that institutionalizing the child is the best, or only, solution. The decision to institutionalize a child is typically made as a last resort—often made in a moment of desperation. Where the potential consequences for the child are so momentous, allowing a parental decision under those conditions to go unreviewed seems unwise. And sadly, the kind of information and advice which parents receive from physicians and other professionals is often based upon ignorance of alternatives to institutions. And in the case of mentally retarded children, it may be based upon startlingly inadequate knowledge about mental retardation itself (21). These factors outweigh the interest in family privacy because the consequences of a wrong decision in the life of a child may be disastrous.

The problem of exacerbating parent-child disputes by formalizing them in a hearing is also troubling. It is not inconceivable that in some cases the confrontation will be traumatic. But neither is it inconceivable that bringing unspoken feelings and concerns into the open may have a therapeutic effect and allow the re-creation of a stronger family foundation. We have few empirical data to assist us in evaluating the consequences of such hearings on long-term family relationships. But two points are clear. First, the hearing process will not be the *cause* of family disharmony; at most it will reflect already existing tensions. There is a clear parallel here to the minor's abortion case. The Supreme Court noted that giving parents total control over their daughter's decision whether to obtain an abortion would be unlikely to "enhance parental authority or control where the minor and the non-consenting parent are so fundamentally in conflict and the very existence of the pregnancy already has fractured the family structure" (22). Similarly, disagreement between parent and child over whether the child should be placed in an institution will have created the dispute which the hearing will only reflect. And while fundamental fairness requires that the child's wishes be fully represented by his attorney in a truly adversarial hearing, the vigorous advocacy of opposing points of view need not descend into an emotionally wounding battle. The hearing can be designed and conducted in a manner which minimizes the trauma to the child and enhances his sense that his objections to institutionalization have been fully considered and that he has been treated fairly.

In conclusion, the policy questions presented are complex and at the same time delicate. But two basic functions can be served by a commitment hearing system. The first is *individualization* of the child's admission decision and treatment or habilitation planning. A full exploration of the facts about a given child and his situation can sharpen the fact-finding process and decrease the likelihood of errors. A companion requirement of an individual treatment or habilitation plan will also assure that careful attention is paid to the individual child's needs. The second basic function is providing *accountability* to the system. While it is painful and annoying for any of us to have our professional conduct reviewed by others, judicial review, if properly administered and received, can enhance the carefulness and thoughtfulness of professional decision-making. To the extent that professionals view commitment hearings as an opportunity to improve the delivery of services, the procedures are likely to serve that function.

Once the decision has been made to institute a system of hearings for the commitment of mentally ill and mentally retarded children, several important legal questions remain to be answered. Each of these issues will have a major impact on how the commitment system for children works. Many substantive and procedural questions present themselves, such as whether the child will be entitled to a jury trial, whether the hearings will be open or secret, etc. This paper will focus on four of the most important questions: the standard of commitment, periodic review, voluntary admission of adolescents, and disposition when the child cannot return to his home.

Standard of Commitment

When the court (or other impartial tribunal) has heard the evidence on the condition and needs of the child, upon what standard is it to base its decision? In cases involving the civil commitment of mentally ill adults, psychiatrists and lawyers have vigorously debated the proper standard for commitment. The standard adopted by most state legislatures before the 1970s (and still preferred by many psychiatrists) (23) allowed commitment of a patient who was dangerous to himself or to others *or* who was in need of treatment and lacked sufficient insight into his condition to choose treatment for himself. In recent years, a number of courts have struck down such statutes on the ground that the "in need of treatment" portion of the standard exceeded the state's constitutional power (24). These rulings suggested that the state could commit those who were dangerous to themselves or to others, but that treatment of the nondangerous could only take place on a voluntary basis. The Supreme Court noted the issue, but explicitly chose not to decide it in *O'Connor v. Donaldson* (25). Even without a final ruling by the Supreme Court, many states have now chosen to limit commitment of mentally ill adults to the those who are dangerous (26).

Whatever one's views on this controversy involving adults (I personally favor the dangerousness standard), the question of the appropriate standard for children remains. One option is for states to decide that only children who are dangerous to themselves or others may be committed

(27). This has the advantage of limiting institutionalization to those cases in which it is most clearly necessary. A different approach would allow greater latitude in the commitment of children than is permitted with adults. For example, one state which limits commitment of adults to cases involving "likelihood of serious harm to oneself or others," allows the court to order residential treatment of a child when it finds "1) that as a result of a mental disorder or developmental disability the minor needs and is likely to benefit from the treatment or habilitation services proposed; and 2) that the proposed commitment is consistent with the treatment needs of the minor and with the least drastic means principle" (28). This more flexible standard allows the child to be committed when the court is convinced that he needs the treatment, will benefit from it, and the treatment cannot be provided in a less restrictive or intrusive manner.

On public policy grounds, this latter standard may be preferable because it allows intervention for a mentally ill child in need of treatment but who does not (yet) manifest dangerous behavior. The state must still show that treatment is really required, and that such less drastic measures as outpatient therapy are not likely to be effective with this child. It may be argued that even with these safeguards, the standard is still unconstitutional. No court has yet ruled on that issue, but the Supreme Court has repeatedly stated that "the power of the state to control the conduct of children reaches beyond the scope of its authority over adults" (29). This greater power over children may be sufficient to allow involuntary mental health treatment when need for that treatment is demonstrated.

Periodic Review

One of the evils of the parental "voluntary" admission system is that it does not require periodic evaluation of the child's continuing need for treatment. This has several unfortunate consequences. It may allow the child to become "lost," particularly in understaffed facilities. It is an especially troubling problem in cases of mentally retarded children whose parents have essentially "abandoned" them to the institution (30). The lack of periodic review may also allow the changing treatment needs of the child to go unnoticed over long periods of time. Where periodic judicial review is required, the treatment team will regularly have occasion to reconsider the child's needs. And finally, the lack of periodic review may give the child the impression—whether correct or incorrect—that he has been forgotten and that his institutional confinement will last indefinitely.

Whether the decision to require periodic review is mandated by courts in constitutional rulings or chosen by the legislature, the question of how frequently to provide such review will prove difficult. A balance must be struck between hearings conducted so infrequently that the child's case is not reviewed as circumstances change, and hearings conducted so frequently that no change has taken place and the proceedings become mere formalities. There is also a concern on the part of many child psychiatrists that hearings not be scheduled so frequently that they unduly interfere with the treatment process. Another factor to be considered is the child's concept of time, because clinicians have confirmed that younger children are unable to grasp fully the meaning of long intervals (31). An appropriate balance might be to have the first commitment period viewed as evaluative, and therefore no longer than a month or six weeks. Subsequent periods of renewed commitment could be longer, such as three or four months. Another possibility would be to provide hearings more frequently for very young children—every two or three months—than for teenagers (every four or six months). In no case should the child's commitment period be longer than six months, and in no case should it be longer than that provided to adults.

The Voluntary Minor Patient

As noted above, the term "voluntary admission of a child" has come to mean a child whose parents placed him in the institution. I have argued that such a system is unacceptable as a matter of constitutional law and public policy. But there are adolescents who truly wish to enter a residential facility voluntarily. Whether this should be allowed, and under what circumstances, is a difficult issue. The problem with allowing children an unlimited right to seek voluntary admission is that the safeguards of a hearing system could be denied to those children whose "voluntariness" has been obtained by coercion. Obviously, children are subject—and vulnerable—to a greater array of subtle and overt pressures than are adults. Therefore, some check on the minor's voluntariness is essential. New Mexico has developed a statutory scheme which allows a child 12 years of age or older to become a voluntary patient on his own initiative. He must then consult with an attorney appointed to represent him. The lawyer will explain his rights and then will ascertain whether the child really wants to remain in the residential facility. If the child does wish to stay, the lawyer will inform the court of this fact, and the child may be treated as a voluntary patient. The child is then free to leave treatment at any time (he is under no commitment order) unless the facility or his parents decide to seek his commitment. The voluntary child retains the right to periodic review, and his voluntariness will be recertified at regular intervals (32).

This system is still untested in practice, and will only remain acceptable if abuses do not develop. It is not available to children younger than 12 or to mentally retarded children, on the grounds that their voluntariness is even more suspect. The system attempts to balance the child's legal rights with his developmental abilities and his treatment needs.

Children Who Cannot Return Home

A serious practical problem will arise in some cases in which the court determines that the child does not need institutionalization. Finding that the child does not meet the statutory requirements for commitment (see Standard of Commitment above) is not equivalent to a finding that the child can return to his family's home. In some cases, the family may simply be unwilling to let the child return. In other cases, the hearing may produce evidence of problems in the home which make it unsafe or unwise to return the child to his family (e.g., child abuse or incest). Drafters of child commitment statutes will have to confront these problems.

One approach would be to allow the commitment court to order alternative placement of the child when the parents are unwilling to allow the child to return home. This would allow the child to go to other relatives, a foster home, a group home, or the like without the necessity of putting the parents through the ordeal and stigma of a neglect proceeding (33). It is important, however, that such a provision *not* be made available to deprive parents of custody who want to keep their child. Parents must not lose their procedural and substantive rights to due process in a neglect proceeding under the guise of mental health or retardation placement. But where the parents are willing to have the child live away from the family home, a practical mechanism should be available so the child will not have to be sent to an institution whose services he does not need or to a home which is unwilling to take him in.

IMPLEMENTING A COMMITMENT SYSTEM FOR CHILDREN

Any new legal system which significantly revises the way in which social institutions operate will prove difficult to implement (34). The juvenile commitment systems under discussion radically alter the relationships between parents, children, and mental health and mental retardation professionals. They will also add new actors—lawyers and judges—to this already complex system of relationships. It should not be surprising if the transition proves difficult in some states.

One important factor in this process will be the role played by the child's counsel. The attorney should not unnecessarily interfere in the relationships between his client and the client's parents and doctors, nor should he or she unnecessarily impede the process of treating the child. On the other hand, the lawyer must not be seduced into substituting his or her own judgment about the child's best interest for that of the judge or the child. The attorney's job is to ascertain what the child wants to do (when the child is able to communicate his wishes) and to present that position persuasively to the court. Nothing in the Canons of Ethics prohibits the lawyer from counseling with the client about the advisability of a particular course of action, but once the child has chosen, the lawyer's job is to represent and advocate, not to second-guess (35).

As the preceding paragraph suggests, the attorney is faced with a task of some delicacy. To advise, counsel, interpret, and represent the child adequately will require lawyers who possess considerable sensitivity. In addition, for the lawyer to be effective he or she will have to know a great deal about mental health or mental retardation and the possible forms of treatment for children. Each of these considerations argues for a system of specialized professional attorneys who operate in the mental health/mental retardation system on a full-time basis. To ask a lawyer in private practice to handle such a case by appointment on rare occasion raises the possibility of poor legal services for the child and unnecessary disruption of the mental health or mental retardation system because of the lawyer's inexperience and lack of expertise. Having capable and knowledgeable lawyers representing children is in the best interest of all parties. Therefore, the creation of a specialized mental health and mental retardation advocacy service seems advisable (36).

An equally important factor in the implementation of a commitment system is the role of the mental health or mental retardation professional. If professionals acting as service providers view the commitment hearings as nothing more than a formalistic impediment to their professional work, they may create a self-fulfilling prophecy. Hearings will advance the cause of individualization and treatment only to the extent that professionals allow them to do so. Their expert testimony will be required to guide the court's judgment. And their patience and understanding will be required to assist their minor clients in understanding the legal process and in adjusting to the court's orders. At first glance, a spirit of cooperation and shared enterprise may seem inconsistent with the adversarial model which is the core of the hearing system. But diligence in advocacy does not require that adults of different professions cannot work together to make the system serve the needs of children.

REFERENCES

1. *E.g., Institutionalized Juveniles* v. *Secretary of Public Welfare,* 459 F. Supp. 30 (E.D. Pa. 1978); *J. L. & J. R.* v. *Parham,* 412 F. Supp. 112 (M.D. Ga. 1976); *In re Roger S.,* 19 Cal. 3d 921, 569 P.2d 1286, 141 Cal. Rptr. 298 (1977). *See* note 14, *infra.*

2. *E.g.,* N.M. Stat. Ann. § 43-1-16.1 (Supp. 1979).

3. *E.g.,* Teitelbaum & Ellis, *The Liberty Interest of Children: Due Process Rights and Their Application,* 12 Fam. L.Q. 153 (1978), *reprinted* in 2 Mental Disability L. Rptr. 582 (1978); Ellis, *Volunteering Children: Parental Commitment of Minors to Mental Institutions,* 62 Calif. L. Rev. 840 (1974); Bezanson, *Toward Revision of Iowa's Juvenile Commitment Laws: Thoughts on the Limits of Effective Governmental Intervention,* 63 Iowa L. Rev. 561 (1978); Mental Health Treatment for Minors, *Legal Issues in State Mental Health Care: Proposals for Change,* 2 Mental Disability L. Rptr. 459 (1978).

4. *E.g., Comment by the American Psychiatric Association, the American Society for Adolescent Psychiatry, the American Academy of Child Psychiatry, and the American Association of Psychiatric Services for Children,* 3 Mental Disability L. Rptr. 74 (1979).

5. Ellis, *supra* note 3, at 840 n. 1.

6. U.S. Public Health Service Publication No. 51 (1951).

7. 1919 Mont. Laws, Ch. 102, § 9.

8. WOLFENSBERGER, W. (1975). The Origins and Nature of Our Institutional Models, Syracuse, N.Y.: Human Policy Press.

9. *E.g., Wyatt* v. *Stickney,* 344 F. Supp. 373 (M.D. Ala. 1972), *aff'd sub nom. Wyatt* v. *Aderholt,* 503 F.2d 1305 (5th Cir. 1974).

10. *E.g., Halderman* v. *Pennhurst State School & Hospital,* 446 F. Supp. 1295 (E.D. Pa. 1977).

11. *E.g., Nelson* v. *Heyne,* 355 F. Supp. 451 (N.D. Ind. 1972), *aff'd,* 491 F.2d 352 (7th Cir. 1974).

12. *Planned Parenthood* v. *Danforth,* 428 U.S. 52 (1976).

13. *In re Gault,* 387 U.S. 1 (1967).

14. *Parham* v. *J.R.* — U.S. —, 61 L.Ed. 2d 101, 121 (1979).

15. LIDZ, T., FLECK, S., & CORNELISON, A. (1965). *Schizophrenia and the Family.* New York: International Universities Press. Ellis, *supra* note 3, at 850-63 and sources cited therein.

16. Teitelbaum & Ellis (1978), *supra* note 3, at 190-97 [2 M.D.L.R. at 598-601]; *see also* A. Turnbull & H. R. Turnbull, (1978). *Parents Speak Out: Views from the Other Side of the Two-Way Mirror,* Columbus, Ohio: Charles Merrill.

17. Teitelbaum & Ellis, *supra* note 3, at 197 n. 187 [2 M.D.L.R. at 601 n. 187].

18. *Mathews* v. *Eldridge,* 424 U.S. 319, 335 (1976).

19. *See* studies collected in Teitelbaum & Ellis, *supra* note 3, at 180-86 [2 M.D.L.R. at 593-96].

20. For a more complete discussion, see Ellis, *supra* note 3, at 850-52; Teitelbaum & Ellis, *supra* note 3, at 190-97 [2 M.D.L.R. at 598-601].

21. KELLY & MENOLASCINO, *Physicians' Awareness and Attitudes Toward the Retarded,* 13 Mental Retardation 10 (December 1975).

22. *Planned Parenthood, supra* note 12, at 75.

23. *Comment by the American Psychiatric Association,* 2 Mental Disability L. Rptr. 519 (1978); *see also* A. Stone, *Mental Health and Law: A System in Transition* 43-82 (1975); *but see* Kahle & Sales, *Comment on Civil Commitment,* 2 Mental Disability L. Rptr. 677 (1978), reporting that a majority of psychiatrists surveyed favored limiting commitment of adults to those who are dangerous to themselves or others.

24. *E.g., Lessard* v. *Schmidt,* 349 F. Supp. 1078 (E.D. Wis. 1972), *remanded* 414 U.S. 473 (1974), *on remand,* 379 F. Supp. 1376 (1974), *remanded,* 421 U.S. 957 (1975), *on remand,* 413 F. Supp. 1318 (1976); *Suzuki* v. *Quisenberry,* 411 F. Supp. 1113 (D.C. Hawaii 1976); *Kendall* v. *True,* 391 F. Supp. 413 (W.D. Ky. 1975).

25. 422 U.S. 563, 573 (1975).

26. *E.g.,* Cal. Welf. & Inst. Code §§ 5200-5213, 5250-5268 (West 1972 & Supp. 1979); N.M. Stat. Ann. § 43-1-11 (C) (Supp. 1979).

27. *E.g.,* N.C. Gen. Stat. §§ 122-58.1 *et seq.* (Supp. 1977).

28. *Compare* N.M. Stat. Ann § 43-1-11 (C) (Supp. 1979) *with* N.M. Stat. Ann. § 43-1-16. (G) (Supp. 1979).

29. *Prince* v. *Massachusetts,* 321 U.S. 158, 170 (1944).

30. *See* Hammond, Sternlicht & Deutsch, *Parental Interest in Institutionalized Children: A Survey,* 20 Hospital & Community Psychiatry 338 (1969); Downey, *Parents' Reasons for Institutionalizing Severely Mentally Retarded Children,* 6 J. Health & Human Behavior 147, (1965).

31. GOLDSTEIN, J., FREUD, A., & SOLNIT, A. (1973). *Beyond the Best Interests of the Child,* New York: Free Press pp. 40-49.

32. N.M. Stat. Ann § 43-1-16 (Supp. 1979).

33. Mental Health Treatment for Minors, *supra* note 3, at 476; Ellis, *supra* note 3, at 890 ff.

34. BARDACH, E. (1977). The Implementation Game: What Happens After a Bill Becomes a Law, Cambridge, Mass.: M.I.T. Press. (describing and analyzing the process of implementing California's adult civil commitment statute).

35. For a more complete discussion of the lawyer's role, *see* Ellis, *supra* note 3, at 881-90. For a discussion of the lawyer's responsibility in representing an incompetent client in juvenile court proceedings, *see* Institute of Judicial Administration—American Bar Association, Juvenile Justice Standards Project, (Tent. Draft 1976). *Standards Relating to Counsel for Private Parties* 78-82 (L. Teitelbaum, reporter).

36. Mental Health Advocacy Service, *Legal Issues in State Mental Health Care: Proposals for Change,* 2 Mental Disability L. Rptr. 269 (1977).

17

PERSONAL INJURY TO CHILDREN: THE COURT SUIT CLAIMING PSYCHIC TRAUMA

LENORE C. TERR, M.D.

The civil suit claiming psychic injury to a child is an area of forensic child psychiatry rarely reported upon in the literature, yet it is a field which frequently requires expert psychiatric testimony. Psychic injury often follows a serious accident, assault, or episode of medical malpractice. The child victim may have been physically injured with concomitant psychic injury, or the entire post-traumatic result may be emotional. In such cases, several additional people may have been injured, some of whom died or were mutilated.

This chapter will present a general overview of the effects of psychic trauma upon children and a review of the legal principles involved. Thirteen personal injury cases in which the author was consulted as a child psychiatrist were reviewed and will serve as illustrations of the principles discussed. Table 1 summarizes the injuries in the 13 cases and the time intervals prior to legal action, psychiatric evaluation, and psychotherapy.

PSYCHIC TRAUMA IN CHILDREN

Freud's (9) definition of psychic trauma, "an extensive breach being made in the protective shield against stimuli," remains the best working concept we have. The psychoanalytic literature which followed Freud contained many further theories, such as "strain trauma" (13), "cumulative trauma" (12), and "retroactive trauma" (20), which departed from Freud's original meaning. In the field of child psychiatry, the term "trauma" was applied repeatedly to such events as the birth of a sibling,

249

hospitalization, surgery, and chronic parental rejection. Believing that trauma theory had become unwieldy, A. Freud (6), urged a return to Freud's original definition. The American Psychiatric Association's DSM III Draft (1978) defines a traumatic event as "the stressor . . . must be of sufficient magnitude that it would be expected to produce significant symptoms of distress in most individuals, and is also outside the range of such common normal human experiences as simple bereavement, chronic illness, business losses, or marital conflicts."

In a study of 23 kidnapped children of Chowchilla (22), I found early and later symptoms and signs of psychic trauma. The Chowchilla group were ages 5 to 14, of both sexes, of Chicano, Caucasian, and American Indian backgrounds, and from lower and middle class homes.

Early effects observed were: 1) Immediate fears of death, separation, and further trauma; 2) Misidentification of perpetrators and/or hallucinations; 3) Attempts to regain ego mastery by retrospectively searching for omens, portents, or signals which could have warned the child of impending disaster; 4) Mild to minimal denial; and 5) Absent were vegetative nervous system effects, tantrums, extreme passivity, or amnesia.

Late effects observed were: 1) "Traumatic play" (repetitive, monotonous, compulsive play which creates, rather than relieves anxiety; 2) "Reenactment" (single or multiple episodes in which parts of the traumatic experience or connected fantasies are reperformed by the child with no conscious connection to the traumatic episode; 3) Personality change on the basis of frequent reenactment, exaggeration of preexisting traits, or chronic anxiety; 4) Four types of traumatic dreams (non-remembered panic dreams, exact repetitions of the traumatic event, modified repetitions, and disguised dreams); dreams of death to the child himself and "predictive dreams"; 5) Fears of further trauma (similar to Rado's "traumatophobia" (19), fears of the "mundane" (the dark, being alone, strangers, being outside, vehicles, etc.), and a general distrust of the world and its inhabitants; 6) Cognitive errors such as time distortions, misidentifications, and overgeneralizations; and 7) Daydreams at will in older children, but no intrusive flashbacks.

In earlier studies of trauma in childhood, interesting findings have been reported. A. Freud and Dann (7) reported a sense of mutual protectiveness and lack of rivalry or competition in a group of child survivors of concentration camps. Dillon and Leopold (4) noted frequent enuresis in litigated cases involving head injuries to children. Lifton (17) described "survivors' guilt" in individuals who had been children at the time of the atomic bomb attack on Hiroshima. The same type of guilt has been noted by Lacey (14) in the child survivors of a coal-mining disaster which wiped-out their school in Aberfan, Australia. In general, survivors' guilt is seen only when some individuals die who were exposed to the same or similar trauma to which the surviving child was exposed. Newman (18) reported a pervasive sense of death in the children who were evaluated after the Buffalo Creek flood.

Three older concepts about trauma must be reappraised critically: 1) Fenichel's (5) idea that traumatic neurosis includes, "readiness to become overwhelmed traumatically" (p. 117), implying that the weak, the disturbed, the constitutionally poorly endowed will develop psychic effects from a traumatic event. In the light of recent literature on sensory deprivation and disaster (extensive review of the literature by Hocking (11), it has been shown that *any* normal person can develop traumatic aftereffects if the event is sudden enough, unexpected enough, and threatening enough. This does not mean that family and developmental history need be ignored in trauma cases. It simply means that the entire posttraumatic symptom complex cannot be "blamed" upon a pretraumatic emotional illness.

2) A. Freud and Burlingham's (8) and Solomon's (21) opinions that caretaking adults' reactions will determine children's traumatic responses. This factor has been eliminated, at least initially, in cases where the child undergoes the traumatic experience away from parents, guardians, or adult friends (sexual assault, attacks by dogs, Chowchilla kidnapping, and accidents in which the child was alone). In the author's experience, such children are able to recall severe initial post-traumatic psychic effects *prior* to their first parental contact. These observations bring into question the emphasis in the older literature upon parental reaction as it affects youngsters' postraumatic symptomatology. Certainly an aberrant parental reaction may worsen the child's psychic response, but it is doubtful that the parental reaction causes the child's psychopathology.

3) The idea of "secondary gain" interfering with treatment of any patient undergoing a lawsuit. Fenichel (5) states, "obtaining financial compensation or fighting for one creates a poor atmosphere for psychotherapy . . ." (p. 126-127). This point of view taken literally has led many psychiatrists to refuse psychotherapy prior to the settlement of civil suits. Leopold and Dillon (15) studied a group of survivors from a marine explosion and concluded that litigation had had little effect upon treatment outcome. Their group, who by maritime law were sure of receiving compensation, became more psychiatrically disturbed three years after the explosion than they had been initially. "Secondary gain" could not

have created a worsening of symptoms; instead, their conditions worsened because their posttraumatic reactions created more anxiety the longer they continued.

SUMMARY OF THE THIRTEEN CASES

The cases I have included in this chapter can be divided into three categories: those in which the child sustained physical injury during the accident, those in which the child was traumatized only emotionally, and those in which the child was an indirect participant. There is only one indirect participant case in which it was necessary to establish that a 4-year-old child, who had been the sole witness to an accident, had remembered it accurately (Doris, Case 7). In seven of the remaining 12 cases (Case 1, 2, 3, 8, 9, 10, 11) there was no physical injury other than scratches, cuts, or bruises (psychic trauma alone).

Five cases were associated with serious physical injury (psychic trauma plus physical injury). In one of these (Lisa, Case 12), the child was injured in an automobile accident which killed her two brothers and two of her cousins. Lisa required facial plastic surgery. She has a large disfiguring scar on her leg. Coleen (Case 6) sustained severe burns of her face, neck, and chest from flammable pajamas. Linda (Case 4), a girl born with Turner's syndrome who was hit by a car, required skin grafting to her lower thigh. Jennifer (Case 5) injured her vagina, uterus, and abdomen when she stepped over an out-of-control high pressure hose in an attempt to stop the water. Carolyn (Case 13) was nearly killed by a vicious dog that slashed open her trachea. The psychiatric evaluation of these five injured children was directed not only towards the possibility of posttraumatic stress response syndrome, but also towards the repercussions upon a child of a permanent disfigurement, sexual injury, prolonged hospitalization, and/or mourning for dead family members.

Eleven of the 13 cases are plaintiff's cases, that is, the report was prepared for the attorney representing the injured party. Two of the cases were referred by defense attorneys, that is, attorneys representing an automobile insurance company (Mark, Case 1), and a major television network (Gladys, Case 11). In all instances, the referrals were screened by phone by the author before agreeing to the evaluations. Eight cases were referred by attorneys, two by pediatricians, two by other psychiatrists, and one by a social worker.

The data upon which this report is based were collected while the

TABLE 1

Time Intervals in Lawsuits Studied

Name	Accident Type	Accident Date	Psychiatric Evaluation	Re-Evaluation	Legal Settlement Or Trial	Psychiatric Treatment
1. Mark	Passenger in auto	1970	1973	.	1974	1970-71 (4 months)
2. George	Bike struck by car	1966	1967		1967	0
3. Jay	Pedestrian hit by car	1973	1974	1977, 1978	1978	0
4. Linda	Pedestrian hit by car	1973	1975		1975	0
5. Jennifer	Waterhose	1975	1975		1978	0
6. Coleen	Pajama fire	1967	1974		Pending	1975 (12 months)
7. Doris	Witness to brother's fall	1968	1973	1975 (2 times)	1975	0
8. Christine	Schoolyard rape	1975	1975	1976, 1977	1977	0
9. Greg	Slapped by M.D.	1967	1969		1970	0
10. Jim	Gas explosion	1968	1969		1973	1972 (3 weeks)
11. Gladys	Sexual assault	1974	none requested		Trials: 1976, 1978	Some Rx, but dates not known
12. Lisa	Passenger in auto	1974	1976		1977	0
13. Carolyn	Attacked by dog	1973	1978		1979	Begun 1978, continued post-trial 3 mos.

author was a faculty member at Case Western Reserve University Medical School, Cleveland, Ohio, and at the University of California San Francisco Medical School.

Personal injury lawsuits concerning psychic injury concern three practical issues: 1) Was someone directly or indirectly at fault? (liability); 2) Was permanent emotional damage done, or is there a high probability of future emotional problems related to the accident? (damages); and 3) Can the party being sued pay? (collectability). Attorneys determine collectability early in their consideration of a case. They rarely ask child psychiatrists to help settle issues of liability, although these are often of social importance and will be discussed in this chapter. In general, most requests for psychiatric evaluation in civil suits relate to the determination of damages.

Liability

Of the 13 cases of civil suits on behalf of children in my files, the question of liability was brought up by the attorneys in two cases (Cases 8 and 11). In two other civil suits in which the issue of liability was not posed to me (Cases 7 and 9), courtroom discussion of liability could have also raised important health and social questions. In the first case, Gladys X. vs. PDQ-TV, Gladys, 8, brought legal action against a TV network for showing a homosexual rape with a mop handle during a "family hour" documentary. Gladys had been vaginally assaulted with a bottle a few days after the TV program by a group of older girls, whose leader had heard about, but probably had not seen, the TV show. Gladys' parents sued PDQ-TV claiming that their child would not have been assaulted in such a fashion if not for the TV program. The case was initially dismissed on grounds of freedom of speech, was reviewed by the California Supreme Court which ordered a retrial, and was lost by Gladys again in the lower court. In the second trial, the judge ruled that PDQ-TV would have had to present the program with the intent of inciting others to such attacks in order to be liable for the assault upon Gladys. The author served twice as a consultant to PDQ-TV's lawyers. The attorneys wished to understand the outlook of a local child psychiatrist about the possible internal motivations for such an attack and about the effects their program might have upon both normal and emotionally disturbed youngsters (liability issues). It is ironic to note that amicus curiae briefs were submitted by eminent medical and psychiatric groups in this case, but the TV network's attorneys worked on the liability issues with one local child psychiatrist.

Another interesting case involving liability is Christine S. vs. Largetown, California Board of Education, et al. Christine had been "kicked out" of a 9th grade dance because she was discovered holding a cigarette. Despite Christine's protests that her parents were not at home and that she had no transportation, she was ordered twice by teachers to leave the school building. The 14-year-old girl was then raped anally and vaginally by a gang of youths in the school parking lot. If this case had proceeded to trial (and interestingly enough, it did not because Christine was too upset following her deposition to be able to testify again), liability questions would have been posed to the author. Does a school have responsibility to provide some protection for youngsters coming to its functions? Does it have "in loco parentis" obligations? In determining at trial whether a school is so obliged, the child psychiatrist is asked to provide an expert opinion about the needs of youngsters as related to schools.

The following cases are illustrations of those in which important liability questions were *not* asked of the author, yet the lawyers later responded that they could have asked such questions with effective results. Doris M., at age four, had been the sole witness to a horrifying episode in which her baby brother leaned against a closed window in their slum apartment, and fell out of the building. Although the author was asked only to qualify Doris as an accurate witness, the liability question might have been asked. What activities of a normal child of a given age would make him susceptible to danger from slum conditions? (Parenthetically, the damages question might also have been asked: Was Doris M. psychically harmed by witnessing such a fall? She indeed was.)

Greg S., a 4-year-old boy suffering from cerebral palsy, was slapped by an orthopedic surgeon about 15 times. The surgeon had attempted to saw off a hip-length cast, first stating, "I'm going to cut this right here" (pointing to the child's groin). Greg, fearing castration, screamed and attempted to squirm out of the way of the saw. The doctor then pummelled Greg's face in the presence of the boy's grandparents. Although the author was asked to report about damages, not liability, the attorney for Greg S. later noted that bringing up the liability question would have allowed courtroom discussion of the mismanagement of a child in a physician's office. Aside from lawsuits, in my clinical practice I have heard several complaints by parents that their children were manhandled in doctors' offices. Courtroom testimony is one way to combat this occurrence. It is a form of "professional liaison" which makes a distinct impression!

Damages

The use of the child psychiatrist expert witness to help assess damages is the most practical and the most frequently used expert testimony in civil suits involving psychic trauma. There are two types of damages: special and general. Special damages include total costs of diagnostic studies and treatment to date and future medical expenses, if they are "reasonably certain" to occur. General damages are awarded for pain and suffering, humiliation, and inconvenience.

To fully assess special damages, a child psychiatrist is asked if there is "reasonable certainty" of future expenses and/or suffering. Estimates about future medical expenses are based upon the child's status during evaluation. For example, if there are serious injuries to sexual organs in early childhood, there is often "reasonable certainty" of problems with adult sexuality in the future. Seven-year-old Jennifer (Case 5) was injured at her apartment complex when she stepped over an out-of-control high pressure water hose in an attempt to stop the water. Her vagina and cervix were torn, requiring emergency surgery. When she recovered physically she allowed no gynecological examinations, nor was she able to discuss the injury or the anatomy involved. I reported that Jennifer will "probably" have difficulty accepting her body as an adolescent because currently she has difficulty doing so. There is a likelihood that her problem will worsen in adolescence and adulthood. Coleen, age eight (Case 6), was burned on her chest, neck, face, and pelvis in a pajama fire. Not only was Coleen profoundly depressed and suicidal throughout latency, but it was possible to prognosticate worsening of symptoms in adolescence and adulthood. Growth of her breasts would require several new plastic surgery procedures, and by adolescence she would begin to understand and resent the significance of her inability to bear children.

Because prognostication is a particularly difficult aspect of the psychiatric report in civil suits, a checklist may help, at least in part (see Table 2). There is no way at this time to prognosticate with "certainty," but the modifier "reasonable" is helpful. Bear in mind that each individual case is different, and therefore may not apply to this list, and that the need for specific prognostication is a legal, not a medical requirement. "Reasonable certainty" is the legal test for determination of specific damages and future general damages. Some indications for "reasonable certainty" of future expenses and/or suffering in civil suits are indicated in Table 2.

TABLE 2

Indications of "Reasonable Certainty" of Future Expenses and/or Suffering

1) Likelihood of worsening of a physical or emotional condition because of further expected developmental phases or physical development. For instance, if more plastic surgery would be required, or if more emotional significance would attach to the injury at a later date, it would be reasonable to assume further pain and suffering in the future.

2) Longstanding posttraumatic personality change with concomitant problems with relationships.

3) The presence of the longest lasting symptoms of stress response syndrome: loss of trust, well-established fears of the "mundane," fears of reexperiencing trauma, frequent or terrifying dreams, serious reenactments, or continuing "traumatic play."

4) "Survivors' guilt" and/or suicidal depression.

5) Longstanding poor school performance postaccident. This must be documented with school records from before and after trauma.

PROGNOSTICATION AND LONG-TERM FOLLOW-UP

In 13 civil suits claiming psychic trauma to children, I was asked to assess future damages in 10 of these (Cases 2, 3, 4, 5, 6, 8, 9, 10, 12, 13). Eight exhibited a "reasonable certainty" of future emotional disturbance (4, 5, 6, 8, 9, 10, 12, 13) and two were considered to show a "possibility" of future disorder (Cases 2 and 3). Follow-up of at least one year was available in seven of these. Two years after settlement of her civil lawsuit, Linda, a 10-year old with Turner's syndrome who had been hit by a car (Case 4), continued her postaccident closeness with her mother and unwillingness to leave the house to socialize. Coleen, eight years old (Case 6), who was burned in a pajama fire continued suicidal and severely depressed 10 years after her accident. Christine, age 14 (Case 8), who was raped in her schoolyard, maintained her belligerent personality and her fantasies of revenge two years after the asault. Jim, age 11 (Case 10), who survived a gas explosion in front of his house, remained "weird" according to his mother, and he often indulged in staring spells at age 19. Carolyn, age eight (Case 13), who began psycho-therapy with the author at age 13, five years after an attack by a dog, remains cautious in the neighborhood, afraid that dogs might run into her house, and prone to dreams of being bitten and dying.

The two patients for whom the author prognosticated "possible" future difficulty were both followed up. Five-year-old George, hit on his bike by an automobile, cried and defecated initially. After the accident he was beset with fantasies about little green men who were about to poke his buttocks. George's post-traumatic difficulties appeared to the author to lie in the exacerbation of Oedipal castration fantasies. If he could be helped toward closure of the Oedipal phase, perhaps he would suffer no further abnormality. The lawsuit was settled one year post-accident. His mother was contacted for follow-up 10 years after the accident. George had progressed normally through adolescence and had experienced no further difficulties with anxiety about injury or damage.

On the other hand, Jay, an 8-year-old pedestrian who had been hit in a crosswalk by an automobile, manifested poor school performance and fear of crossing streets one year postaccident. The author felt that there was a "possibility" of future difficulty, but that this was not "reasonably certain." In Jay's case, the attorneys chose to wait five years prior to settling his lawsuit. During that time Jay was reevaluated twice by the author. He suffered an exacerbation of repeated nightmares at age 11 and never recovered his excellent pretraumatic school performance. In retrospect, he could have been given the "reasonably certain" prognosti-cation. The "possible" prognostication moved his lawyer to delay settle-ment until the long-term outcome was more evident.

Prognostication about future need for therapy is only one element in the awarding of damages. Damages related to pain and suffering, humil-iation, and inconvenience can be determined in part through the psy-chiatric report and/or testimony. A large portion of the eventual settle-ment or jury award rests upon the pain, suffering, and humiliation "intangibles."

DELAYS IN EVALUATION, TRIAL, AND TREATMENT IN CHILDREN'S CIVIL SUITS

Age of Majority and Statute of Limitations

In cases involving children, the statute of limitations allows the child plaintiff to wait to file the complaint until one year after the age of majority is reached (California Code of Civil Procedures § 352, 1976).

All but three states, Florida, Louisiana, and Connecticut, have statutes of limitations similar to California's in regard to age of majority (1).

The delays which result from the prolonged period prior to filing a lawsuit can be tragic. For example, Coleen, who had been burned in 1967, was evaluated in 1974 and had not yet completed her lawsuit in 1977. During that waiting period, she had made three suicide attempts. She had received social work counselling in her small community, but her lawyer stated that no local psychiatrist had been willing to treat her because of the pending lawsuit.

Delay Prior to Psychiatric Evaluation

Because of the delay on the part of parents to seek legal counsel following an accident to their child, and because of the long waiting period prior to the time cases must be filed, civil cases are often seen by child psychiatrists many years after the trauma. In Table 1, the waiting periods for the author's 13 cases are summarized. Note that only two cases (5 and 8) were evaluated the same year as the accident. Three cases (6, 7, and 13) came to the psychiatrist five years or more postaccident, and interestingly, these were among the most severely affected victims in the group. A waiting period of one to three years is the most usual (Cases 1, 2, 3, 4, 9, 10, 12). The children who were interviewed psychiatrically three to seven years after trauma all suffered posttraumatic physical problems. Mark, seen three years after an auto accident, had developed ulcerative colitis three weeks after the accident, and his attorney waited to observe its progress. (There were no further attacks in three years.) Doris, who had witnessed her brother's fall from a window, did not come for evaluation until her traumatically retarded brother's first five years of life had been carefully observed and recorded. Coleen was not psychiatrically evaluated until seven years after she was burned because the attorneys wished to allow full prognostic and therapeutic efforts by the plastic surgeons who were treating her. Similarly, Carolyn was not referred for psychiatric evaluation until her attorney understood her plastic surgery status after her attack by a dog.

On the other hand, the cases which were referred for psychiatric evaluation during the same year or one year post accident were those in which the accident caused psychiatric symptoms only, rather than physical damage (Cases 2, 3, 8, 9). The one exception, Jennifer (Case 5), was discussed in the Chapter 14 (The Child as a Witness).

Not infrequently, trial attorneys wait until the very last minute prior to a trial to contact a child psychiatrist for expert testimony. This creates a very difficult situation for the child and for the potential expert witness.

Delays Prior to Settlement or Trial

Even after psychiatric evaluation has been completed, the trial or settlement may be postponed, often necessitating reevaluation of the child. Cases 3 and 10 represent particularly long periods between initial evaluation and final legal settlement. In both cases the lawyer wished to watch the child's progress prior to making any agreements with the "opposite side."

Treatment: Often Delayed, Frequently Eliminated

Of 13 cases evaluated psychiatrically, only five received any psychiatric treatment (1, 6, 10, 11, 13); two of these were inadequately treated (6 and 10). Coleen (Case 6) attempted suicide after "counselling" treatment, and Jim remained "strange and dreamy" according to his mother eight years following his accident. He had undergone only three weeks of psychiatric inpatient treatment and no outpatient treatment.

Often it is not feasible for the psychiatrist who evaluates the child for the lawsuit to also conduct the psychotherapy. Some children come from far distant towns to be evaluated near their attorney's office. Such trips would not be possible more than once or twice (Cases 6, 9, and 12). Furthermore, some parents are interested in the evaluation, but not at all interested in obtaining treatment for their child. This fact becomes evident when the evaluation is complete and the parents turn down the idea of psychotherapy (Case 12). Additionally, many parents cannot afford private psychotherapy, and would be unable to do so until the case has been settled (Cases 2, 3, 4, 5, 7, 8, 10). Finally, some cases are evaluated for the defense, not the plaintiff (Cases 1 and 11) and, as such, would not be appropriate for the "defense psychiatrist" to take into treatment.

It is sad to note that in long-term follow-up of seven of the settled plaintiff cases (2, 3, 4, 8, 10, 12, and 13), only one of these children (Carolyn, Case 13) received psychotherapy after they had won their cases and had received payment of damages. Jim (Case 10) used his money to buy a small business, but he continued to be psychiatrically disturbed in adulthood. George (Case 2) and Christine (Case 8) received such small settlements, that after the attorneys' and physician's fees were paid, there was no more money available for psychotherapy.

Linda's (Case 4), Greg's (Case 9), and Mark's (Case 1) settlements have remained untouched in trust.

The only child for whom the author has been able to provide long-term psychotherapy is Carolyn (Case 13). Her parents can afford private treatment and they understood the need for initiating psychotherapy *prior* to the settlement of her lawsuit. The therapy which began prior to the trial continued afterward for three months.

THE PATIENT'S RIGHT TO TREATMENT

In the study group of 13 children involved in civil suits related to accidents, attacks, or medical malpractice, each child showed signs and symptoms of posttraumatic stress syndrome. Those who had been physically injured showed psychic responses to loss of function and disfigurement. How is it, then, that only one child has undergone long-term psychotherapy? First, the delays inherent in the legal process account for these children's late initial arrival in the psychiatrist's office. Their interest, and their parents' interest in obtaining treatment is blunted by years' delays. Second, some children (e.g., Coleen) are denied psychiatric treatment because the psychiatrists do not wish to treat those who are in the midst of a lawsuit. Finally, parents often have other ideas in mind for their children's use of the damages payments, and it is the parents and the courts who control the funds until the child attains majority. Courts which award financial compensation to children require that the money be put into a guardianship or trust account until the child reaches age 18. This is true not only in California and Ohio where this study was done, but in most other states. Parents may request the Court to release money for purposes approved by the Court. Since the damages payment has been originally recommended, at least in part, for psychotherapy, the funds could be released from the trust account for that purpose, provided it can be shown that the parents cannot afford to pay for therapy on their own. Still, such money, once secured in trust, was not released by this series of parents.

It is interesting to note that the child's rights vs. parents' rights issue might arise in civil lawsuits involving children. In only one case in this series, that of Lisa (Case 12), did the child wish psychotherapy and did the parents refuse. The child did not sue the parents for the right to treatment, nor was this suggested by any participating party. Rather, Lisa, as a compromise, accepted the idea of counselling by the parish priest, a condition which the parents also endorsed. Unfortunately, it was not possible to obtain long-term follow-up after the compromise between Lisa and her parents was reached: the attorney with whom the author had prepared the case left the firm which continued to represent Lisa.

CIVIL SUITS AND CONFIDENTIALITY OF PREVIOUS PSYCHIATRIC RECORDS

In California, a plaintiff who claims injury to himself relinquishes the right of confidentiality of all previous medical records relevant to the issues raised. For instance, let us hypothesize that a child psychiatrist has treated Mary from age eight to 10 for obsessive-compulsive neurosis. Then at age 14 Mary is hit by a truck and suffers both physical injuries and psychic effects. She becomes a plaintiff against the trucking company, and the trucker's attorneys subpoena Mary's earlier child psychiatric records. Such records are no longer protected by rules of confidentiality because if a patient becomes a plaintiff, he/she automatically relinquishes this right. The well-known cases of Lifschutz (16) and Caesar (3) represent attempts of treating psychiatrists to protect their patient's records in such instances. In neither case was the psychiatrist able to prevail in protecting his patient's file, since the patients had automatically given up their right to confidentiality when they sued. There were concessions made by the courts in both instances, however. In their opinion on Lifschutz, the California Supreme Court maintained that if either side or the expert witness disputes the relevancy of the files, they can be submitted in confidence to the judge who will decide which portions of the record are relevant. (The California psychiatrist could make this request to the judge on his/her own without legal counsel.) In Caesar, likewise, the Court maintained that it must be shown that the subpoenaed medical file is relevant to the lawsuit. In a more recent decision, Britt vs. Superior Court of San Diego County (2), the California Supreme Court maintained that the plaintiffs' automatic waivers of confidentiality do not automatically put all the medical records up for discovery; the plaintiffs waive only those records which were directly relevant to their lawsuit. Each state has its own statutes of confidentiality which must be consulted. The Caesar and Lifschutz cases, however, gained national attention and may have influenced other jurisdictions.

Returning to 14-year-old Mary, if this hypothetical truck accident victim claimed only physical injury and no psychic injury, the psychiatrist who treated her from age eight to 10 might be able to quash the subpoena of her file on the grounds that the psychiatric record is not relevant to the issue of the lawsuit. Note that the practicing psychiatrist, in order to quash the subpoena, would need his/her own attorney if neither participating attorney were willing to move to quash the subpoena. Furthermore, Mary's psychiatrist might on his/her own ask that the record be submitted in confidence to the judge who would decide which portions of the record were relevant to Mary's truck accident.

DEALING WITH THE ATTORNEY

Psychiatrists working with personal injury attorneys should establish a verbal contract at the onset. Prior to accepting the case, the attorney's reputation may be informally checked with a reputable attorney from the same area. Before seeing the patient, the psychiatrist needs to know precisely what questions the attorney wishes answered. Is the report to deal mostly with damages? Is the report to concern itself with finding of fault? The report of the original evaluation will be a legal document for negotiating settlement or preparing for trial. It will very likely be read by the family, and perhaps by the child. (George, Case 2, read his report as a teenager and laughed about the "green men," whom he had repressed.) The evaluation and report must be objective, complete, and frank so that the parties can plan their lawsuit realistically. Psychiatric theory must be explained as it applies to the child's injury. The report is sent directly to the attorney who originally made the request, and he/she in turn often sends copies to the family, the opposition, or another expert examining the child.

Often it is necessary to meet in person with the attorney prior to writing the report, or prior to the taking of the psychiatrist's deposition. Communication by phone and/or in consultation meetings is necessary in developing a well planned case. Unless otherwise arranged in advance, it is customary to bill the attorney, not the patient, for his/her client's interviews and the time required to write the report or prepare the case.

THE TRIAL: A RARITY

In the series of 13 cases reported in Table 1, only two cases (Gladys X v. PDQ-TV, and Carolyn) ever came to trial. Gladys's case, in fact, was tried twice, but I was not called to appear as a witness because the legal issues of freedom of speech and "incitement" determined both trial outcomes without necessitating expert psychiatric testimony. The only case at which I testified at trial was that of Carolyn (Case 13). Of 12 cases which are now concluded, 10 ended with pretrial settlements. Psychiatric reports were required in all but the Gladys vs. PDQ-TV case. Pretrial depositions were taken in four of the cases (Cases 8, 9, 10, 13).

It is interesting to note that almost all of this type of civil suit are settled out of court. Franklin et al. (10) found that in 1961 in New York State, of 193,000 cases of victims who sought to recover damages caused by someone else's fault, only 7,000 reached trial, and of these, 2,500 reached verdict. Instead of anticipating a trial in cases of child victims, the social worker or psychiatrist can proceed with careful evaluation and treatment. A complete report, much the same as one presented to colleagues, but with no abbreviations or psychiatric "jargon," will suffice in the majority of these cases.

REFERENCES

1. AMERICAN JURISPRUDENCE TRIALS (1966), 4:602-603. San Francisco: Bancroft-Whitney Co.
2. Britt v. Sup. Ct. San Diego County, 30 Cal. 3d 844; 574 P 2d 766 (1978).
3. Caesar v. Montanos, 542 F2d 1064 (1976).
4. DILLON, H. & LEOPOLD, R. (1961). Children and Post-Concussion Syndrome. J.A.M.A., 175:86-92.
5. FENICHEL, O. (1945). The Psychoanalytic Theory of Neurosis. New York: W. W. Norton & Company.
6. FREUD, A. (1967). Comments on Trauma. In Psychic Trauma, S. Furst (Ed.). New York: Basic Books, pp. 235-245.
7. FREUD, A. & DANN, S. (1951). An Experiment in Group Upbringing. In The Writings of Anna Freud, 4:163-229. New York: International Universities Press, 1968.
8. FREUD, A. & BURLINGHAM, D. (1943). War and Children. New York: Medical War Books, Ernst Willard.
9. FREUD, S. (1920). Beyond the Pleasure Principle. Standard Edition, 18:7-64. London: Hogarth Press, 1953-1974.
10. FRANKLIN, M., CHANIN, R. & MARK, I. (1961). Accidents, Money and the Law: A Study of the Economics of Personal Injury Litigation. Columbia Law Rev., 61:1-10.
11. HOCKING, F. (1970). Extreme Environmental Stress and Its Significance for Psychopathology. Am. J. Psychotherapy, 24:4-26.
12. KHAN, M. M. R. (1963). The Concept of Cumulative Trauma. The Psychoanalytic Study of the Child, 18:286-306. New York: International Universities Press.
13. KRIS, ERNST (1956). The Recovery of Childhood Memories in Psychoanalysis. The Psychoanalytic Study of the Child, 11:54-88. New York: International Universities Press.
14. LACEY, G. (1972). Observations on Aberfan. J. Psychosom. Res., 16:257-260.
15. LEOPOLD, R. & DILLON, H. (1963). Psycho-anatomy of a Disaster: A Long Term Study of Post-Traumatic Neuroses in Survivors of a Marine Explosion. Am. J. Psych., 119:913-921.
16. In re Lifschutz, 2 Cal. 3 415; 85 Cal. Reporter 829; 467 P 2d 557 (1970).
17. LIFTON, R. (1967). Death in Life; Survivors of Hiroshima. New York: Random House.

18. NEWMAN, C. (1976). Children of Disaster: Clinical Observations at Buffalo Creek. *Am. J. Psych.,* 133:306-312.
19. RADO, S. (1942). Pathodynamics and Treatment of Traumatic War Neurosis. *Psychosom. Med.,* 4:362-368.
20. RANGELL, L. (1967). The Metapsychology of Psychic Trauma. In *Psychic Trauma,* S. Furst (Ed.). New York: Basic Books, pp. 51-84.
21. SOLOMON, J. (1942). Reactions of Children to Black-Outs. *Am. J. Orthopsych.,* 12:361-362.
22. TERR, L. (1979). Children of Chowchilla: A Study of Psychic Trauma. *The Psychoanalytic Study of the Child,* 34:552-623.

18

LEGAL ISSUES IN THE PRACTICE
OF CHILD PSYCHIATRY

SANDRA G. NYE, J.D., M.S.W.

An understanding of the law as it regulates the practice of child psychiatry requires exploration of several basic legal concepts. The psychiatrist/patient relationship is both a clinical and a legal entity. It is hoped that clinical exigencies will determine most treatment decisions. Even as economic exigencies must be the determiner at times, so also may legal mandates or restrictions influence the course of treatment delivery. Legal issues arise in every professional or commercial relationship, and in many interpersonal ones as well. The child psychiatrist juggles medical, mental health, and family law constantly. To some extent, the psychiatrist is always at risk for legal involvement—if not direct liability. Psychiatry is much safer for the psychiatrist when practiced with some sophistication in its legal aspects.

LEGAL NATURE OF THE PSYCHIATRIST/PATIENT RELATIONSHIP

The legal nature of the relationship of the psychiatrist and patient is that of a personal service contract. This is the case irrespective of whether or not the word "contract" is ever spoken between them, whether or not the services are paid for, and whether or not there is any written agreement. The agreement between psychiatrist and patient that the psychiatrist will deliver treatment services and patient will receive these services may be expressed or implied. The terms of the contract are likely to include the nature of the services to be delivered; the time, place and frequency of service delivery; the cost (if any) and arrangements for payment; the nature of the patient's participation in the treatment process—and any other details of the respective rights and responsibilities.

Essential to the validity of the contract is what is referred to as a "meeting of the minds." Simply, this involves a mutuality of expectations —an understanding between the parties as to what is to be done by whom. The contractual concept of "meeting of the minds" has special relevance to the psychiatrist/patient contract. In the ordinary course of events, an individual has total freedom to choose whether or not and with whom to enter into a contractual relationship of any nature. Mutuality of expectation requires that the person consenting to treatment— contracting for treatment—be informed as to what he/she is agreeing to do or have done. It has been suggested—and is very likely true—that a large percentage of claims by patients against physicians arise out of a lack of mutuality of expectations. The patient's assumptions as to what he/she will receive or is expected to contribute to the treatment process may bear little or no relationship to those of the physician. When the patient doesn't get what he/she thinks he/she bargained for, dissatisfaction may well be expressed in a legal proceeding. A meeting of the minds is the basis for "informed consent," without which the physician may not—in a voluntary treatment situation— treat the patient.

An uninformed consent is a legal nullity. For a consent to be valid, three major requirements must be met.

The consentor (the patient and/or the parent) must be informed as to:

1) *The nature of the condition being treated.* There is some concern about the effect on patients and their families who are exposed to psychiatric diagnoses. Under some circumstances, it might suffice to inform the consentor descriptively as to the condition being treated. It is to be noted, however, that if a diagnosis is to be recorded and disseminated —as to a third party payor or a state mental health department—the consentor has an absolute right to know what that is so that he/she can make an informed choice as to whether or not to permit this to occur.

2) *Treatment alternatives possible for the condition being treated and the probable success of the treatment.* The consentor should be informed as to the particular advantages of the various treatment alternatives, including availability and cost.

3) *Foreseeable risks* of the several alternatives, including side effects, and *benefits.* The consentor must be helped to consider the "risk/benefit ratio" in determining upon a course of action. It is entirely appropriate to "sell" the treatment modality preferred by the psychiatrist so long as the patient has been properly informed as to risks and alternatives.

CHILDREN AND CONTRACTS

Who May Enter into a Contract

Historically, the law has viewed adults as the only legal persons. A minor—one who had not achieved the status of adult—was a legal non-person and was generally devoid of legal capacity to act on his/her own behalf. The contractual capacity rule was a commercial concept which evolved as protection for children (who were generally assumed to be lacking in education and judgment to make wise business decisions) from exploitation by unscrupulous adults. Inasmuch as a minor lacked capacity, with certain significant exceptions, to enter into a contract, any person attempting to contract with a minor did so at risk of the minor's later avoidance of his/her contractual obligations. The minor might have some liability to return the goods contracted for, if possible, but he/she could otherwise back out, leaving the adult party to the contract to absorb his/her losses.

The contract rule of minor noncapacity dovetailed neatly with the legal view of children as chattels—the property of their parents. As chattel holders, parents had the right to the services, including earnings, of their children, and to their custody and control. The concomitant right of the child was to support and maintenance from the parent. The rule, if applied without exception, imposed an undue and inappropriate hardship on those minors who were, for one reason or another, not supported and maintained. Recognizing that some minors had to provide their own support and maintenance or not survive, the law created an exception to the contractual capacity rule and conferred capacity on a minor to contract for his/her "necessaries," i.e., food, shelter, clothing and—presumably—medical care for life threatening conditions (1).

An emancipated minor—one who had left his/her parent's home, was self-supporting, and/or was married—achieved adult status as to contractual capacity. It must be remembered that emancipation is an economic doctrine by which parents are relieved of the legal obligation to support a child who is no longer living within their control and providing services (2). Mere unilateral leaving home does not emancipate a minor. The parents must actively or, by failing to object, passively consent to the leaving, thus emancipating—freeing—the child from his/her economic ties to the family. Upon emancipation, a minor acquires the common law rights and responsibilities of adulthood. An unemancipated minor, having no capacity to enter into a contract or otherwise enter into a legal transaction, could not contract for or consent to medical treatment. Only a parent or guardian had the prerogative to consent on behalf of the child. Long before the enactment of any statutes governing medical practice, the common law rule conferring upon minors the capacity to consent for "necessaries" could be invoked to allow a physician to treat a child on his/her own consent in a life and death situation.

The common law concepts of parental prerogative, minor noncapacity, emancipated minor, and the "necessaries" exception probably sorted out most consent issues, though not all of them. A physician who treated a minor on the "necessaries" contract theory might still be subject to a tort action for technical battery (3). Aside from any contractual issues, touching the person of another without consent is a battery; thus medical treatment of a child without parental consent is technically battery—even when it is for the child's best interest. If the parent of an unemancipated minor objects to treatment of a child who required it, a physician who treated the child would be gravely at risk for law suit. Although the irate parent might be hard pressed to establish damages (proves his/her economic loss by reason of the physician's treatment), and so might be unlikely to recover any sizeable sum from the physician, the physician would still be subjected to the stress and expense of defending the action. Furthermore, punitive or exemplary damages (to teach a lesson to persons who interfered with parental authority) were always a possibility. In some jurisdictions, to protect well-intentioned clinicians from meritricious tort lawsuits for battery, a doctrine of implied consent arose (4). The law assumed that, in the case of a person who was unable to give consent by reason of his/her condition, consent would have been given if the person were able; consent to treat was "implied." Likewise, in the absence of parental consent because the parent was not available, consent to treat a child would be implied if the condition requiring treatment was life-threatening or so serious that delay for purpose of obtaining parental consent was likely to endanger the child's health.

MEDICAL PRACTICE ACTS AND CAPACITY TO CONSENT TO TREATMENT

Within the past century or so, the common law of the physician/patient relationship has been codified to some extent by medical practice statutes enacted in every state. These statutes establish who may practice medicine and upon whom medicine may be practiced. Typically, they permit a physician to deliver medical services only to certain described persons, thus prohibiting delivery of services to anyone else. Therefore, irrespective of the common law status a minor may have, whether emancipated or not and whether or not the "necessaries" rule might apply, the physician may or may not be legally permitted by statute to deliver services under certain conditions. In a sense, medical practice acts confer consensual capacity on those persons whom a physician is permitted to treat.

Practice acts vary from state to state. The typical statute will permit a physician to treat consenting persons of a certain age or over, as well as minors who are married or pregnant, and will also provide that parents of a minor child may consent to treatment of the minor (5). The statute may add that a physician may treat without consent in the event of an emergency (which may be variously defined). Some statutes may provide that a physician who treats in any emergency will not be liable on account of lack of consent (6). Most states (but by no means all) confer upon minors of a certain age (usually 12 years or over) capacity to consent for treatment of venereal disease and substance abuse, for birth control services and for treatment of conditions relating to pregnancy (7). We are beginning to witness statutory authority for minors to consent to mental health care as well (8).

OBTAINING TREATMENT FOR MINORS WHEN PARENTS FAIL OR REFUSE TO PROVIDE IT

There has been much written in recent years concerning the minor's right to consent to—or refuse—medical treatment. The law of parental authority has been predicated on the assumption that parents have their children's best interests at heart and will act beneficently on their behalf. Probably this is so in a majority of cases, but we know that it is by no means universally true. Recent legal trends have recognized that children have constitutional rights and that the state has a compelling interest in the welfare of children which will support intervention into and abrogation of parental authority over children when necessary to protect a child or when the welfare of the community requires (9).

Thus is has come about that the law has variously conferred upon minors limited capacity to consent to medical treatment and related services. Most states recognize some right in minors to obtain some form of treatment under some conditions. Where such capacity has not been legislated, or where a child does not have the desire, maturity or capability to act on his/her own, it has often proved tragically difficult to treat. The usual recourse in such cases is to the Juvenile Court.

Parental failure to provide a child with necessary medical treatment has been looked upon as neglect (10). The position of courts has varied from jurisdiction to jurisdiction as to the necessary prerequisities for court intervention. It is generally held that the state may intervene, take guardianship of a child, and order treatment over parental objection for life threatening conditions. In cases where life is not at risk, there is considerable lack of consensus as to what conditions are required to override a parent's refusal to permit treatment.

In the Jehovah's Witness cases, blood transfusions have been ordered over parental objections notwithstanding the argument of parental prerogative and the constitutional issue of religious freedom (11). In two New York cases in which both parent and child declined to consent to potentially beneficial but nonlifesaving surgical procedures for the child, the respective courts arrived at apparently opposite conclusions. One court refused to order repair of a harelip and cleft palate in a child who had apparently made a good social adjustment despite his infirmity and who concurred with his mother in refusing surgery (12). In another case, however, there was a contrary holding in which the court ordered surgery for a facial deformity stating that the state had a "paramount duty to insure (the child's) right to live and grow up without disfigurement— the right to live and grow up with a *sound mind* in a sound body" (13) (emphasis added). Whether psychiatric treatment would be ordered in the face of parental refusal to consent might well be determined by the seriousness of the psychiatric disturbance and the danger inherent in it to the child or others (14).

An additional source of treatment decision-making has been provided by P.L. 94-142, part of the federal Education for All Handicapped Children Act of 1975. School systems are required by law to provide clinical services necessary to correct conditions which interfere with a child's learning. If psychiatric treatment is deemed necessary for a child and the parent(s) refuse to permit it, extrusion from school may follow due process procedures with the result that the child may be deemed to be educationally neglected. Juvenile court intervention would be appropriate in such an instance.

CHILDREN OF DIVORCED OR SEPARATED PARENTS

It seems fairly clear from the above that, absent a statute conferring capacity upon a minor to consent to psychiatric treatment, it is within the parent's prerogative to do so. In an intact family, or in a separated family where there has been no court order as to child custody, both parents have coequal rights as guardians. Each may make decisions as to the child's activities; each has an equal right to "possession" of the child, and each—or either—may singly consent to medical treatment of the child. In a separated or divorced family, where there has been a custody order, the custodial parent has the right to the "care, custody, control and education" of the child, unless there is a specific clause in the order to the contrary. It is to be noted that although the custodial parent has the primary right to consent to treatment for the child, most medical practice acts do not make a distinction as to custodial and noncustodial parents. If the statute merely states that "a parent" has capacity to consent to a child's treatment, a physician may ordinarily rely upon either parent's consent for ordinary medical care. Where long-term therapy, surgery or hospitalization is required, the custodial parent's consent should be obtained. The psychiatrist, aside from the obvious clinical problems raised, would be well advised to decline to treat without the custodial parent's consent.

As to who is responsible for payment for the treatment, as between the careprovider and the parent of the child, the parent who contracts for the child's treatment is primarily liable, notwithstanding any order directing that the noncustodial parent pay for any or all medical care. Any dispute between the parents as to support obligations must be settled between them, if necessary in the divorce court. The psychiatrist is not obliged to become a party to that dispute. Modern divorce law holds that both parents are coequally responsible for the support and maintenance of their children. Thus, if the contracting parent does not have the wherewithal to pay, the psychiatrist who finds himself/herself forced to resort to lawsuit for collection may choose to join both parents in the action (15).

CONFLICTS OF INTEREST IN THE TREATMENT PROCESS

In the vast majority of cases, the psychiatrist treats a child under a contract with the parents. Where a parent, or any other third party, contracts for clinical services on behalf of the patient, the psychiatrist may be faced with a dilemma as to whom his/her major duty is owed. So long as the parent's goals and inclinations are congruent with the child's treatment needs, there is no problem. By virtue of the very nature of the therapeutic process, this is not always likely to be the case.

Where parent's wishes and child's treatment needs conflict, the psychiatrist's primary duty is to his/her patient. The obvious "kicker" is that the parent has the right to terminate the treatment if he/she is not satisfied with what is occurring. The double bind for the psychiatrist is apparent: to alienate the parent may result in the treatment being interrupted or withheld; to conform to the parent's wishes when contrary to the clinical needs of the child is malpractice, at best. By and large, this dilemma is best dealt with as a clinical issue, utilizing a clinical approach. Where that doesn't work, the psychiatrist will have to ascertain the latent—as well as manifest—risks to the child, not to speak of the parent/child relationship, in attempting a legal maneuver—recourse to the Juvenile Court—with no guarantee as to outcome.

The best approach to conflict with a parent who is sabotaging or otherwise interfering in a child's treatment is a preventive one. The contract for treatment should spell out with the greatest possible specificity what role the parent will be expected to play, how the psychiatrist will relate to the parent, what behavioral manifestations the treatment process is likely to evoke in the child, the likelihood of alteration of family relationships, the probable (or possible) length of the treatment process—and any other aspects of the relationship and its operation that the psychiatrist can anticipate. All of this is, of course, included in the concept of informed consent. Consent to treatment based on any less information than this can hardly be said to be informed. Although no writing is required to validate the treatment contract, psychiatrists may wish to consider a procedure whereby this information is put in written form so that it may later be referred to.

THE CONTRACT TO EVALUATE AND REPORT

If it is clear that the duty of the psychiatrist to the patient is superordinate to any obligation to the parent who contracts for the treatment and pays for it, it stands to reason that the same rule obtains where the third party contractor is other than the parent. The psychiatrist who is hired by a school or a court may feel somewhat torn as to loyalties. It is important to distinguish, in these contractual relationships, between evaluation and reportorial services and treatment services. If the psychiatrist is hired to perform an evaluation and make a report, the person or persons being evaluated are not patients; the relationship between psychiatrist and evaluation subject is not that of therapist/patient. The psychiatrist owes to the evaluation subject only the duty to do a proper and careful evaluation. Indeed, the psychiatrist's client in this situation is the person or institution who hires him/her to do the evaluation, and it is to that client to whom the duty is owed. It is essential, however, that the subject be fully informed as to the nature of the relationship, that the subject's communications will not be confidential, that a report will be rendered and to whom.

THE NONPARENT THIRD PARTY CONTRACT FOR TREATMENT

Where, on the other hand, the psychiatrist is hired to provide treatment services, the relationship to the individual treated is that of therapist/patient and the primary loyalty and duty are to the patient (16). Two common examples of such an arrangement are the student health service or the court clinical service. The patient always has the right to assume and rely upon the assumption that the treater is providing optimal care based on the patient's needs and that the patient's interests are being served. If any third party is to be given access to the patient's clinical data or to receive reports or direct the treatment, the patient (and his/her parent or guardian) must be informed of this arrangement at the time treatment commences, and this becomes part of the treatment contract. In accepting employment by a third party, it behooves the psychiatrist to have clearly spelled out and agreed upon relative rights and responsibilities of employer, therapist and patient.

CHILDREN AND PSYCHIATRIC HOSPITALIZATION

The recent cases of *Bartley* v. *Kremens* (17) and *J. L.* v. *Parham* (18) have presented to the United States Supreme Court a question particular to psychiatric hospitalization of children, but general to the entire fabric of the parent/child relationship. Given the fact that a child is a person with constitutional rights, who has the right to waive those rights on behalf of the child? Historically, parents had total control over the treatment and living arrangements of their children. The right of a parent to place a minor child in an institution was accepted without question. The issue of a child's constitutional rights was never raised, much less decided. Basic to our constitutional system, of course, is the right to liberty. The state may abridge that right by an exercise of its "parens patriae" powers when an individual is deemed in need of protection and care. The exercise of these constitutional powers may take place only by due process of law.

The various "rights" movements of the sixties produced rights concepts that had either not been previously articulated or had, at most, been around in nascent form. The right to privacy emerged as including a right to control over one's own body—and presumably, by extension, over the mind housed within that body (19). This privacy right marches alongside the rights to freedom of speech and expression and religion. Put them all altogether, and a right to be "original," "different," even "deviant" is constitutionally protected.

Also early in the 1960s was born a revolutionary concept of "right to treatment"—an outgrowth of the right against deprivation of liberty. The theory, briefly stated, is that a person deprived of liberty because of a clinical condition has a right to be treated for that clinical condition; to confine a person and not treat the condition is to deprive that person of his/her liberty without due process of law (20). Corollary to the concept of right to treatment is that of right to refuse treatment. If one has a constitutional right to liberty and privacy, a right to be left alone, does (s)he not also have a right to refuse unwanted treatment—to refuse to consent to treatment? And if (s)he has not consented to treatment, is it not true that the clinician has no right to treat? Operative in this discussion is the "due process of law" mechanism by which the individual's constitutional right may be abridged.

As to children, they are in many ways subject to invasions of privacy and deprivations of liberty from infancy onward. Their parents, not they, have the power to consent to and impose upon them all sorts of constraints—from toilet training to bedtime to injections, foul-tasting medicines and surgery, spinach, Sunday school, secular school, piano lessons, boarding school, camp—and all of this without a murmur as to constitutional infringement. Why, then, are we suddenly faced with a question as to the right of a parent to institutionalize a child for treatment?

Indeed, the subject of constitutional rights of children has only just been tapped. It was only in 1967 that the law recognized that children were persons entitled to constitutional protection (21). This concept is being developed through a series of cases in which the courts are defining and delimiting children's rights. Over time, the law of parent/child relationships has evolved recognizing certain instances in which the old concept of parental immunity from lawsuit by a child can be overturned (27); providing to children a right to be heard on the matter of their custody (23); and allowing state intervention in parental prerogative based on the theories of *parens patriae* and police power in dependency, abuse and neglect situations (24). The right of a parent to institutionalize a child is particularly vulnerable by reason of the tremendous impact such a step must have on the child's future. Some of the arguments against parental prerogative to institutionalize a child have been expressed as follows: the stigma attached will accompany the child through life; with modern data collection storage and retrieval methods, there is no possibility of leaving behind the experience of having been psychiatrically hospitalized; the ramifications will be intense; career, education and social opportunities restricted, and insurance and credit opportunities adversely affected, to name a few; there is sufficient clinical data to the effect that children do not thrive in institutions to cast doubt on the efficacy of institutionalization as a choice in the best interests of children (25).

Parameters for deprivation of personal liberty have emerged in recent years, for better or for worse: a person confined as punishment for wrong-doing is confined by due process of law and may be confined in a most restrictive setting. A person who has not been convicted of a crime and who is deprived of liberty because of illness as a result of which he/she is in need of confinement in order to treat and/or is in danger or endangers others must be confined only to the extent necessary to prevent the harm sought to be avoided and to treat the condition for which he/she is confined: the least restrictive alternative. Child rights advocates insist that if a child requires treatment, habilitation, custodial care—whatever—and if he/she cannot be kept at home and with his/her family, he/she may be placed elsewhere by his/her parents—but that child's freedom can be abridged only to the extent required by his/her condition, and only by due process of law.

The counter arguments range from invocation of traditional parental prerogative to the theory that either the child, or the parent on the child's behalf, can waive any due process requirements that may exist. The child advocates then urge that inasmuch as the law does not recognize the child as having contractual capacity, it does not recognize in the child the capacity of waiver. If the child has no legal capacity to contract away his right to liberty, he cannot waive his right to due process before someone else contracts away that right and he cannot volunteer himself for treatment, at least not without statutory authority.

Both Bartley and Parham are concerned, at bottom, not with treatment issues at all. Their real concern is to further define constitutional rights of children and to add one more piece to the jig-saw puzzle existing in the issue of waiver and substituted waiver of rights. At the time of this writing, the Bartley case has been dismissed by reason of changes in the local law under which it arose and the aging of the children on behalf of whom it was brought. Parham has been argued before the Supreme Court; in a most unusual move, the Supreme Court has asked for additional briefs before rendering its opinion. In a highly controversial opinion, the Court held that parents do have the right to institutionalize their children without a due process hearing because there are safeguards in the clinical system to preclude abuse. However, another round on the state level is still to be fought.

PROFESSIONAL LIABILITY AND TREATMENT OF CHILDREN

Physicians often ask with asperity what right lawyers have to muck about in the professional practices of the medical profession (26). The answer lies in the political role assigned by society to the institution we call "law." The role of law as an institution is to regulate relationships among members of society. Lawyers, as practitioners of the law, then find themselves involved in issues of rights and responsibilities of individuals and groups to each other and the community. The law as regulator of business and personal relationships has evolved into a sophisticated and complex system of rules, methods of their enforcement and sanctions for their breach. When the psychiatrist enters into a professional relationship with a patient, both parties have rights and responsibilities vis-à-vis each other. By reason of the special quality of that relationship—e.g., the psychiatrist is in the position of greater knowledge and power, the patient is dependent for his/her well being on the knowledge, skill and good will of the psychiatrist—the law apportions those rights and responsibilities much to the advantage of the patient. Again because of the high level of trust required in the psychotherapeutic relationship, the law imposes upon the psychiatrist the highest duty towards the patient—that of a "fiduciary" (27).

In addition to any express terms in the therapeutic contract, such as time, place, frequency and cost of treatment, there are implied in the contract two warranties—the implied warranty of confidentiality (28) and a warranty that the psychiatrist is possessed of and will appropriately utilize that level of skill and knowledge which could be expected from the typical member of the profession (29). The law does not imply a guarantee of results of treatment. Unless the psychiatrist is foolish enough to expressly guarantee results, the law interprets the treatment contract as just that—a contract to treat; not a contract to cure (30).

The psychiatrist is in charge of the clinical process and has not only the right but the duty to choose the modality of treatment (31). The psychiatrist determines the hours he/she will work, the location of treatment, and whom he/she chooses to treat. There is no obligation to be available after clinic hours or on weekends. There *is* a duty to provide backup or alternative treatment services—and this may well be referral to the nearest hospital emergency room. Every clinician has a right to take reasonable vacations; some sort of locum tenens arrangement in the psychiatrist's absence satisfies the standard of care so long as the substitute is qualified.

The legal duty owed by psychiatrist to patient arises out of the contractual relationship. Another way to put it is that the clinician owes no duty to one who is not his/her patient. Professional liability arises out of a breach of the duty owed under the contract. There are three major aspects of professional liability: breach of contract, tort liability and premises liability. The breach of contract arises when either the psychiatrist or the patient fails to live up to the express or implied terms of the treatment contract. Tort liability arises when an individual commits a wrongful act other than a breach of contract—either negligently or intentionally—upon another causing that person to suffer damages (which may be monetary or physical or both) for which the law recognizes a remedy.

Negligence in the delivery of professional services is known as "malpractice." A deliberate breach of contract or a deliberate tortious act is not malpractice. A clinician who deliberately, willfully, sets out to harm or otherwise wrong a patient may be liable for his deliberate wrongful act—but not as malpractice. If he/she is accused of a willful wrong, his/her malpractice insurance carrier is not obliged to defend against the claim and is not obliged to pay any damages on account of it. Malpractice insurance protects against *negligent* acts—accidental or careless errors—not intentional wrongs.

Much concern has arisen among medical practitioners over the massive increase in malpractice claims in recent years. Not only the incidence of claims, but also the size of settlements and awards, has increased, driving professional liability insurance rates skyward. No sector of the profession has escaped unscathed, but psychiatrists may take "Dutch comfort" in the knowledge that among the specialties, theirs is the least sued. The reasons for this have been the subject of a lot of speculation. No doubt several elements have combined to produce this result. The special nature of the relationship, and especially the transference phenomenon, is doubtless a factor. Also, the nature of the psychiatric population may mitigate against such activity.

With the patients' rights movement and increased consumer education, the psychiatrist's vulnerability to suit may increase. Panic is uncalled for, even in the light of increased risk; it is estimated that the incidence of claims against psychiatrists is 1.5 claims per 100 psychiatrists per year with most being settled for a small sum or dismissed (32). A lawsuit impugning one's personal character or professional capability is a horrendous experience and even if one wins, it is best avoided. The information in this chapter is by way of forewarning and forearming.

The plaintiff in a malpractice suit is not going to find it easy to win. A disgruntled patient—or parent or guardian of a patient—will be required to establish a certain constellation of elements to sustain his/her case. If the plaintiff fails to do so, the case will be dismissed. Even if he/she manages this feat, the psychiatrist has an opportunity to defend against the claim and win. Every plaintiff has "the burden of going forward" and establishing a "prima facie case." For malpractice to "lie" (legal jargon meaning that there's a case), the plaintiff must prove that

1) the defendant/psychiatrist owed a duty to the plaintiff patient (another way to say this is that there was a psychiatrist/patient contract) ;
2) the defendant was negligent and thereby breached his/her duty;
3) the patient suffered some injury (e.g., physical or financial) as a proximate (direct) result of the negligent breach.
4) the injury would not have occurred but for the negligence of the psychiatrist (33).

A good faith error in judgment is not malpractice. Incorrect diagnosis or treatment *not* arising out of negligence are not malpractice. Nobody expects even a psychiatrist to be 100 percent correct all of the time. Even if the patient suffers the most grievous harm, so long as the psychiatrist acted within the scope of the consent and exercised due care in service delivery, there is no malpractice.

In determining whether or not a clinician is negligent, the law applies as the standard of care "the duly careful member of the profession." What that mythical person would have done will be considered appropriate. Due care includes possession of the reasonable and ordinary qualifications of the profession, diligence and skill in treatment. One holding oneself out to be a specialist is held to a higher degree of skill and knowledge than the general practitioner. Due care will require, for example, returning calls within a reasonable period of time; listening (really hearing!) to a patient's complaints; taking an adequate history and verifying facts; and—as indicated—obtaining consultation or referring.

A physician may withdraw from a case at any time he/she chooses and for any reason so long as he/she gives reasonable notice of intent to withdraw in plenty of time for the patient to find a successor. Sufficient records and information must be provided (with consent) to the successor—to insure proper care. Unilateral severance by the psychiatrist of the treatment relationship, without reasonable notice, at a time when care is still required and continued treatment is not contraindicated, is abandonment. Precipitous discharge from the hospital is also abandonment.

The third major form of professional liability is "premises or equipment liability." A patient who is injured by equipment used by the psychiatrist can sue the psychiatrist, the facility and the manufacturer of the equipment (34). If it is established that the equipment injury is the result of negligence on the part of the psychiatrist or the facility, of course the manufacturer would not be held liable. An example of premises liability would be a child getting hurt while running around unsupervised in the waiting room or on the grounds of a facility while a parent is receiving treatment. The therapist who is aware of the situation, as well as the facility, would probably be liable for any injury to the children while on the facility premises.

There are instances in which a nonnegligent psychiatrist will be liable for the wrongful act of another. This is known as vicarious liability (35). A psychiatrist in charge is clearly liable for the negligence of other professionals and paraprofessionals working under him, and so forth down the line. This is of particular interest to the psychotherapy field because of the pervasiveness of supervision. To put it briefly, the supervisor is responsible for the negligence of his supervisee; the facility is responsible for the negligence of its employees.

Professionals practicing in a partnership are jointly and severally liable for each other's negligence. The implication here is that one must choose one's partners very carefully because one is legally responsible for their professional errors (36).

An attending physician may be responsible for the negligent acts of the substitute who is covering for him in his absence only if the attending professional has been negligent in choosing the substitute (a person less qualified than he/she or if he/she fails to inform his/her patient of the intended substitution in time for the patient to transfer to another professional of his/her own choosing (37). It is particularly important, when utilizing a substitute with less experience or lesser qualifications, to inform the patient of the substitute's position. The patient has the right to be treated by a clinician possessing the degree of skill and experience upon which he/she has been led to rely.

CONFIDENTIALITY, PRIVILEGE AND PRIVACY

Although the concept of psychiatric confidentiality is so ingrained that it seems almost unnecessary to dwell upon it at length, a number of cases have arisen in very recent years concerning rights and responsibilities as to patient information. An overview seems indicated.

Earlier in this chapter, it was mentioned that there is inherent in the psychiatrist/patient contract an implied warranty of confidentiality. The psychiatrist, in contracting to treat a patient, is obliged by reason of that contract not to disclose the patient's confidential information without written informed consent. In addition to the contractual duty, the psychiatrist owes the duty based on the fiduciary, or high trust, nature of the relationship. Many states have enacted statutes imposing and delineating a duty of confidentiality as well.

Disclosure of a patient's confidential communications without his informed consent is grounds for a lawsuit based on breach of contract and/or breach of confidentiality. If the information wrongfully disclosed is of an embarrassing or unflattering nature and results in the patient being held in opprobrium or subjected to ridicule, it may be considered "defamation of character," even if every word of it could be proven true (38). A disclosure in violation of a statute may result in a criminal or license revocation proceeding. In short, it is not only generally good clinical procedure to carefully maintain a patient's confidentiality, it is also good business!

Breach of confidentiality is frequently just plain neglect. Careless handling of records and documents, indiscreet conversation about a patient within earshot of another, elevator and cafeteria chit-chat, are common occurrences. Perhaps equally common and even more reprehensible is what is essentially gossiping—cocktail party conversation or "war stories." Patient confidentiality is often breached in the process of "linking," "networking," and inter-agency cooperation. Casual telephone inquiries and discussions about patients without consent are as inappropriate as gossiping. Agencies may react with hostility to a refusal to discuss a patient who has not given consent. Although inter-professional goodwill is an essential component of service provision, patient's rights cannot and need not be sacrificed to it. If a choice is required between violating professional responsibility to the patient and irritating a co-professional, opting to protect the patient is also protection from liability.

A patient's confidential data may be shared without his/her consent within the clinic/agency or institution for purposes of the patient's treatment. It is generally accepted that supervisors and consultants are considered part of the patient's "treatment team." Any such professional with whom information is shared will have the same duty to maintain confidentiality as the patient's own therapist. Without obtaining informed consent, identified patient information may not be shared for teaching, research or any other purpose.

Informed consent to disclose is exactly the same in nature as informed consent to treat. The consentor must be informed as to what he is consenting; he/she must be instructed as to alternatives, foreseeable risks and benefits. It is elementary that a consentor must know the contents of any record material to be disclosed in order to be informed. A patient who has given an uninformed consent and who later is distressed by the content of the material disclosed will have a breach of confidentiality suit against the discloser. Uninformed consent is no consent at all. The obvious consequence of the informed consent rule is that any patient (or other appropriate consentor) must have access to the record and know what it is to which he/she is consenting if the consent is to be valid.

In the case of a minor patient, without statutory consent authority, the minor lacks capacity to consent to release of information. The parent or guardian must authorize any disclosure. Some statutes which give minors certain consent rights are silent as to disclosure of clinical data. The rule of thumb is that the right to access and consent is a correlate of the right to consent to treatment.

When the patient is a young child, the right of the parent to have access to the child's information is not in dispute. Adolescents, however, present a different clinical situation. Often, perhaps usually or always, parental access to an adolescent's treatment information is contraindicated. At the commencement of treatment, the psychiatrist, adolescent patient and parents should have a very clear understanding as to what, if anything, will be shared with the parents. If a dispute arises around a parent's demand for access and the psychiatrist's unwillingness to permit it based on the patient's clinical needs, the worst thing that could happen would be a lawsuit to compel the psychiatrist to comply. The outcome of such a suit is not certain; the author knows of no reported cases in which such an action was brought. Much would depend on the presentation of clinical evidence and expert opinion as to the needs of the child and the prior agreement with the parents.

Allied to the duty of confidentiality is the concept of privacy. Every person has a common law and constitutional privacy right—the right to have his/her private facts kept private; not to have his/her name or likeness appropriated; and not to have his/her personal activities subjected to observation or intrusion. Identified patient data, clinical case histories, audio and video-tapes, photographs of patients may not be used for any purpose outside of treatment and its direct corollaries without written, specific and informed consent (39).

A third concept having to do with patient information is that of a communication privilege. Privilege is an evidentiary concept which provides an exception to the general principle of law that courts have the right to every man's evidence. The concept has relevance only in the context of the testimonial arena. A testimonial privilege (or shield law) permits those protected by it to withhold testimony or records, notwithstanding a subpoena.

The means by which a witness is compelled to appear in court or for deposition to testify is the *subpoena*. A *subpoena duces tecum* demands production of documents. Although a *subpoena* is a formidable looking document which may not be ignored, it is not to be mindlessly complied with. A lawyer should be consulted for advice when a *subpoena* is received. Frequently, it is subject to being "quashed." Even when it isn't, negotiation can often result in significant limitations on the data which must be disclosed. The psychiatrist's fiduciary and contractual relationship with the patient require him/her to take steps to contest a subpoena where it is not in the patient's interest to disclose. Failure to do so may be considered a breach of duty and subject the psychiatrist to suit (40).

Some—not all—jurisdictions have enacted a psychiatrist-patient privilege. Without such a statute, no privilege exists. It is imperative that the psychiatrist be thoroughly informed as to any privilege existing in his/her jurisdiction. Patient involvement in legal proceedings is far from uncommon, and psychiatrists are not infrequently pulled into these affairs, willingly or not. Patients with legal involvements must be informed in detail as to the existence or absence of a testimonial privilege so that they can make informed choices as to what information they wish to expose to possible discovery.

RECORDS AND RECORDING

With the advent of third-party payments and various types of audits, not to speak of patient access to and general vulnerability of records, there is considerable discussion as to what kind of psychiatric records should be kept, if any! The purposes for which records are kept will determine the type and style of the record.

In the days during which records were kept only as a clinical tool to assure continuity of patient care, there was not too much concern over what was written in them. With the advent of sophisticated data storage and retrieval technology and widespread concern over the misuse of psychiatric records, a new concept of recording is emerging. The new guideline must be, "less is more."

Realizing that a psychiatrist's records may, in a professional liability case be his/her best evidence of proper care, it is recommended that diagnostic and treatment decisions be backed up by record. There should be an accurate log of treatment and medication. Any statutory recording requirements must be met, and there must be enough detail to satisfy accountability requirements for payors. Consistent with these demands and the patient's clinical needs, recording of treatment content should be minimal.

Process recording should not be included in the record of patient care. Nor should the record contain insulting, judgmental descriptions or remarks, hunches or speculations, or unverified material from third parties (including other clinicians and family members). A therapist who has need to write down material of this nature for training, supervision or research purposes should keep it in a separate place, unidentified as to patient name, and clearly designated as the therapist's fantasies or speculations. It must be remembered that material in written form takes on a life of its own. Whereas a clinician reading such material would be able to assess its relevance and value, a nonclinician would not. It is entirely too likely that a judge or other nonclinical reader misapprehend and misconstrue clinical record content, especially when objective, verified statements are all mixed up with speculative material.

There are instances, furthermore, wherein the psychiatrist may be behooved to deliberately omit from a record certain types of data which—although relevant to treatment needs—could be more harmful to the patient if made known to him or others than loss of the information would be. An example would be the report that the patient is the product of incest, or his/her parent is involved in a homosexual affair! Modern recording techniques are available to guide in restructuring clinical record systems. One of the most promising of these from the perspective of economy of time and usefulness as a clinical instrument is the problem oriented record.

How long should psychiatric records be kept? If there is a statutory requirement, it must be met. Otherwise, the record should be kept until it is no longer useful for service needs or for use as evidence of the standard of care delivered. A statute of limitations exists in every state which prevents bringing a lawsuit after a certain time period has elapsed following discovery of a cause of action. For example, the statute of limitations for malpractice may be two years; for a breach of contract action, five years. The statute does not begin to "run" in the case of minors until the minor reaches the age of majority. Thus every record of treatment of a child should be kept at least to the age of majority plus the period of the longest statute of limitations relevant to care given (in most cases, the contract statute).

REFERENCES

1. FOSTER (1974), A "Bill of Rights" for Children.
2. Smith v. Seibly, 72 Wash. 2d 16, 431 P.2d 719 (1967); Cohen v. Delaware L. & W.R.R., 150 Misc. 450, 269 N.Y.S. 667 (Sup. Ct. N.Y. County, 1934). See also Katz, Schroeder and Sidman, Emancipating Our Children—Coming of Legal Age in America, 8 Fam. L.Q. 211 (1974), and Clark, Law of Domestic Relations, p. 24 of (1968).
3. Bonner v. Moran, 126 F.2d 121 (D.C. Cir. 1941); Zoski v. Gaines, 271 Mich. 1, 260 N.W. 99 (1935); Zagman v. Schultz, 19 Pa. D & C 309 (1933). W. Prosser, Handbook of the Law of Torts 35 (4th ed. 1971, at 103).
4. Tabor v. Scobee, 254 S.W. 2d 474 (Ct. App. Ky. 1951).
5. See e.g. Ill. Rev. Stat. C. 91, § 18.1.
6. PILPEL, Minors Rights to Medical Care, 36 Alb. L. Rev. 462, 464 (1972).
7. Pilpel, supra. at note 6, pp. 474-486; Wilkins, Children's Rights: Removing the Parental Consent Barrier, 1 Ariz. L.J. 31 (1975).
8. Ill. Reo Stat Ch 91½.
9. See Note, Judicial Power to Order Medical Treatment for Minors Over Objection of Their Guardians, 14 Syracuse L. Rev. 84 (1962).
10. HOLDER, Legal Issues in Pediatrics and Adolescent Medicine, pp. 114-115.
11. People ex rel Wallace v. Labrenz, 104 N.E. 2d 769, 111 (1952).
12. In re Seiferth, 309 N.Y. 80, 127 N.E. 2d 820, (N.Y. 1955).
13. In re Sampson, 328 N.Y.S. 2d 686, (N.Y. 1972).
14. In re Carstairs, 115 N.Y.S. 2d 314 (1952).
15. Holder, supra at note 10, p. 137.
16. Beadling v. Sirolta, 176 A. 2d 546, N.J. 1961; Union Carbide and Carbon Corp. v. Stapleton, 237 F.2d 229, C.C.A. 6, 1956; Coffee v. McDonnell-Douglas Corp., 503 P.2d 1366, (Cal. 1972).
17. Bartley v. Kremens, 402 F. Supp. 1039 (E.D. Pa. 1975).
18. Parham v. J.L., 412 F. Supp. 112 (M.D. Ga. 1976).
19. Roe v. Wade, 410 U.S. 113 (1973); Eisenstadt v. Baird, 405 U.S. 483 (1972); Greswold v. Connecticut, 381 U.S. 479 (1965). See also Raitt, The Minor's Right to Consent to Medical Treatment: A Corollary of the Constitutional Right of Privacy, 48 48 Southern California L. Rev., 1417-1456 (1975).
20. Birnbaum, The Right to Treatment, 46 A.B.A. J. 499, May 1960; Rouse v. Cameron, 373 R. 2d 451, D.C. C.A. 1966; Pyfer, The Juvenile's Right to Receive Treatment, 6 Fam. L.Q. 245 (1972).
21. In re Gault, 387 U.S. 1 (1967).
22. Katz, Schroeder and Sidman, supra at note 2, pp. 219-299.
23. See Speca and Wehrman, Protecting the Rights of Children in Divorce Cases in

    Missouri, 38 U.M.K.C. L. Rev. 1 (1969); Foster and Freed, *A Bill of Rights for Children*, 6 Fam. L.Q. 318-330 (1972); Inker and Perretta, *A Child's Right to Counsel in Custody Cases*, 5 Fam. L.Q. 32-44 (1971).

24. *State* v. *Perricone*, 37 N.J. 463, 181 A. 2d 751 (1952); *Prince* v. *Massachusetts*, 321 U.S. at 170.

25. PANNETON, *Children, Commitment and Consent: A Constitutional Crisis*, 10 Fam. L.Q. 295-334 (1977).

26. SEDHEV. (1976). Patients' Rights or Patients' Neglect: The Impact of the Patients' Rights Movement on Delivery Systems. *J. Psych. and Law*, 4:333-376.

27. DAWIDOFF, (1973). *The Malpractice of Psychiatrists*, pp. 43-60.

28. *Doe* v. *Roe*, 345 N.Y.S. 2d 560, *aff'd* 33 N.Y. 2d 902, 352 N.Y.S. 2d 626, 307 N.E. 2d 823, 20 A.L.R. 3d 1109 (1977); *Hammonds* v. *Aetna Cas. and Surety Co.*, 243 F. Supp. 793 (N.D. Ohio, 1965).

29. SLOVENKO, (1973). *Psychiatry and Law*, pp. 395-396.

30. Slovenko, *supra*, p. 399.

31. *Derr* v. *Bonney*, 231 P.2d 673 (Wash. 1951).

32. SLAWSON, (1970). Psychiatric Malpractice; a Regional Incidence Case Study. *Am. J. Psych.*, 126:1302.

33. HOLDER, (1978). *Medical Malpractice Law*, 2d ed, p. 101.

34. Holder, *supra* at note 33, pp. 174-199.

35. *See, e.g.*, 204 *J.A.M.A.* No. 2, page 257, April 8, 1968.

36. *Hess* v. *Lowery*, 23 N.E. 156, Ind. 1890; *Walfsmith* v. *Marsh*, 337 P.2d 70, (Cal. 1959).

37. *Holder, supra* at note 33, p. 202.

38. *Smith* v. *Di Cara*, 329 F. Supp. 439 (D.C. N.Y. 1971).

39. *See Slovenko, supra* at note 31, pp. 434-440.

40. GROSSMAN, (1973). The Psychiatrist and the Subpoena. *Bull. Am. Acad. Psych. and Law*, 1:245-254.

INDEX

287